DYNAMICS OF CLINICAL REHABILITATIVE EXERCISE

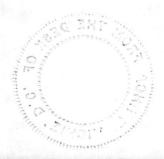

DYNAMICS OF CLINICAL REHABILITATIVE EXERCISE

Stephen M. Ordet, D.C.

Hobe Sound, Florida

Leonard S. Grand, D.C.

Palm City, Florida

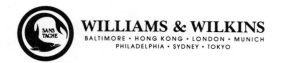

WILLIAMS & WILKINS
BALTIMORE · HONG KONG · LONDON · MUNICH
PHILADELPHIA · SYDNEY · TOKYO

Editor: John P. Butler
Associate Editor: Linda Napora
Copy Editor: Deborah K. Tourtlotte
Designer: Jo Anne Janowiak
Illustration Planner: Lorraine Wrzosek
Production Coordinator: Anne Stewart Seitz

Accurate indications, adverse reactions, and dosage schedules for drugs are provided in this book, but it is possible that they may change. The reader is urged to review the package information data of the manufacturers of the medications mentioned.

Printed in the United States of America

Library of Congress Cataloging-in-Publication Data

Ordet, Stephen M.
    Dynamics of clinical rehabilitative exercise / Stephen M. Ordet,
Leonard S. Grand.
       p. cm.
    Includes index.
    ISBN 0-683-06654-4
    1. Exercise therapy. 2. Chiropractice. I. Grand, Leonard S.
II. Title.
    [DNLM: 1. Exercise Therapy.   WB 541 065d]
RZ255.073 1991
615.8'2—dc20
DNLM/DLC
for Library of Congress   90-13124
                                   CIP

           91 92 93 94 95
1 2 3 4 5 6 7 8 9 10

PREFACE

When we first conceived this text, it was to be a manual for exercises that the average practitioner could utilize in the daily operation of his or her profession. As such, it was to be a book of pictures, with accompanying explanations of procedures, and little else. After all, what more could a busy practitioner use effectively? We presumed that the patient had already been properly diagnosed and, in most cases, been treated for some period of time. We also allowed for the fact that each of the doctors had already studied anatomy, biomechanics, physiology, and pathology for hundreds of hours, although perhaps a long time previously. Therefore, we prepared a "cookbook" of exercise maneuvers that could be simply "plugged" into such a practice.

The more we studied and read about the subject, the less reasonable this approach seemed to be. In fact, we found it necessary to include a certain amount of information on contraindications to certain or all exercises, with respect to specific conditions. We began to add a little anatomy and physiology, just to refresh the reader's memory. Then we realized that a certain amount of pathology and pathophysiology needed to be included, to correlate with diagnostic information and to relate indications and contraindications to the treatment plans. Biomechanical and kinesiological information also forced its entry, since we found the need to ask the questions "why?" for each type of motion and "how?" for each type of program. On top of this we sprinkled a smattering of physics and biochemistry, simply because we desired to reduce all language to that of the basic sciences. This last point is crucial, since, within each subdivision of each healing art, there is a plethora of jargon that is only semi-intelligible to those of other specialties. By reducing all substance and definition that we can to the language of the

basic sciences, we have a common denominator. Other subject areas, such as medicolegal issues and patient-practice management, were omitted for the sake of brevity, but they need to be considered in the whole picture.

We have attempted to break down, then condense, a complex set of data into a coherent and simple format for exercise rehabilitation. We recognize that exercise is not the only form of rehabilitation, but, in this high-tech era, it may be one of the more neglected forms. The reason to use exercise as a therapeutic device is simply explained. No muscle functions independently; rather, each muscle functions in coordination with surrounding muscles. Therefore, an essential part of repairing an injured or weakened joint or muscle is to restore normal mobility to that area. Only then is proper functioning with relation to the surrounding muscles accomplished. If such proper functioning is not restored, the area involved may become permanently disabled. Thus, a proper exercise program is necessary to expedite recovery and reduce the possibility of permanent disability. In the main, we have emphasized exercises that can be performed either by the patient alone, or with minor assistance from a therapist or, eventually, some other party. Despite this, it is not difficult to conceive of a number of variations of each exercise that utilize therapist or machine or both to augment effect. While these are the heart of the text, a good deal of time and effort is put into the explication of means of determining exactly which exercises will be performed and exactly in which manner they will be done. This is a series of clinical decisions, based upon ongoing data accumulation, clinical experience, and sound physical and medical principles. We do not take these decisions lightly, which is why we have not made them for you. However, if you carefully read the early chapters, and perhaps some texts in the aforementioned subject matters, you will be competent to make such decisions. We believe it is important that the physician be in control at all times. This can only be accomplished if one knows what and why he or she is doing (or instructing someone to do) something.

In Chapter 5, we have organized the clinical information around basic condition types, which is probably more useful for the clinician in the diagnostic stages. This is a very important chapter and within it resides the rationale for subsequent clinical decision making. The exercises themselves are generally arranged according to body area. Some exercises are useful for more than one area, and we have arbitrarily placed them in either the first area mentioned or the main area in which they work. This is more useful for the clinician during the treatment phases, in the prescription of the program that will be employed. Their order is not otherwise significant.

It is imperative for the patient to realize the importance of exercise therapy and to be properly instructed in the proper technique of performing maneuvers. The patient should also be instructed on correct utilization with follow-up by the physician to ensure that exercises are being done properly.

The development of an exercise regimen must be as carefully analyzed as any other part of the patient's treatment program. Prior to the prescription of any exercise, it is imperative that the physician know exactly what he or she is trying to accomplish with the specific movement, i.e., what exactly he or she is trying to rehabilitate, and what movement is needed to satisfy the patient's need. All too often exercises are given without proper conceptual consideration, and therefore may be contraindicated.

We view this textbook as a takeoff point for the doctor in guiding the patient through the rehabilitative process. This book will not replace the need for proper medical or chiropractic diagnosis and treatment. It is a guide to determine which exercises are best suited for the rehabilitation of the patient's condition. We hope to provide the clinician with proper therapeutic intent and a basis for the enactment of that intent. It is unlikely that any two clinicians will arrive at exactly the same programmatic determination with a given patient. However, their differences should be rational and, usually, inconsequential. It is our contention that a well thought out program will usually provide the expected results within the expected time frame. This means that the patient will be adequately evaluated both in the beginning and during the process to determine what those expectations ought to be. Not all patients can be returned to preinjury status, but "how far?" and "how soon?" are legitimate questions one needs to answer. We must emphasize that we follow the Hippocratic dictum, *primum non nocere*. This means that no exercise should be performed to the point or in such a manner so as to cause or increase pain or risk further injury. Actions that tend to do so must be eliminated as contraindicated or restricted by the doctor so as not to exacerbate the problem. Other than this, many of these exercises can and are designed to be performed by the patient on his own, at home.

For the sake of completeness, we feel that we must first note the obvious, that we are both male practitioners. As a result, we usually refer to the third person in the masculine gender. When this is the case, we mean to imply the neutral third person, which can be masculine or feminine. Lastly, we do not mean to imply that this is "the last exercise book you will ever need." Actually, we hope it is the first, the primer if you will, on rehabilitative exercising.

FOREWORD

For anyone who wishes to take notice, it is abundantly clear that health care delivery in U.S. is changing rapidly and drastically. Surely, it is fair to say that for the past century, the attention of health care providers in general has been largely directed toward alleviation of symptoms and toward crisis care. During this same time, health care was, generally, reasonably affordable for most people. This is no longer true, undoubtedly for a variety of reasons; however, I have little doubt that one significant reason for the extremely high cost of health care today is the massive infusion of "high-tech medicine" into the health care process.

Finally, belatedly, the decision-makers of our country and also, grudgingly, many members of the health care system are turning toward preventive health care and toward rehabilitative care that are oriented toward habit and life-style change for the express purpose of decreasing the incidence and severity of disease and disability.

Within this setting, the authors, Drs. Stephen M. Ordet and Leonard S. Grand, have undertaken to write a book that, in my opinion, is sure to become a standard text in the offices of many chiropractic, medical, and osteopathic physi-

cians, as well as of others who engage in the practice of manual medicine.

I am impressed with authors' ability to provide highly practical rehabilitative procedures without concomitant dependence on expensive, high-technology equipment, the latter having become the latest "must have" in rehabilitation centers across the country. This book takes patient rehabilitation out of the exclusive domain of the rehabilitation specialists and provides the typical practitioner the opportunity and the ability to perform much needed rehabilitative services in the office and in the patient's home.

This text is comprehensive and provides an excellent refresher in the basics of relevant anatomy and physiology. Also, it clearly and concisely provides well-designed and well-thought out exercise procedures that can be put to use in the office on Monday morning. I compliment the authors. Their work is a fine addition to the literature on rehabilitation.

James Winterstein, DC, DACBR
President
The National College of Chiropractic
Lombard, Illinois

CONTENTS

3
Pathology and Pathophysiology

4
Clinical Considerations for Rehabilitative Programs

5
Program Design and Implementation

6
Specific Conditions by Body Area

7
Cervical Spine

8
Upper Extremities

9
Upper Back and Thorax

1

Functional Anatomy and Biomechanics

Anatomy is the science of the structure of the animal body, and the relationship of its parts (1, p. 2). In this chapter we will discuss the anatomical relationships of and in the body, as it will be used throughout this text. We will also concentrate on the functional anatomy and biomechanics of the joints and their movements, which will form the basis for the rehabilitative exercise principles we advocate. It is not a text on anatomy, and one may wish to refer to an accepted anatomy text for a more detailed study.

Figure 1.1 is a diagram of the body illustrating the planes of the body and the terms of direction and position, which will be the standard of reference throughout this text. The median sagittal plane (Fig. 1.2) bisects the midline of the body. The midcoronal (frontal) plane (Fig. 1.3) intersects the body laterally halfway between the ventral and dorsal aspects. The midtransverse plane (Fig. 1.4) bisects the body horizontally across the ventral axis, approximately halfway between the top of the head and the bottom of the foot. All similarly named planes will be parallel to these midline planes, in accordance with their name. For instance, all frontal planes are parallel to the midfrontal one, but may be anterior or posterior to it.

The development of the skeletal system begins in the embryo as cartilage or membranous fibrous tissue. Primitive cells form

the mesoderm, appearing early between the ectoderm and the endoderm. The mesoderm, which develops rapidly, forms the connective tissues, bone, muscles, blood, and the vessels of the body. The notochord, a very primitive backbone, begins as an early condensation of mesodermal cells. At birth the human body contains approximately 270 bones. Fusion of various bones of the body begins at infancy, continues through puberty, and sometimes to age 30, until the skeletal system reaches the optimal number of 206 bones. The growth of long bones occurs at the epiphyseal endplates. This growth cycle lasts through puberty, until the epiphyseal endplates mature and fuse. The remaining secondary ossification centers consolidate as the adult forms matures, somewhere between the 14th and 25th year (1, pp. 280–3).

The axial skeleton consists of the cranium and vertebral column (Fig 1.5). The vertebral column is formed by an individual series of bones called vertebrae. At birth the vertebral column consists of 33 vertebrae divided into five regions. They are the seven cervical vertebrae, 12 thoracic vertebrae, five lumbar vertebrae, five sacral segments, and four coccygeal segments. The vertebrae in the cervical, thoracic, and lumbar areas remain distinct throughout life and are known as the "true" or movable vertebrae. By adulthood, the five vertebrae of the sacrum and the four vertebrae of the

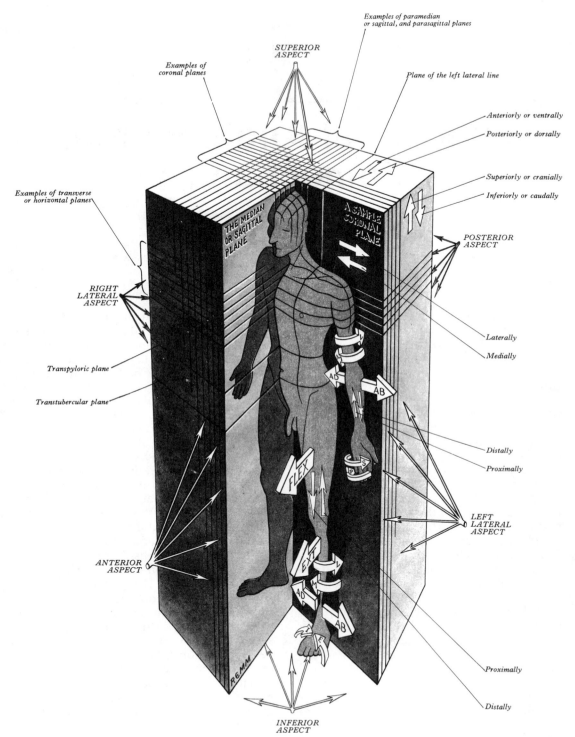

Figure 1.1 Planes of the body. (Reprinted with permission from Williams PL, Warwick R, Dyson M, Bannister LH, eds: Gray's Anatomy. 37th ed. New York:Churchill Livingstone, 1989.)

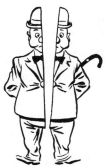

Figure 1.2 Median sagittal plane. (Reprinted with permission from Basmajian JV: Primary Anatomy. 8th ed. Baltimore:Williams & Wilkins, 1982.)

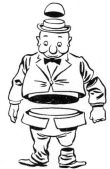

Figure 1.4 Midtransverse plane. (Reprinted with permission from Basmajian JV: Primary Anatomy, 8th ed. Baltimore:Williams & Wilkins, 1982.)

coccyx fuse to form the sacrum and coccyx, respectively, and are known as "false" or fixed vertebrae (1, pp. 324–5). However, the sacrum and coccyx can together move freely. The vertebral column consists of four curves, separated into specific anatomical regions. The cervical curve is a secondary curve, convex ventrally, with its most cephalad apex at the dens and continuing caudad through the second thoracic vertebra (1, pp. 329–30). The thoracic curve is one of the two permanent or primary curves, convex dorsally, emanating from the middle of the second thoracic vertebra. It continues through to the middle of the 12th thoracic vertebra. The lumbar curve is a secondary curve, convex ventrally, beginning in the middle of the 12th thoracic vertebrae. This lumbar curves continues through to the vertebral-sacral angle. The pelvic (sacral) curve is a primary curve, concave caudally and ventrally, beginning at the vertebral-sacral angle and continuing to the tip of the coccyx.

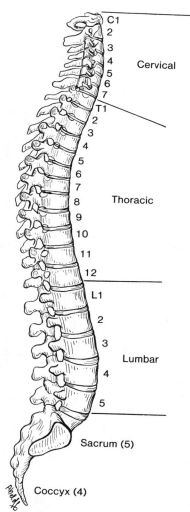

Figure 1.5 Vertebral column. (Reprinted with permission from Basmajian JV: Primary Anatomy, 8th ed. Baltimore:Williams & Wilkins, 1982.)

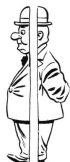

Figure 1.3 Midcoronal plane. (Reprinted with permission from Basmajian JV: Primary Anatomy, 8th ed. Baltimore:Williams & Wilkins, 1982.)

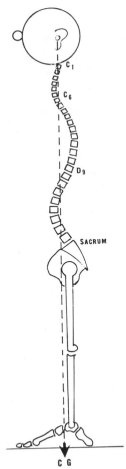

Figure 1.6 Normal physiological postural curves. (Reprinted with permission from Cailliet R:Soft Tissue Pain and Disability. Philadelphia:FA Davis, 1977.)

A normal vertebral column, with normal curves, has an index of 95, ranging from 94 to 96. If the vertebral column has exaggerated curvatures, then there is an index of less than 94, indicating a difference between the actual height of the column and its fully extended length. A vertebral column with reduced curvatures, almost straight, will have a Delmas Index of greater than 96. Delmas has shown by use of this index that a column with increased curvatures is of the dynamic type, while a column with reduced curvatures is of the static type (2, p. 20).

The vertebral column can be subdivided into anatomical motor units (AMUs), which consist of two vertebrae separated by an intervertebral disc (Fig. 1.7). They are heavily supported by ligamentous tissue. The anterior portion of the motion segment is primarily for weight bearing, whereas the posterior portion is primarily for gliding or movement (3, pp. 41–54). According to Kapandji (2), one may consider a biomechanical link between the anterior and posterior portions of the AMU. If the articular processes are the fulcrum, then the anterior portion would allow direct and passive absorption at the intervertebral disc (IVD), with indirect and active absorption at the paravertebral musculature. The AMUs, together with supporting ligamentous and

Figure 1.6 is a representation of the normal physiological postural curves of the spinal column, with the head directly above the pelvis. The thoracic kyphosis is approximately $30°$. The curvatures of the spinal column are significant in their ability to increase the resistance of the spinal column to axial compression forces. An engineering principle states that the *resistance of a curved column is directly proportional to the square of the number of curvatures plus one.* The importance of this principle is further elicited by the Delmas Index, as follows:

$$\frac{\text{actual length of vertebral column from S1 to the atlas}}{\text{fully extended length of vertebral column from S1 to the atlas}} \times 100$$

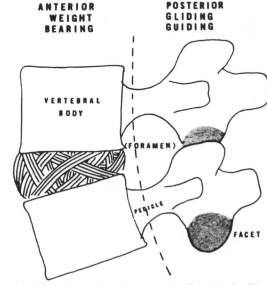

Figure 1.7. Anatomical motor unit. (Reprinted with permission from Cailliet R: Soft Tissue Pain and Disability. Philadelphia:FA Davis, 1977.)

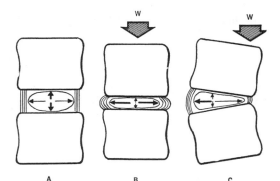

A   B   C

Figure 1.8 Intervertebral disc compression forces. (Reprinted with permission from Cailliet R: Low Back Pain Syndrome. Philadelphia:FA Davis, 1968.)

muscular tissues, make up the functional motor units (FMUs). The IVD is composed of two portions; the central portion is the nucleus pulposus, and the outer portion is the annulus. The nucleus pulposus acts as a swivel within the FMU, allowing six types of motion: flexion, extension, lateral flexion, gliding in the sagittal plane, gliding in the frontal plane, and right and left rotation (2, p. 30). Figure 1.8 is a representation of how compression forces affect the IVD in a healthy and a diseased state. The amount of the compression on the IVD increases caudally toward the sacrum. The cervical vertebrae are the smallest of the true vertebrae, which gain in size as they descend toward the lumbosacral joint.

The sacrum is formed by the ossification and fusion of five vertebral bodies, which form a larger triangular bone (Fig. 1.9). The union of these segments is usually not completed until sometime between the ages of 25 and 30 (1, p. 315).

The coccyx is formed by the ossification and fusion of the four remaining caudad vertebral bodies (Fig. 1.9).

The cranium is composed of 14 bones forming the face, and eight more that form the skull (Fig. 1.10). With the exception of the mandible, the bones are joined together by immovable articulations. Initially the cranial sutures (i.e., joints) are separated by fibrous tissue forming a syndesmotic articulation. Later in life the fibrous tissue ossifies and forms a synostosis (4, p. 25). The temporomandibular joints (Fig. 1.11) are synovial joints with two discs separating the upper and lower compartments.

The bony thorax is formed on the dorsal side by the 12 thoracic vertebrae and the posterior portions of the 12 ribs. The ventral surface is formed by the sternum and costal cartilages. The lateral border of the thorax is formed by the lateral portions of the 12 ribs (Fig. 1.12). There are, of course, numerous soft tissue supporting structures adjacent to this skeletal outline.

The appendicular skeleton is anchored

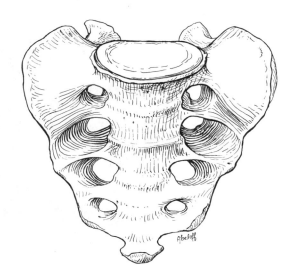

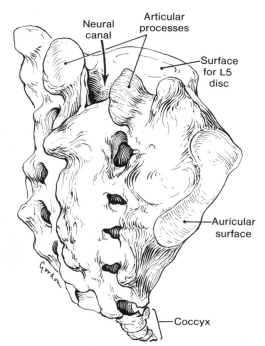

Neural canal

Articular processes

Surface for L5 disc

Auricular surface

Coccyx

Figure 1.9 Sacrum. (Reprinted with permission from Basmajian JV: Primary Anatomy. 8th ed. Baltimore:Williams & Wilkins, 1982.)

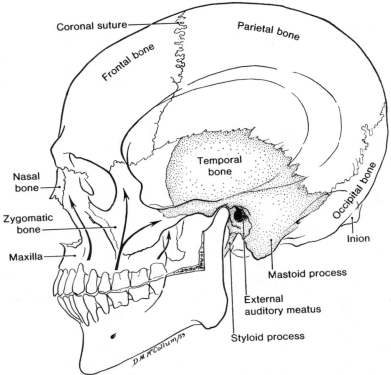

Figure 1.10 Cranium. (Reprinted with permission from Basmajian JV: Primary Anatomy. 8th ed. Baltimore:Williams & Wilkins, 1982.)

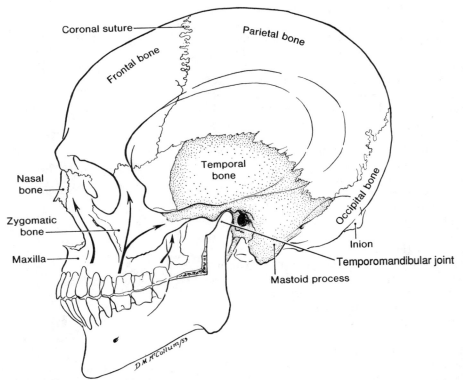

Figure 1.11 Temporomandibular joints. (Modified from Basmajian JV: Primary Anatomy. 8th ed. Baltimore:Williams & Wilkins, 1982.)

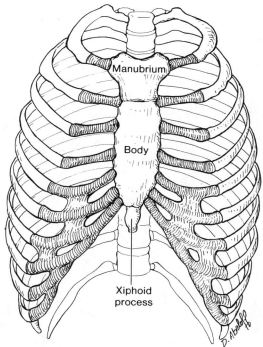

Figure 1.12 Thorax. (Reprinted with permission from Basmajian JV: Primary Anatomy. 8th ed. Baltimore:Williams & Wilkins, 1982.)

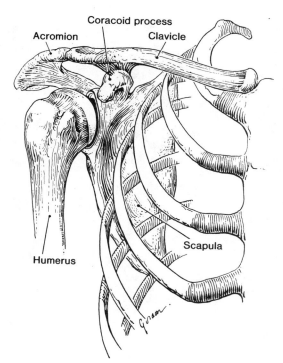

Figure 1.13 Anterior shoulder joint. (Reprinted with permission from Basmajian JV: Primary Anatomy. 8th ed. Baltimore:Williams & Wilkins, 1982.)

anteriorly, posteriorly, and laterally to the axial skeleton, forming the bilaterally symmetrical upper and lower extremity girdles and extremities. Each limb is composed of numerous bones, decreasing in size and increasing in dexterity as they become more distal, and a considerable amount of soft tissue structures, depending upon body type, conditioning, and gender.

The upper extremity begins with the shoulder girdle, a structure whose anteriormost component is the clavicle (Fig. 1.13). It articulates medially at the sternum and laterally at the acromion of the scapula. The dorsal portion of the shoulder girdle is formed by the body of the scapula (Fig. 1.14). The humerus, the largest bone of the upper extremity, articulates proximally at the glenoid cavity, an osseous fossa of the scapula, and distally with the ulna and radius of the lower arm (Fig. 1.15). The ulna and radius articulate with each other near their proximal and distal ends, along their axis by virtue of a fibrous membrane, and at their distal ends with the carpal bones of the wrist.

Figure 1.16 displays the articulations of the carpal bones with the metacarpals and distal phalanges.

The formation of the pelvic girdle begins with the right and left ilia, which, together with the ischium and pubis, form the bony pelvis (Fig. 1.17). These three distinct os-

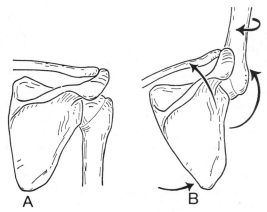

Figure 1.14 Posterior shoulder joint. (Reprinted with permission from Basmajian JV: Primary Anatomy. 8th ed. Baltimore:Williams & Wilkins, 1982.)

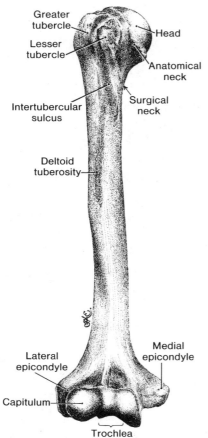

Figure 1.15 Humerus. (Reprinted with permission from Basmajian JV: Primary Anatomy. 8th ed. Baltimore:Williams & Wilkins, 1982.)

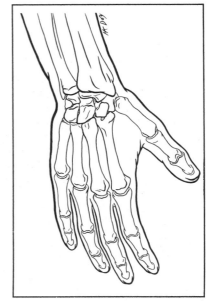

Figure 1.16 Wrist and hand articulations. (Reprinted with permission from Clarkson HM, Gilewich GB: Musculoskeletal Assessment: Joint Range of Motion and Manual Muscle Strength. Baltimore:Williams & Wilkins, 1982.)

seous entities join to form the acetabulum. During the developmental phase, the ilium, ischium, and pubis are joined by cartilage. At puberty they fuse, forming one solid half of the pelvic girdle. The lower end of each ilium forms into a ring, the obturator foramen, which forms the pubis anteriorally and the ischium posteriorally. The femur, the largest bone of the body, articulates proximally at the acetabulum (an osseous fossa in the ilium), and distally with the tibia at the knee joint (Fig. 1.18).

The distal end of the tibia forms the medial malleolus on its medial side. The fibula articulates with the tibia in three areas at the proximal end, and once distally with the foot. The part of the fibula that extends inferiorly and laterally to the tibia forms the lateral malleolus. The ankle articulation is at the calcaneus and talus tarsal

bones. All of the tarsal bones articulate with each other and distally with the metatarsals, which, in turn, articulate with the phalanges of the foot distally (Fig. 1.19).

It should be understood that muscles move bones, nerves innervate muscles, and most of the soft tissue structures cross the joint lines described. This is why we have addressed the issues of chronic disarticulation and chronic joint instability as neuromuscular problems.

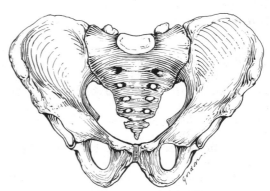

Figure 1.17 Bony pelvis. (Reprinted with permission from Basmajian JV: Primary Anatomy, 8th ed. Baltimore:Williams & Wilkins, 1982.)

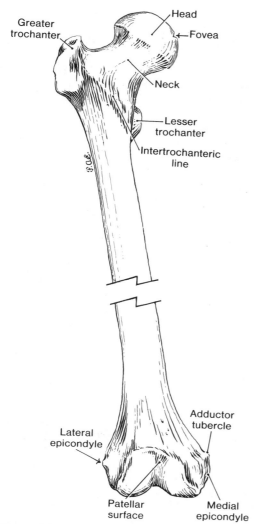

Figure 1.18 Femur. (Reprinted with permission from Basmajian JV: Primary Anatomy. 8th ed. Baltimore:Williams & Wilkins, 1982.)

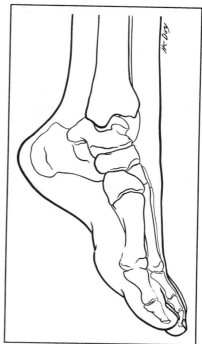

Figure 1.19 Ankle and foot. (Reprinted with permission from Clarkson HM, Gilewich GB: Musculoskeletal Assessment: Joint Range of Motion and Manual Muscle Strength. Baltimore:Williams & Wilkins, 1982.)

Articular System

Figure 1.20 is a schematic representation of the developmental formation of a joint.

Joint classification is shown in Table 1.1. In order to be more precise throughout this text in relation to joint movements and their relation to axial movements, an engineering method is used to describe ranges of motion. Background and descriptions are provided so that the reader can appreciate that this method is deeply ingrained in the scientific literature. Using this mathematical description facilitates interdisciplinary communications not easily accomplished

Table 1.1. Joint Classifications

Joint Composition	Action	Types
Fibrous	Synarthrosis; immovable	Syndesmosis Sutura Gomphosis
Cartilaginous	Amphiarthrosis; slightly movable	Synchondrosis Symphysis
Synovial	Diarthrosis; freely movable	Uniaxial Ginglymus Trochoid
		Biaxial Condyloid Ellipsoid
		Multiaxial Arthrodial Enarthrosis Sellaris

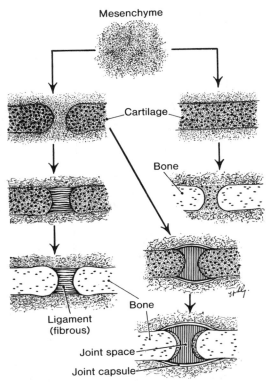

Mesenchyme

Cartilage

Bone

Bone

Ligament
(fibrous)

Joint space

Joint capsule

Figure 1.20 Developmental formation of a joint. (Reprinted with permission from Basmajian JV: Primary Anatomy, 8th ed. Baltimore:Williams & Wilkins, 1982.)

using only anatomical terminology. The authors will equate the systems so that readers unversed in this method can relate it to systems they already utilize.

Cartesian Geometry

I have resolved to quit only abstract geometry, that is to say, the consideration of questions which serve only to exercise the mind, and this, in order to study another kind of geometry, which has for its object the explanation of the phenomena of nature.
—Descartes (5)

Rene Descartes (1596–1650) developed a system for defining the position of points in space. He brought the analysis and understanding of both curvilinear and rectilinear motions out of the realm of the geometer and into the realm of the algebraist, and beyond. About the same time, Pierre de Fermat was working on the same problem and made significant contributions to this new analytical, or coordinate, geometry. This enabled the mathematician (or the physicist) to apply the function to the curve and

allowed for the mathematics to outstrip our concept of the physical world. They showed that there is an equation to describe the set of points of each curve depicted on the graph and that each equation that has n variables (where n is a positive integer) can be depicted in an n-dimensional Cartesian space (5, p. 164). For our purposes, we need only apply that portion of the system that is important for the study of body kinematics. It is a set of rectangular axes, also called Cartesian coordinates, that are three mutually orthogonal (at right angles) axes that intersect at a common point. This point is the 0 point on each axis. The axes increase in dimension in a direction that corresponds to the right-hand screw rule (see below). The increasing side of the axis is positive, and the decreasing side is negative. Each point in space is located by its perpendicular projections upon the three axes, taking its sign and value from the point at which those projections intersect the axes. We represent that point, P_i, by its coordinates (x_i, y_i, z_i) in space, as described above.

If we make the first point P_1, with coordinates $(x_1, y_1,$ and $z_1)$, and then mark a second point, P_2, with coordinates $(x_2, y_2,$ and $z_2)$, we can denote the components of displacement between the two points as d, with the value $(x_2 - x_1, y_2 - y_1, z_2 - z_1)$. We can also note the displacement of these points from the origin (or intersection of the axes), and see that it is the same value as the coordinates themselves, since the origin is at $(0, 0, 0)$. The distance between any two points is the square root of the sum of the squares of the differences between their coordinates (i.e., their displacements from each other). The actual physical distance between each of these points and the origin(s) is the square root of the sum of squares of the differences between each of the components.

$$s = \sqrt{(x_2 - x_1)^2 + (y_2 - y_1)^2 + (z_2 - z_1)^2}$$

We could just as easily define this coordinate system as the intersection of three orthogonal planes. This now begins to look a little more familiar; but it does not lend itself well to mensuration, which is necessary when computing motions, forces, and the like. If the human figure in anatomical position is superimposed upon these axes (Fig. 1.21), the Cartesian coordinates can be

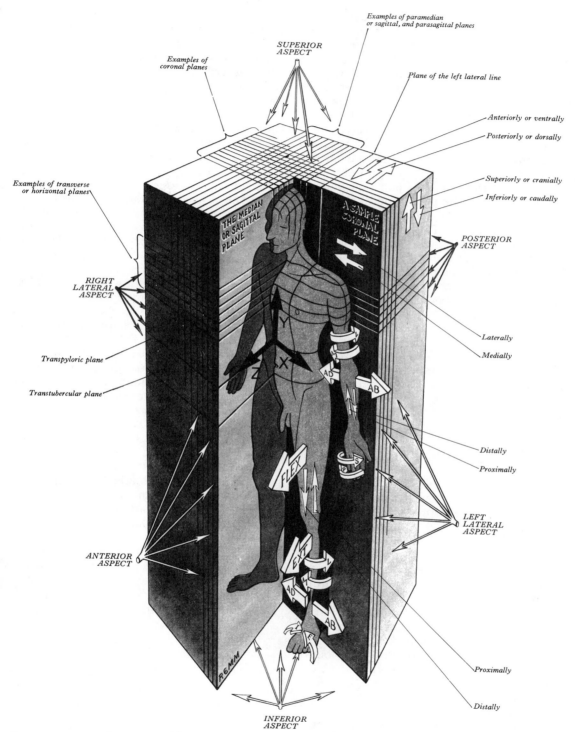

Figure 1.21 Anatomical representation of human body on Cartesian axis. (Modified from Williams PL, Warwick R, Dyson M, Bannester LH, eds: Gray's Anatomy, 37th ed. New York:Churchill Livingstone, 1989.)

related to the planes of the body. The plane formed by the yz axis corresponds to the frontal (sagittal) plane. The plane formed by the xz axis corresponds to the transverse plane. The plane formed by the xy axis corresponds to the frontal (coronal) plane. It should also be noted that motion in the frontal plane would rotate about the z axis; motion in the sagittal plane would rotate about the x axis; and motion in the transverse plane would rotate about the y axis. If we drop a perpendicular line to each of the planes from point P, we produce the projection of the line OP upon that plane. The angle which the projection of the segment OP upon the xy plane makes with the x-axis is labeled θ_x. The angle which the projection of the segment OP upon the xy plane makes with the y axis is labeled θ_y. The angle which the projection of the segment OP upon the xz plane makes with the z axis is labeled θ_z. It is fairly arbitrary upon which planes one makes these projections, as long as the angles with each axis are defined.

Next, we need to show another way to relate the components along each of the axes by the appropriate trigonometric functions. The component of the distance along each of the axes is defined below:

$$x_2 - x_1 = s \times \cos \theta_x$$
$$y_2 - y_1 = s \times \cos \theta_y$$
$$z_2 - z_1 = s \times \cos \theta_z$$

Now, by altering our thinking slightly, we can see how to express nonlinear motion within these coordinates. Such motions as parabolas and circles follow that function through space with a set of points describing curvilinear paths. The linear motion through the coordinate system is referred to as translational and the nonlinear motion as rotational or angular. To describe motion about the x axis, which would be in the yz or sagittal plane, we would label the angle formed with the starting point as θ_x. To describe motion about the y axis, which would be in the xz or transverse plane, we would label the angle formed with the starting point as θ_y. Lastly, with motion occurring about the z axis, which would be in the xy or frontal plane, we would label the angle formed with the starting point as θ_z. The positives on the axes are determined by the right-hand screw rule (Fig. 1.22). Therefore, an angle

created by motion following this rule would be a positive angle, and an angle created by motion in the opposite direction would be a negative angle.

Two types of quantities are encountered when describing all physical relationships and motions, whether one is talking about the solar system or the musculoskeletal system. A scalar quantity is a measurable value without the attribute of direction-in-space. A vector quantity is a measurable value possessing this attribute. This vector concept does not reach its full significance until one considers three-dimensional space, but it has importance and more ease of operation in one- or two-dimensional space. Simply putting a " + " or a " − " sign on a number, which could be graphed in one-dimensional space, creates a vector quantity, since $+7$ is graphed exactly opposite of -7. Their absolute value, 7, is the same, but their directions are diametrically opposed. The absolute value of a number is the value of the number without regard to the sign. The absolute value of a number, written 1×1, would be a scalar quantity, while the designation of direction with a sign creates a vector quantity. The vector so created is a one-dimensional entity. One might label the line upon which it travels the x axis. If this line were to take a turn, requiring then two axes to describe the position of any point on it, one would then label a second axis the y axis and make it perpendicular to the x axis. The combination of points on this line would form a two-dimensional vector, all of the points of which would lie in a plane described by the two axes.

Theoretically, the pure motions of the joints of the body (i.e., flexion, extension, etc.) describe an arc within a single plane. This is not generally the case, however, and such motions produce points on the arc

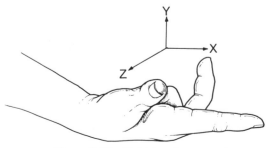

Figure 1.22 Right-hand screw rule.

that fall outside the plane formed by the two axes. This necessitates the formation of a third orthogonal axis, the z axis, which can be used to describe points in real body motion. Such motion is virtually always in three dimensions, that is, cubical space, by virtue of the design of and constraints within the joints, the external forces exerted upon this motion, and the usual lack of attention to the tasks at hand. In our exercises, naturally, we will attempt to isolate specific tissues with specific motions, but even this may result in a planar motion. The vectors so formed by such motions can be described in a few different ways, all boiling down to distances and/or angles. The displacements are easily defined once the orthogonal axes have been put into place. The angles always refer to the angular displacement from one of the axes. For example, if we refer to the flexion motion at the shoulder joint, we may be talking about yz plane motion about the x axis. (Fig. 1.23). This is only true of pure motion; it is rarely true in real life situations but can be made artificially true in experimental or testing conditions. One can describe the motion as r degrees of flexion, or of flexion in the sagittal plane. However, these data can have little done to them. If the motion is described in terms of displacements of the body parts, such as the radial tuberosity or the lateral humeral condyle, or in terms of the θ_x angular motion, one has much more to work with.

This concept obviously can be carried through to any number of dimensions, including far more than the consensus standard of three. However, this goes into abstract mathematics and has no vital bearing on the problem at hand. When there is more than one vector to consider, one can combine their effects upon graphic displacement by a special addition process that considers each orthogonal component and/or each angular component, paying attention to direction and sign. This process is known as resolution of vectors. If we were to work in the opposite direction and attempt to break the vectors into their orthogonal or angular components, we would then be speaking of the composite displacements that make up the vector summation. This is necessary when one finds the aplanar motion discussed above. Obviously this is not necessary when working with scalar enti-

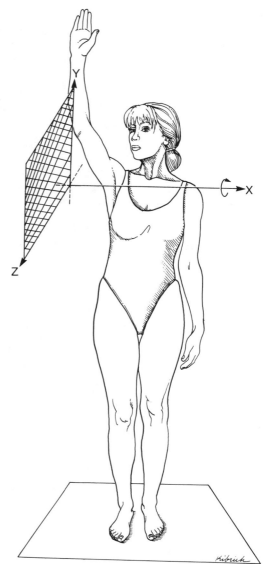

Figure 1.23 yz plane motion about the x axis (shoulder flexion).

ties. As you see from above, some knowledge of geometric, algebraic, and trigonometric principles is required. Without getting too deeply enmeshed into the proofs and formulations, suffice it to say that the motions, tests, and procedures to follow are described from this frame of reference, utilizing these mathematical tools. This will bring the material in this textbook into the realm and under the purview of the relationships and syntax of the language of science itself, mathematics. In so doing, one may communicate accurately with scientists of all ilk and all nationality, without being bogged down in specious dogma or linguistic colloquialism.

The following is an example of how the cartesian method will be utilized, along with the standard anatomical listing of ranges of motion.

Joint	ROM	Anatomical	Cartesian
Elbow flexion	135°	sagittal plane	Θx (yz plane)
Shoulder abduction	180°	frontal plane	$\Theta 2$ (xy plane)

The kinds of movements permitted by the joints are gliding and angular movements, circumduction, and rotation (Fig. 1.24).

Arthrodial joints permit only gliding movements, as between the carpals and tarsals.

Angular movements, found in uni-, bi-, and multiaxial joints, either increase or decrease the angle between two adjacent bones. Examples of this type of movement are flexion, extension, abduction, and adduction.

Circumduction is a combination of flexion, extension, abduction, and adduction. It is found in multiaxial joints. This is the type of motion seen in the shoulder and hip joints.

Medial and lateral rotation, internal and external rotation, and lateral flexion occur when a bone moves around a central axis, without deviating from that axis (see Chapter 2).

The movements permitted by the various joints are dependent on two factors: the type and shape of the articulating surfaces, and the restraining ligamentous structures of the joint.

Ligamentous tissue is passive in nature and does not have the ability to contract. Ligaments are composed of primarily collagenous fiber bundles of tissue. The functions of the ligaments within a joint are to restrict movement, to limit motion to a specific axis, and to limit the normal range of motion within the joint. Ligamentous tissue has the capacity to expand under a load and to return to its original size once the load has been removed (1, p. 474). There is a large capillary matrix supply to ligamentous tissue. The central artery disappears, sometimes as early as the third decade, resulting in ligamentous tissue nutrition from the surrounding capillary network (6, p. 56). This allows for the degeneration and weakening of ligamentous tissue, and must be considered in rehabilitative programs.

Articular capsules consist of an external

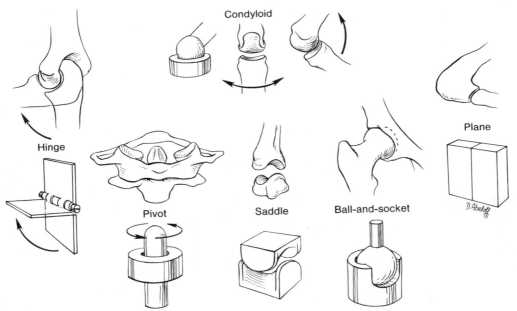

Figure 1.24 Types of joints. (Reprinted with permission from Basmajian JV: Primary Anatomy. 8th ed. Baltimore: Williams & Wilkins, 1982.)

fibrous tissue and an internal layer of tissue called the synovial membrane. The articular capsule forms an encasement around the freely movable joints. The synovial membrane surrounds the inner surface of the fibrous capsule, forming a synovial cavity. Loose connective tissue is found within the synovial cavity along with a thick viscous synovial fluid. There is normally just enough synovial fluid to lubricate the synovial surfaces, to permit free joint motion. When there is trauma, the amount of synovial fluid may increase, causing increased pressure within the joint and subsequent pain.

Synovial tendon sheaths enable the tendons that pass through fibrous and bony tunnels to glide freely over these prominences. Synovial bursae are found in the connective tissue between various muscles, ligaments, tendons, and bones. They enable the free gliding of tendons and muscles over bony or ligamentous prominences.

Table 1.2 displays the various joints of the body, the type of joint, and the movement allowed.

There is a surprising lack of conformity and even decision as to how the motions of the pelvis are to be named. Kapandji discussed a motion of the sacrum, relative to the pelvis, which he called nutation (and counternutation) (2, p. 64). The nutation motion represents a rotation about the x axis (positive θ), or an anterior/inferior motion of the sacral base. This motion has an analog in the anterior nodding of the head (occipitoalantal motion) upon the neck. Nutation in the sacrum is accentuated by the "backward tilt" of the pelvis (2, p. 70). This pelvic motion, which is called tilting, has a normal angulation (angle between the line joining the anterior border of the sacral promontory and the superior border of the pubic symphysis and the horizontal line) of about 60^0 (2, p. 74). In forward tilting of the pelvis, the line connecting the superior iliac spines, posterior to anterior, moves inferiorly on the anterior side of the pelvis (2, p. 106). This motion is essentially accom-

Table 1.2. Joints of the Body

Joint	Composition	Joint Type	Joint Action
Temporomandibular	Synovial	Ginglymus	Diarthrodial, uniaxial
Vertebral column	Cartilaginous	Synchondrosis	Amphiarthrodial
Sternoclavicular	Synovial	Condyloid	Diarthrodial, biaxial
Ribs	1st—cartilaginous, synovial	Arthrodial	Diarthrodial, biaxial
Coracoclavicular	Fibrous	Syndesmosis	Synarthrodial
Acromioclavicular	Synovial	Condyloid	Diarthrodial, biaxial
Shoulder	Synovial	Ball-and-socket	Arthrodial, multiaxial
Elbow	Synovial	Ginglymus	Diarthrodial, uniaxial
Radial-ulnar	Synovial	Trochoid	Diarthrodial, uniaxial
Radial-carpal	Synovial	Condyloid	Diarthrodial, biaxial
Midcarpal	Synovial	Condyloid	Diarthrodial, biaxial
Metacarpophalangeal	Synovial	Condyloid	Diarthrodial, biaxial
Sacroiliac	Synovial (1), fibrous	Gliding, syndesmosis	Diarthrodial, biaxial, synarthrodial
Symphysis pubis	Cartilaginous	Symphysis	Amphiarthrodial
Hip	Synovial	Ball-and-socket	Arthrodial, multiaxial
Knee[a]	Synovial	Ginglymus	Diarthrodial, uniaxial
Tibiofibular, superior	Synovial	Gliding	Diarthrodial, biaxial
Tibiofibular, inferior	Fibrous	Syndesmosis	Synarthrodial
Ankle	Synovial	Ginglymus	Diarthrodial, uniaxial
Intertarsal	Synovial	Gliding	Diarthrodial, biaxial
Tarsometatarsal	Synovial	Gliding	Diarthrodial, biaxial
Intermetatarsal	Synovial	Gliding	Diarthrodial, biaxial
Metatarsophalangeal	Synovial	Condyloid	Diarthrodial, biaxial
Interphalangeal	Synovial	Ginglymus	Diarthrodial, uniaxial

[a] The medial and lateral femoral condyle articulations with the menisci are condyloid joints. The articulation of the patella and the femur is partially arthrodial.

plished by a positive θ (i.e., x axis rotation) in the sagittal plane, upon the axis through the femoroacetabular joints. We have labeled this anterior tilting of the pelvis to be flexion, just as anterior nodding of the head is called flexion. It should be noted that hip flexion normally causes extension (or posterior/backward tilting) of the pelvis. However, when the legs are fixed, pelvic flexion moves the anterior superior iliac spines in an anterior and inferior direction, while extension moves the posterior superior iliac spines in a posterior and inferior direction. It is generally agreed that the rotation of the pelvis in the frontal plane (θ_z) will be labeled pelvic obliquity (7, p. 30). It should be noted that this conceptual language is in accordance with the subluxation listing precepts as espoused by Alfred States, D.C., and others (8, pp. 13, 113–43).

Muscular System

Three types of muscle systems are found within the body, categorized according to their function and cell morphology. Skeletal muscles, also known as the voluntary or striated muscles, are controlled by the will of the body. Smooth or involuntary muscles function without conscious will. Cardiac muscle has many characteristics found in skeletal and smooth muscles but functions involuntarily.

Skeletal muscle finds its attachment to bone by either a fibrous tendinous attachment or by way of the muscle fibers themselves making a direct connection with the periosteum of the bone. Customarily, the proximal attachment of the muscle is called the origin, and the distal attachment the insertion. Muscles whose specific action produces a desired motion are termed "prime movers" or "agonists" (4, p. 117). A muscle whose contraction prevents an undesired movement is termed a "synergist" (4, p. 117). A muscle that acts to oppose the primary muscle is termed an "antagonist." A muscle that is part of a larger group of muscles that, with or without gravity, immobilizes part of the group is termed a "fixation muscle" (9, p. 48). A classic example of these various muscle actions is found in the wrist flexor/extensor motion. In wrist extension the wrist extensors are the agonists, and the wrist flexors are the antagonists. If, while keeping the hand and fore-

arm on the same plane, the fingers are flexed, then the wrist extensors provide a synergistic action by contracting just enough to prevent wrist flexion.

A muscle contracts when it shortens or attempts to shorten. A muscle relaxes when it lengthens or attempts to lengthen. Isotonic contraction occurs when the muscle shortens during the contraction, while isometric contraction occurs when there is no shortening of the muscle fibers during contraction (9, p. 48). This is discussed in detail in Chapter 2. All musculature tissue contains white fibrous tissue composed mainly of collagen. Tendinous tissue contains the same collagenous fibrous tissue without muscle fibers. Tendinous tissue can be formed into bundles or sheets; the latter is termed an aponeurosis. The flat tendinous fibers that form an aponeurosis tend to give increased strength to an area, as seen in the abdominal wall. However, because aponeurotic tissue is poorly vascularized, healing of this tissue is slow; some believe that, after an incision, an area will never regain normal strength (7, p. 816). Muscle tendons are involved in the contraction or relaxation of the muscle in a limited fashion only. The involvement of the tendons is to dampen the contraction and relaxation of muscle and prevent "jerky" movements (9, p. 48). The muscle belly is the part of the muscle that is not tendon. If the tendinous attachment of a muscle begins either inside the muscle or at one end, the muscle is defined as pennate. In unipennate muscle (e.g., the semimembranosus) all of the muscle fibers are attached to the tendon from one side. If the muscle fibers attach to the tendon on both sides, it is a bipennate muscle (e.g., the rectus femoris). Pennate muscles are found where, anatomically, there is a small space, and power is a requirement. This type of muscle may be seen going from the forearm to the wrist and hand.

Two laws define the operation of muscle action. The law of approximation states that when a muscle contracts, it allows the origin and insertion of the muscle to come together. The law of detorsion states that during muscle contraction the origin and insertion of a muscle come together on the same plane, decreasing any spiraling of the muscle fibers. The laws of approximation and detorsion are seen in the sternocleidomastoid muscle (9, p. 50). It also appears that during muscle contraction, if the synergistic muscle is not functioning properly, then the amount of spiraling of the muscle fibers will be affected. Wolff's law of bone repair, which states that extra bone is deposited during the remodeling of bone at the stress sites and removed in areas where stress is not applied, may also contribute to the failure of synergistic functioning of muscles.

The nervous system controls the various movements of the muscles within the body automatically, in the normal person. This automatic neurogenic control of the muscles is termed cybernetic regulation. This regulation of the muscles via the nervous system can be further broken down into positive and negative feedback (9, p. 54). Positive feedback, a pathophysiological state, occurs when the neural impulses cause an increase in muscular action, as when a muscle responds to an increasing resistance to maintain a position. During positive feedback, the antagonistic musculature is not functioning, thereby causing a so-called "runaway" condition. If a person holds a vessel, keeping the arm extended at 90°, and water is added to the vessel, the action of the muscles to maintain that position is via positive feedback. Negative feedback, like normal reflexes (see Chapter 2) or gastrointestinal functioning, occurs when a muscle is activated to restrict or "fix" a muscle to prevent the further action of another muscle. The principle of positive and negative feedback may be applied when evaluating which muscles must be rehabilitated after an injury. If the antagonistic or synergistic muscle is affected, which then affects the agonist muscle, then rehabilitative exercises for the agonist muscles is counterproductive and may increase the disabling condition.

Muscles never work independently, but rather in a group. This is termed the mass action of muscles (9, pp. 63–7). This action is best realized in postural mechanics, where if a muscle group were to act independently of another group, then proper posture would not be possible. Throughout this text, exercise determination must consider this fact, realizing that in establishing a program of rehabilitation, much more than the injured muscle must be taken into consideration.

This chapter has provided a description of the anatomy needed to understand the intent of this text, to enable the physician systematically to develop a rehabilitative exercise program for the injured patient. At the beginning of subsequent chapters, specific local anatomy will be described and illustrated.

References

1. Williams PL, Warwick R, Dyson M, Bannister LH, eds.: Gray's Anatomy. 37th ed. New York: Churchill Livingstone, 1989.
2. Kapandji IA: The Physiology of the Joints. 2nd ed. New York: Churchill Livingstone, vol 3, 1982.
3. Cailliet R: Soft Tissue Pain and Disability. Philadelphia:FA Davis, 1977.
4. Basmajian JV: Primary Anatomy. 8th ed. Baltimore:Williams & Wilkins, 1982.
5. Kline M, Thomas Y: Mathematics and the Physical World. New York:Crowell, 1959.
6. Steindler A: Kinesiology of the Human Body. 4th ed. Springfield, IL:Charles C Thomas, 1973.
7. Cailliet, R: Low Back Pain Syndrome. Philadelphia: FA Davis, 1972.
8. Kirk CR, Lawrence DL, Valvo NL: States Manual of Spinal, Pelvic and Extravertebral Technics. 2nd ed. Lombard:National College of Chiropractic, 1985.
9. Basmajian JV, Wolf SL: Therapeutic Exercise. 5th ed. Baltimore:Williams & Wilkins, 1990.

2

Histology and Exercise Physiology

There are more than 430 voluntary (skeletal) muscles in the body (1, p. 289). Skeletal muscles are made up of numerous muscle fibers, ranging in size from 10 to 100 μm in diameter. Each fiber is separately wrapped by a fine layer of connective tissue called the endomysium, and each collection of fibers, called a fasciculus, is similarly wrapped in a connective tissue layer known as the perimysium. These fibers usually extend the entire length of the muscle and are typically innervated by only one neuromuscular junction, which is located approximately in the middle of the fiber. Each muscle is about 75 to 80% water, 15 to 20% protein, and 5% other substances, such as phosphates, urea, lactic acid, calcium, magnesium, phosphorus, various enzymes and pigments, ions of sodium, potassium, and chloride, amino acids, fats, and carbohydrates (1, p. 290; 2, p. 241).

Each muscle fiber contains from several hundred to several thousand myofibrils. Every myofibril has about 1500 thick myosin filaments and about 3000 thinner actin filaments, lying side by side within it. Furthermore, each myosin filament has tiny cross-bridges, arranged in a helical pattern along the longitudinal axis of the filament, projecting outward in a hexagonal configuration, toward the actin filaments, which surround it on six sides. Meanwhile, the actin filaments consist of two long fibrillar actin molecules, spirally wound

about each other, with reactive sites regularly along its longitudinal axis. The most abundant proteins in the muscle fibers are myosin (52%), actin (23%), and tropomyosin (15%), and 700 mg of the conjugated protein myoglobin (Mb) are incorporated into each 100 g of muscle tissue (1, p. 290). Other proteins include enzymes and various structural entities (2, p. 241). Myoglobin is a large iron-carrying molecule, analogous to hemoglobin, which is responsible for providing additional oxygen for the muscle in the following reversible reaction:

$$Mgb + O_2 \leftrightarrow MgbO_2$$

and for facilitating the transfer of oxygen to the mitochondria. This is a temporary solution to the mild hypoxia that occurs when the muscle vigorously contracts and diminishes the blood flow to itself (2, pp. 45, 174).

Muscle Fiber Types

Muscle fibers with a higher concentration of this respiratory pigment appear reddish to the eye, while those without it appear pale, or whitish, to the eye. Two types of skeletal muscle fibers have been identified and classified, according to their contractile and metabolic characteristics. Fast-twitch fibers produce quick and forceful contractions. This is due to their enhanced ability to transmit electrochemical action potentials, their high activity level of myosin ATPase, and the rapid release and uptake of calcium ions (1, p. 298). They have an intrinsic contraction speed and tension development two to three times faster than their slow-twitch counterparts. These fibers rely principally on a well-developed, short-term glycogenolytic system for energy transfer. They are more likely to be utilized in short-term, forceful muscular contractive activities, like sprints and baseball pitching, by producing rapid energy supplies through anaerobic pathways. The slow-twitch fibers produce energy more through aerobic pathways; their characteristics are opposite those described for fast-twitch fibers.

Furthermore, the concentrations of mitochondria and myoglobin are far greater in this type of fiber. Such fibers are more suited for long-term, endurance type activities. In those activities in which both aerobic and anaerobic capabilities are required, such as soccer, racquetball, swimming, or middle distance running, both types of fibers are activated. It has also been shown that endurance type exercise programs enhance myoglobin storage in animals, although this effect in humans is not yet fully proven (1, pp. 218, 301). So far, it seems that the genetic coding is the predominant determinant in the fiber composition one exhibits in any muscle. There may be hope, though, since, at the highest levels of performance, it seems that either muscle type is at least functionally trainable in the other's capability. This effect occurs only in those specific muscles trained, so, if one switches activities, one would probably need retraining.

Endurance athletes exhibit a majority of relatively normal sized slow-twitch fibers in the muscles that they use for their athletic endeavors. Power and speed athletes, on the other hand, usually exhibit a predominance of enlarged fast-twitch fibers. These fibers may be 45% larger than those of comparable endurance athletes or sedentary people. These latter fibers also have a considerably increased glycogen content. This actual increased individual fiber size is known as hypertrophy, in which the diameters of the fibers increase, and they gain in total numbers of myofibrils and various nutrient and metabolic substances (3, p. 91). These intermediate metabolites, such as adenosine triphosphate (ATP), phosphocreatine, and glycogen, help to nourish the increased motive power of these muscles.

Comparative Muscle Vascular Flow

Whether the activity is aerobic or anaerobic, there needs to be an adequate blood supply and venous and lymphatic drainage from the area being used. When the body requires an oxygen uptake of 4.0 liters/min, muscle oxygen consumption increases almost 70 times over the resting rate, to about 11 ml/100 g/min (1, p. 290). This requires redirection of large quantities of blood through the active tissues. The blood influx follows the rhythm of the exercise, decreasing during the contraction phase and increasing during the relaxation phase. Conversely, the egress of vascular fluids (blood and lymph) is assisted by the contraction phase and delayed during the relaxation portion of this cycle.

Furthermore, a complementary dilatation of some 4000 capillaries/mm^2 of muscle cross-section accompanies this pulsatile flow (1, p. 291). The increased capillary density associated with training is responsible, in part, for the improved exercise capability. Studies have shown upwards of 40% increased capillary density, paralleling the similar amount of increased oxygen uptake, in endurance athletes (1, p. 291). This is due to increased heat removal ability as well as to the obvious increased flux of nutrients and waste products that can reach and be eliminated from a much larger surface area, as a result. Isometric contractions (or any type at least 60% of maximum power) will occlude blood supply, sometimes to the extent that anaerobic glycolytic reactions are required to maintain it.

Muscle Histology

It is thought the some sort of interaction between the cross-bridges and the reactive sites provides the necessary force for the translational energy to move the actin filaments. Under electron microscopy, this myofibril appears as a series of alternating dark and light bands. The light bands contain only actin filaments and are called I bands, since they are isotropic to polarized light; the dark bands contain interdigitating myosin and actin fibrils and are called A bands, since they are anisotropic to polarized light. The combination of an A and an I band is called a sarcomere, which, in a resting state, is about 2 μm in length. Actin filaments are attached to each other at the so-called Z line or Z membrane. This membrane attaches myofibrils to each other across the muscle fiber, causing the respective sarcomeres of adjacent myofibrils to lie side by side. When a muscle fiber is stretched beyond its natural length, the ends of the actin filaments pull apart, leaving a light area in the center of the A band, called the H zone, which is an abnormal finding. Actin filaments are about 2.05 μm long, compared to the 1.60 μm of the myosin filaments. Therefore, in normal muscle function (i.e., contraction), the ends of the actin filaments are usually slightly overlapped. Neither type of filament needs to change its length during this process. All of these large, polymerized protein mole-

cules are suspended in a fluid matrix, sarcoplasm, containing the normal intracellular constituents, such as potassium, magnesium, phosphate, and protein enzymes. Many mitochondria are also present, in close proximity to the actin filaments of the I bands, suggesting that actin filaments play a major role in energy utilization. There also exists in this matrix an extensive endoplasmic reticulum, the sarcoplasmic reticulum, whose organization is essential to the control of muscle contraction, especially in rapidly contracting muscles. This reticulum contains transverse (T) tubules and longitudinal tubules (which lie parallel to the myofibrils) that terminate in a bulbous cistern on each side, abutting a very small T tubule and forming what is called a triad at that juncture. These triads occur at points where the actin and myosin filaments overlap, therefore creating two such triads per sarcomere. The T system (collection of T tubules) creates a

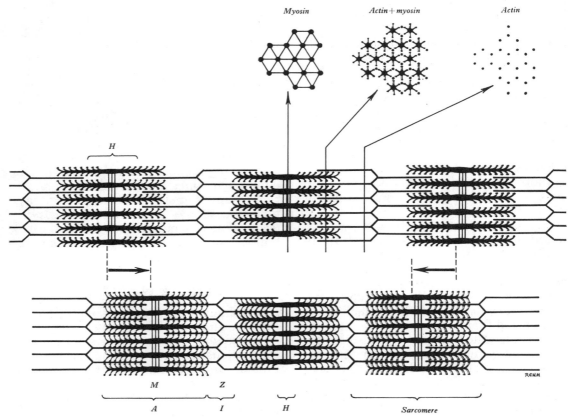

Figure 2.1 Muscle histology. (Reprinted with permission from Williams PL, Warwick R, Dyson M, Bannister LH: Gray's Anatomy. 37th ed. New York:Churchill Livingstone, 1989.)

DYNAMICS OF CLINICAL REHABILITATIVE EXERCISE

means of communicating from the external to the internal portions of the muscle fiber. The T system opens to the exterior rather than the interior of the cell, and therefore contains extracellular fluid. The T system also transmits action potentials from the exterior to the interior of the muscle fiber. See Figure 2.1 for a diagram of the above-described muscle histology.

Basic Muscle Neurophysiology

The normal resting potential of skeletal muscle fibers is about the same as that of nerve fibers, about 80 to 90 mV. The spike potential generated by their excitation has about the same voltage as nerve fibers, but it lasts for 5 to 10 msec, rather than 0.5 msec as do nerves. Muscle fibers can be much more easily stimulated at the site of the neuromuscular junction than elsewhere; these sites of increased excitability are referred to as motor points. The average conduction velocity in skeletal muscle fibers is about 5 m/sec, similar to that in very small myelinated nerve fibers. There is about a 3-msec initial period of latency between stimulation and contraction. The impulse is then conducted along the tubule systems and back out through the sarcoplasm to the membrane, to complete the circuit of local ionic current flow. It is believed that the flow of electrical current through the walls of the longitudinal tubules causes them to release calcium ions into the sarcoplasm, which then very rapidly diffuse into the interior of the myofibrils, initiating the contraction process. These calcium ions are reabsorbed within a few milliseconds as the action potential passes, thereby allowing the muscle to relax. This latter process is an active one, requiring ATP for its completion. Actin filaments appear to be negatively charged at their reactive sites, while the cross-bridges attach ATP, which also has a high electronegativity. This causes the filaments to repel each other and represents the resting state. This electrochemical balance is shifted in the presence of a small amount of calcium, and calcium further potentiates the release of ATPase from the myosin. Additionally, the actin filament also contains another protein called tropomyosin, which alters the behavior of the actin filament with respect to the myosin filament. Other filament proteins can inhibit or suppress ATPase activity and modify the binding characteristics of myosin with actin.

Ratchet Theory of Muscle Contraction

H. E. Huxley, in an article published in "Scientific American" in 1965, proposed this theory, suggesting that the cross-bridges provided a ratchet type mechanism that caused forceful movement of the actin filaments along the myosin filaments. This has since been expanded. The negative charge of the ATP bound to the cross-bridges has no attraction to the negative charge of the actin filaments, in the resting state. Since the shank of the myosin filament is also negatively charged, it is assumed that the cross-bridges project straight outward from it. Calcium ions, when released, now tend to bind with the negative reactive sites on both filaments, pulling them together. This also neutralizes the repulsion of the bridges from the myosin, causing them to bend inward, which pulls the actin filament and shortens the muscle. The folding in of the bridges causes the ATP to split immediately to ADP, due to ATPase activity of the myosin filament. This breaks the calcium-linked associations, but the actin filament has already been drawn parallel to the myosin filament. Each succeeding event, occurring as described above, along the myosin filament pulls the actin filament another notch further. Energy from other sources, such as high-energy creatine phosphate, recreate the ATP molecule, bending the cross-bridges outward again. Thus, the process can begin again with other calcium ions, moving as a "ratchet" does.

Electrostatic Solenoid Theory of Muscle Contraction

As appealing as the ratchet theory is, it does have a significant gap in it. As the myofibrils contract they also expand in diameter, actually increasing their interfilamentous distances by as much as 50 Å. Since it is unlikely that the small calcium ions could chemically bind across such distances, it is likely that some sort of electrostatic forces account for the actions occurring during muscle contraction. If we assume the same electronegativity of both actin and myosin filaments, there is still no attraction occurring at rest. However, if calcium ions bind the myosin molecules, they become relatively electropositive, allowing for a degree of attraction. It is also assumed that the filaments cannot approximate each other, which seems to be true. Since the linear forces of attraction occur mainly at the ends of the myosin filaments, not at the ends of the actin filaments, the contraction should theoretically tend to taper off, which it does. The electrical potential difference that could cause a full-strength skeletal muscle contraction is only 70 mV less than the action potential itself (3, p. 84).

Muscle Contraction Mechanics

At full stretch, the actin filaments are fully outside the myosin filaments (i.e., no overlap), and the tension developed by the activated muscle is zero. As the sarcomere shortens the tension rapidly increases, while the actin gradually overlaps the myosin. At about 2.2 μm the actin has already overlapped all of the cross-bridges but has not reached the center of the myosin. This is the point of maximum tension, and it is maintained for a short distance farther, to about 2.0 μm. Then, as the actin ends begin to overlap, the tension decreases almost as rapidly as it rose. The decrease in tension is probably caused by the backward pull of the cross-bridges on the actin filaments. The curve for the contraction of the whole muscle varies from this. This is mainly due to the large amount of connective tissue contained in it and to the lack of synchronicity or direction of the totality of sarcomeres in the muscle. The force of maximum contraction is a function of the resting position (i.e., length) of the muscle. The greatest force of contraction is obtained when the muscle begins at its normal resting length. As the length decreases, so does the maximum force of contraction, down to the minimum of zero at about 60% of its normal resting length (3, p. 85). When the muscle is stretched prior to contraction, there develops a proportionately increasing resting tension in it. That is due to the elastic forces of the connective tissue, of the

sarcolemma, the blood vessels, the nerves, and so forth, pulling the two ends of the muscle toward each other. This actually results in a decrease of the contractile tension during an active contraction. With no load on it, a muscle contracts fully in about 0.05 sec (3, p. 85).

This velocity is inversely proportional to the amount of the load on it. At a load equal to the maximum force of contraction, the velocity approaches zero. The larger the load, the more reaction sites between the filaments that need to be utilized, therefore the less available for the contraction itself. This may account for the decreasing velocity with increasing load. The shortening of a muscle enables the muscle to move objects against force, thereby performing work. The amount of oxygen and other nutrients increases when one is performing work, over and above that of an isometric contraction, the "Fenn" effect. It is not certain why this occurs, even though it seems as if "it ought to." Perhaps it relates to the increased breakdown of ATP when one tries to overcome a load, and the possible increased numbers of reactive sites that must be activated. The "efficiency" of an engine is represented mathematically by the percentage of energy input that is converted to work, instead of heat. This is less than 20 to 25% in a muscle (3, p. 86). The maximum efficiency is obtained when the muscle contracts at a moderate velocity (about 30% of maximum) (3, p. 86). If it contracts too slowly, large amounts of maintenance heat are released during the process of contraction. If it contracts too rapidly, a large proportion of the energy is necessary to overcome the viscous friction within the muscle itself. Later, we will relate these contraction-length concepts to the type of contraction made. Once again, this will permit us to define and create specific clinical decisions.

Characteristics of the Muscle Twitch

An isometric contraction is one in which the muscle does not shorten during contraction (3, p. 86). An isotonic contraction occurs when the muscle shortens but the tension on the muscle remains constant. Isometric contraction obviously does not require the sliding of myofibrils along each other. In an isotonic contraction, a load is moved, thereby changing its inertia (i.e., causing an acceleration). This, then, causes a momentum to accrue to the load, causing the need for stopping the inertia thus gained. Such a contraction will necessarily last much longer than an isometric contraction of the same muscle. Lastly, isotonic contractions create external work and, therefore, use much more energy. In comparing rapidity of contractions, one usually performs isometrically, because it is so rapid that even the inertia of the recording system is no factor. Most contractions are a mixture of the two types. For example, in running, the isometric contractions mainly keep the legs stiff when striking the ground and the isotonic contractions work mainly to move the limbs. In contracting against a load, muscle fibers need to shorten an extra 3 to 5% to make up for the stretching of the noncontractile elements, such as tendons, sarcolemmal ends of the muscle fibers, and even membranes of the myofibrils (3, p. 87). These components that stretch are known as the series elastic component of the muscle, and will be discussed in detail later in this chapter.

Comparison of Different Muscle Twitches

Skeletal muscles range in size from the tiny stapedius muscle of the ear (a few millimeters long and about 1 mm in diameter) to the substantial quadriceps muscle. Even the fibers themselves can range from 10 to 100 μm in diameter (3, p. 87). Energetics also vary from muscle to muscle. All these physical and chemical characteristics combine to create very different types of muscle contractions. Durations of contractions of muscles may vary as follows: an ocular muscle—0.01 sec, the gastrocnemius—0.033 sec, and the soleus—0.10 sec. Such differences in muscular contraction time reflect the functions of their respective muscles. The faster contraction of the eye muscle is necessary to maintain fixation of the eyes upon specific objects. The medium contraction of the gastrocnemius is necessary to accommodate both the strength and speed required by leg muscles while running. The slower contraction of the soleus

is imperative for the maintenance of posture against gravity. The "all or nothing effect" (discussed in detail below) occurs in muscles, much like it does in nerves. This means that the action potential either spreads over and stimulates an entire fiber or fails to stimulate it at all. The force of contraction, however, can vary, depending upon the initial state of contraction of that muscle. The presence of proper nutrients and/or the state of fatigue also modify the contraction. If the muscle is in a warmed state, it will contract even more strongly than at normal rest.

Fatigue and Muscle Tone

The residual degree of muscle contraction in skeletal muscle, after the promoted (i.e., synchronous discharges) action potentials have ceased, is called muscle tone. It is believed that muscle tone results from direct cord neuronal influences. This tone is then modified by supraspinal influences and monitored and controlled, in part, by special sensors in the muscles and tendons. These special sensors, as well as the concept of muscle tone, are discussed in more detail below.

As the result of very strong or long-term contraction of a muscle, the contractile and metabolic elements of the muscle become unable to maintain the same work output. Even though the neurological elements, including the action potential itself, continue to function normally, the contraction continues to weaken, causing muscle fatigue. This can be caused far more rapidly than normally by the interruption of blood supply to the muscle, thus curtailing its nutrient flow. An extreme fatigue can result in a rigid, continuous contraction, for many minutes, even without subsequent neurostimulus. This so-called physiological contracture is believed to evolve from a peculiarity of the contractile process. Recalling that ATP is actually required to maintain a state of separation between the actin and myosin fibrils, it is quite reasonable that their depletion (as in extreme fatigue) would result in rigid binding of the proteinaceous filaments. The subject of fatigue is both interesting and somewhat complicated and will be dealt with in considerable detail below.

Mechanical Systems

Most of the laws and principles of basic physics rely on certain mathematical assumptions. One of these is that we are dealing with rigid bodies, when we discuss the forces acting upon them or the motions which they are allowed. This is, of course, not true, and some higher mathematical principles can allow for the deformation and/or elasticity of the bodies themselves. However, for our purposes, it is a useful model discussing the motions of joints and the summary action of the motor units that produce them. A lever is actually one of the basic forms of machine that enable man to extend his power into the environment. The use of such a machine as a lever is said to afford an individual a mechanical advantage in performing a task not ordinarily able to be done without it. Simple examples of a lever are the use of a branch to move a boulder, a catapult, or the use of a crowbar to pry apart two pieces of wood nailed together. A dictionary definition of machine, quoted in the Life Science Library book of that name, is "any device consisting of two or more resistant, relatively constrained parts, which, by a certain predetermined intermotion, may serve to transmit and modify force and motion so as to produce some given effect or to do some desired kind of work" (4, p. 10). This definition can be applied to human motion and action, certainly as an engineering concept. Simple machines, such as a lever, do not strictly adhere to this definition because they may not require two distinct parts, but they do follow the definition in spirit. The Greek genius, Hero of Alexandria, around the time of Christ, defined five simple devices around which all mechanical machines are based. These are the lever, the wheel and axle, the pulley, the wedge (later called the inclined plane), and the screw. We can find examples of these all around us and within us, in the workings of our bodies.

The lever is probably the world's oldest machine and basically consists of two parts—the rigid bar (i.e., body) and a fulcrum (or pivot point) about which the action takes place. The load is that to which one desires to impart the force, and the effort is the force that is necessary. There are three basic types of levers. A type I lever has the fulcrum between the effort and the load. A type II lever has the effort between the fulcrum and the load. A type III lever has the load between the effort and the fulcrum. The quadriceps, acting as an extensor at the knee, is a type I lever; the biceps, acting as a flexor at the elbow, is a type II lever; and the lateral deltoid, acting to abduct the brachium, approximates the action of a type III lever. This latter example is difficult to find in the body by itself and depends upon the center of mass of the bone being moved. In this example, if the center of mass of the brachium is below the deltoid tubercle, this would more properly be termed a type II lever. If the center of mass of the brachium is above the deltoid tubercle, it could properly be termed a type III lever. When one carries a weight, such as pieces of lumber, across the arms, a type III lever is exhibited, but this is not an intrinsic action of the body, but an adaptive one to an external load. Type II levers magnify the effort, while type III levers magnify the distance. This means that, in type II levers, the effort is greater than the load itself; in type III levers, the distance traveled at the point of effort is greater than the distance the load must travel. It should be noted that the angular motion is the same in all instances. Since we are concerned with such angular motion in both muscle testing and exercise, we need to discuss its basic principles. These concepts are discussed below.

Historical Concepts of Physics

Some basic definitions and concepts of physics are pertinent to this discussion. Kinetics is the study of motion, and kinesiology is the study of motion in biological organisms. The concept of force is implicit in kinetics because, when there is motion, it is logical that there is a mover, or what might be labeled operative cause. This concept doubtless arose in early thinkers out of both the constant and regular motion of the heavenly bodies as well as the effort required to move an object on the earth itself. A working definition of force could be that which changes the state of rest or motion of matter (4, pp. 126–7). Philosophers in the Middle Ages noted that when the impetus to the motion ceased, the motion gradually (or rapidly) ceased as well. This doctrine of impetus was taught during the 14th and 15th centuries in Europe, and it influenced

Galileo's early thinking (4, p. 121). In his experiments with free (or nearly free) falling objects, he discovered the principle of acceleration due to gravity, and its measure as a constant. His second major discovery along these lines was that the gradually decreasing impetus would be essentially undiminished were it not for resistive forces. Galileo might have taken his thoughts and conclusions much further were it not for his preoccupation with the heavenly bodies.

The Dutch scientist, Christian Huygens, realized that, if unaccelerated (deceleration, or slowing down, is a form of acceleration) motion is the norm, in the absence of external force, then uniform motion in a circle is not free motion, because it requires acceleration to prevent linear motion. This is stated rather elegantly in Newton's first law (below). The significance in physics is the realization that anything but motion in a straight line requires a constant readjustment, or acceleration, applied to it. The implication for this text is that very few motions taken by or forced upon the human body are exactly linear. Therefore, whether in life situations or during exercising, constant change is required in order to obtain such motion. This change is not possible without the exertion of some force upon the mass being accelerated. This force then produces a stressor which, if properly applied, has therapeutic and rehabilitative impetus. However, if this force is improper in timing, in space, or in energy, it can be destructive. This is our premise and this is what requires apt clinical judgment.

Robert Hooke, in 1676, set forth his principles on the deformation of springs under loading. These principles, in modified form, are similar to those necessary to evaluate body motions versus resistance, particularly when working on certain mechanically, hydraulically, or electrically loaded machinery. As discussed in detail below, the musculofascial system contains elastic elements that do not exactly correspond to this law, but it works as a first approximation. Furthermore, it leads one to consider that there is some mathematical relationship that governs the mechanisms of muscular actions. Gradually, it became apparent that there were other forces than that of gravity to account for motion. Beginning with Galileo, the concept of inertia began to emerge.

Towards the end of the 17th century, the groundwork was set for Sir Isaac Newton to formulate the principles of the physics of motion, which lasted until Einstein at the beginning of the 20th century. Newton first had to distinguish between mass and weight. Simply stated, mass is the measure of the quantity of molecular material (matter) present, whereas weight is the measure of the force required to move it against the acceleration of gravity, or the force with which a body is attracted toward the earth. Momentum is a secondary concept, produced by the product of mass and velocity. Inertia indicates a body's tendency toward continued motion in a given direction. Speed is the distance a body travels in a given period of time. Velocity is the speed of an object in a particular direction. Acceleration is the rate of change of velocity, over time. Newton's laws, in a shortened form and simply stated are:

1. A body tends to remain at rest or moving uniformly in a straight line, unless that state is changed by the action of external force upon it. This is the Law of Inertia.
2. The rate of change of momentum of a body is proportional, and responds directionally, to the external force imposed upon it. This is expressed mathematically as $F = ma$, where F = force, m = mass, and a = acceleration. By specifying direction, Newton emphasized the fact that force, acceleration, velocity, and momentum are all vector quantities.
3. In an isolated system of two bodies, the instantaneous accelerations of the bodies are always in opposite directions and their magnitudes are in a constant inverse ratio to their masses. (In common parlance, every action has an equal and opposite reaction. This says, actually, that there is a conservation of linear momentum in ideal collisions, i.e., no external forces.)

All this motion implicitly refers to a state of rest, somewhere and somehow, and an absolute frame of reference must be assumed. We generally refer to the rectilinear, three-dimensional, orthogonal Cartesian coordinate system when we represent and study motion graphically.

A revolution in thought (and paradigm) was introduced by Einstein, Heisenberg,

Schroedinger, Planck, and others in this century. For those situations in which relativity applies, the only absolute is the speed of light (even this has recently been challenged by particle and plasma physicists), and there is no fixed coordinate system, because there are actually four dimensions, with the addition of time. Furthermore, Heisenberg (via his uncertainty principle) essentially proved that one cannot accurately predict both position and time of a body in space. That is the bad news. The good news is that this does not seem to have applications except at speeds nearing the speed of light, and either in very large or in subatomic particle universes. Therefore, we can continue to apply the classic laws of physics, at least for now.

There are additional concepts necessary for a more complete understanding of the physics involved in human motion. In 1847, a young Prussian physician by the name of Helmholtz enunciated a principle far ahead of his time, that of conservation of energy. Energy is the capacity for doing work (4, p. 275). There are basically two kinds of energy: potential, which is the energy of position, and kinetic, which is the energy of motion. This and the laws of conservation of mass and linear momentum, which follow from Newton's laws, hold true in the universe at large, but not necessarily for a closed system that interacts with something exterior to it. That is, they hold true except under conditions in which relativity applies and to the extent that E = mc² is not involved. This latter equation is one of Einstein's other great physics contributions, involving the interchangeability of mass and energy in certain circumstances, although the sum total of the two remain constant. The conservation of mass and energy are the two great scalar laws of physics; the other laws mentioned involve vector quantities.

Other derivative concepts apply to this discussion. Impulse (I) is a change of momentum ($mv_2 - mv_1$). From Newton's second law, $I = F(t_2 - t_1) = Ft$, along the line of the force. In a collision between two bodies, they develop an impulse of the same magnitude but of opposite vector force. As a working definition in physics, work is $W = Fs$, where F is the force exerted and s is the distance moved along the line of the force. Therefore, from a physics standpoint,

if there is no motion or net change in position, no work has been performed. This means that an isometric contraction in an exercise would produce no actual work, although a great deal of energy could be expended. Power is the rate of doing work. Therefore,

$$P = W/t = Fs/t = Fv$$

and clearly power and work are vector quantities, because they are dependent upon force and its direction. However, although both represent the product of two vector quantities, this is nullified by the fact that the vectors must be in the same direction to have meaning. Kinetic energy is also a scalar quantity, even though $E = \frac{1}{2} mv^2$ depends upon velocity, a vector. This is because, when the vector quantity is squared, the concepts of positive and negative are meaningless.

Applications of Basic Physics Concepts

Returning to the simple lever system discussed above, some basic physics are relevant to its application in any model. Regardless of type, a lever system (i.e., rigid body) is said to be in equilibrium, under the action of external forces, if the sum of the moments of the forces about that axis is zero. The moment of the force (or torque) equals the product of the force and its distance from the potential axis of motion. Therefore, a moment of force can be defined as the measure of the effectiveness of a force in producing a rotation about an axis (4, p. 160). Essentially, this refers to rotational equilibrium about the fulcrum point. The perpendicular distance between the force and the axis is known as the moment arm. The law of moments is expressed as

$$F_1 d_1 = F_2 d_2$$

where F_1 = the force on either side of the fulcrum and d_1 = the distance of that force from the fulcrum. The above equation is true when the body is in equilibrium; otherwise an inequality is present.

Two parallel forces acting in concert in opposite directions about an axis produce what is referred to as a couple, whose resultant torque is exactly additive. The above all refers to parallel forces, or the trigonometric vector sums in parallel directions. This law was first articulated, in some form, as far back as Archimedes in ancient Greece, then by Leonardo da Vinci, both on essentially intuitive levels. The center of gravity of a body is the discrete point through which the weight of the body always appears to act. The moments of force are often defined with respect to the distance of those forces from this point, in the absence of a separate fulcrum. When a separate fulcrum is present, the weight, acting through the center of gravity, acts as another distinct force, whose moment arm is the distance between the center of gravity and that fulcrum.

Now, the center of gravity, where the weight appears to act, is not the same as the center of mass, the discrete point from which there appears to be an equal amount of mass on all sides. A force acting through the center of mass will produce translational motion (i.e., in a straight line), whereas motion through the center of gravity may produce rotational motion (as the application of any couple to a body tends to do), with or without translational motion. This means that when there are a set of forces acting through the center of mass of a body, one may simply consider their vector sum in the determination of the resultant purely translational motion which that body undergoes. Translational motion is rectilinear motion, but most motions (especially in the human body) have rotational components. In fact, most body motions, particularly in the extremities, involve the motion of a rigid body (i.e., a limb) about a fixed pivot point (i.e., a joint) at some distance from its center of mass or center of gravity. Just as the velocity in translational motion is defined as the change in distance traveled per unit of time,

$$v = \Delta s / \Delta t$$

the angular velocity in rotational motion is defined as the change in angle traversed per unit of time,

$$\omega = \Delta \theta / \Delta t$$

and, just as acceleration in translational motion is defined as the change in velocity per unit of time,

$$a = \Delta v / \Delta t$$

the angular acceleration is defined as the change in angular velocity per unit of time

$$\alpha = \Delta \omega / \Delta t.$$

The concept of conservation of linear momentum was discussed above, from Newton's third law. Now, the concept of conservation of angular momentum can be added. This, too, is a vector quantity; therefore, conservation of mass and energy are the only scalar laws governing the physical universe at the level we all experience. All of the laws of conservation have some implicit assumptions, which is why they only serve as models to explain reality. Examples of this are how we continually create frictionless surfaces, massless lines, and dimensionless points in physics, in order to derive these equations. Nevertheless, the models still help to explain most of that which we perceive and allow the creation of such engineering marvels as the highly technological instrumentation to simulate and assist in repairing the structures and functions of the human organism. Some of these advances are mentioned in Chapter 12 to indicate the realms of possibility in rehabilitative medicine. But first, let us consider what we can do without the bulk of high technology available today, at often bulkier prices.

Lever Systems of the Body

Muscles attach to bone at two distinct places, their designated origin and insertion spots. The origin of a muscle is essentially the spot from which motion originates, that is, the fulcrum of the motion. The insertion is the spot at which the force causing the motion inserts, or exerts its effect. Theoretically, the origin is a fixed point, like the origin of the Cartesian coordinate system. This is not true in real body motions, unless an attempt is made to anchor or buttress that point, or joint, in space. Real motions of joints, especially those with multiple degrees of freedom, have multiple axes of motion, often with one or more of these axes skew to the coordinate axes. This is typically seen in normally performed shoulder motion. Depending upon the plane(s) of motion and the angle(s) of rotation, there could be as many as four joint areas, fulcrums, and sets of motions occurring simultaneously. These joints could include the sternoclavicular, acromioclavicular, glenohumeral, and scapulocostal joint areas.

Therefore, when performing a specific exercise, the joint area often needs to be braced to produce a semblance of specificity in joint motion. While experimenting to determine normal joint motions by electro-goniometry, we found that it is crucial where one determines to be the origin, end-point, and axis of a particular motion. If we presume to be able to do this, the Cartesian coordinate system can be applied to testing/exercising to make it mathematically reproducible and kinesiologically able to be studied. In each exercise suggested in this book, this system is superimposed over the motion and clinical directions are given to relate this to the vast body of available scientific knowledge.

We can use the biceps and triceps of the upper arm as examples of the lever system in action in the body. Assume that the biceps has a rather large cross-sectional area of about 6 inches^2, producing a maximum force of contraction of about 250 lb (3, p. 90). The actual tension placed upon the muscle fibers amounts to 3.6 kg/cm^2, according to Recklinghausen (5, p. 70). In this case the triceps is the antagonist muscle and the biceps is the agonist muscle. To compute the resultant vector forces, use the

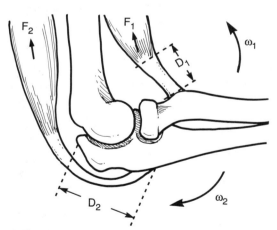

Figure 2.2 Relationships between forces and moment arms in agonist and antagonist muscles. F_1 = force of contraction of biceps; F_2 = force of contraction of triceps; D_1 = distance of site of action on biceps from fulcrum; D_2 = distance of site of action on triceps from fulcrum; ω_1 = angular velocity in direction of flexion; ω_2 = angular velocity in direction of extension.

diagram in Figure. 2.2 as an example of how the relative forces and distances account for the final position of the lever arm. Remember that in each resting position there is a state of equilibrium, brought about by the resolution of the vector forces in such a way as to preserve angular momentum and in accordance with Newton's second and third laws.

The Physics of Muscle Types

There are two types of muscle fibers, parallel and pennated, the former directed toward the line of action of the muscle and the latter oblique to that line. The total tension depends upon the physiological cross-sectional area, which is much larger in a pennated muscle than the anatomical area, which suffices for a parallel muscle. The individual fiber pull in a pennated muscle depends upon the angle of the fibers and is a function of the cosine of that angle. The total work a muscle can perform depends predominantly upon its mass. This means that a more dense but shorter muscle, such as the gastrocnemius, may be able to do the same work as the less dense but longer muscle, such as the sartorius, if they have approximately the same mass. The difference is that the gastrocnemius will be able to lift a larger weight and the sartorius will be able to move weight a greater distance. Since work is the product of force and distance, they can do the same work. The gastrocnemius is essentially a pennated muscle, whereas the sartorius is essentially a parallel muscle. The power of the parallel sartorius is less, because it took longer to perform the work over the greater distance, whereas the pennated gastrocnemius is more powerful. In summary, there are two main types of muscles in the body, long ones that contract a great distance and short ones with greater cross-sectional areas that provide great strength over short distances. Each muscle has some characteristics of one or both types, providing for the variety of movements required by the human body.

The parallel muscle is designed more for speed, therefore, and the pennated one for power. To take advantage of this, the muscle attaching closest to the center of the joint would probably be pennated, since it would take more power to move that lever with the shorter moment arm. Therefore, when testing and/or exercising muscular tissue, the closer to the joint center the load is placed, the more pennated fibers are involved. When speedy isokinetic contractions are applied to the joint musculature, it is parallel fibers that respond, for the most part. One must also remember that the pennated fibers do not move the lever as far, so the starting and finishing positions of the exercise or test also help to determine which fibers are implicated. In terms of the leverage factors themselves, the muscles that supply power are attached at a greater distance from the center of motion and the muscles that supply speed are attached at a lesser distance from the center of motion. The reason for this is that the muscles closer to the center of motion have less actual distance to move the lever arm to acquire a larger angular displacement. This means that the angular velocity is greater. Therefore, this muscle can cause a greater effect in a shorter time and is useful when speed of contraction is required. The larger body joints, especially where weight bearing may take place and where speed and strength are required, are usually provided with both types of muscles (5, p. 72). Examples of this are the elbow, with biceps and brachialis, the knee, with biceps and hamstrings, and the foot, with gastrocnemius and soleus. The maximum rotatory force occurs, of course, when the tendon is perpendicular to its insertion site; at this point, the insertion is about 2 inches anterior to the fulcrum at the elbow. Since the total length of the forearm lever is about 14 inches and the moment arm of the force is about $\frac{1}{7}$ of the moment arm of the resistance, the load capable of being moved is about $\frac{1}{7}$ that of the force exerted. This load is about 36 lb ($\frac{1}{7}$ of the 250-lb maximum force), and includes the actual weight, at the center of gravity of the forearm, of the forearm itself. This is diminished as the arm straightens and the ratio of rotary force to total force decreases, and the distance of the force moment arm decreases.

Kinesiological Considerations

As one observes joint motion, one notes that the radial acceleration that is imparted to the joint member(s) tends to cause the joint space to increase as well. This separa-

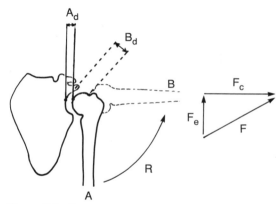

Figure 2.3 Representation of kinetics of motion on relative joint spacing. A = initial arm position; B = final arm position; R = angular acceleration of arm; F_c = centrifugal component of force (i.e., x axis); F = vector force applied by muscular action; F_e = deviation component of force (i.e., y axis); A_d = separation of joint in position A; B_d = separation of joint in position B.

tion of the joint components is partly due to the axially directed centrifugal force generated by the radial motion. In addition, this is usually augmented by a loading of the limb (i.e., moment arm) in the same externally directed longitudinal axis. The resultant force vector, acting in accordance with Newton's second law, causes the joint to separate and the restraining elements to be proportionately stressed (Fig. 2.3) Either a load or a motion in excess of the tensile strength of one or more of these latter elements is usually sufficient to dislocate the joint. In plain English, the action of throwing a baseball causes, at various points along the motions involved, either separation or compression of the implicated joints. The centrifugal forces would cause separation, since they are directed outward, and the centripetal forces would cause compression, since they are directed inward.

As a result, muscular action always has two intents. The first muscle, group, or set of fibers is responsible for causing the radial motion. A second muscle, group, or set of fibers is responsible for maintaining joint integrity by dampening the centrifugal acceleration initiated by the action of the first muscle group (5, p. 67). In fact, this may even be accomplished by some complex internal neuromuscular mechanism within the sets of fibers of a single muscle. The first component is known as the rotatory action and the second one as the stabilizing action. Both actions are part of normal body kinesiology, and they are carefully balanced by parts of the brain so that action takes place without injury. In fact, consideration of these respective roles may be quite helpful in diagnosis and treatment of joint injuries (Figs. 2.4 and 2.5).

The relative proportion of the two components is a function of the angle of insertion of the tendon of the muscle(s) at the bone. This angle is calculated as the angle formed by the mechanical axis of the muscle in interaction with the lever arm of the bone into which it inserts. The rotatory component is proportional to the sine of this angle, or the portion whose vector is perpendicular to the axis of the lever arm (the bone into which the muscle is inserted). The stabilizing component is proportional to the cosine of this angle, or the portion whose vector is parallel to the axis of the lever arm (Fig. 2.4) As the lever arm rotates (e.g., flexes) toward perpendicularity (90° of motion) with the muscle axis, the sine of the angle approaches 1, its maximum, and the muscle action is maximally rotatory. Conversely, as the arm approaches a 0° (or 180°) angle with the muscle-tendon axis, the cosine nears 1, its maximum, and the motion is virtually all stabilizing.

$$F_r = F \sin \alpha$$
$$F_s = F \cos \alpha$$

Therefore, a way to increase the effectiveness of a muscle's action, whether in nor-

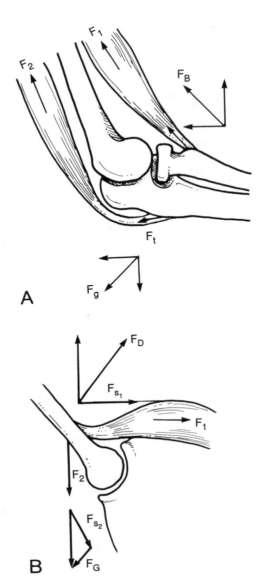

Figure 2.5 **A.** Agonist/antagonist joint stabilization. F_1 = tension in biceps; F_2 = tension in triceps; F_B = effective pull of biceps; F_G = effective pull of gravity; F_t = effective pull of triceps. **B.** Gravity field providing joint stabilization. F_1 = tension in deltoid; F_2 = force of gravity; F_{s_1} and F_{s_2} = respective joint stabilization components of F_1 and F_2; F_D = effective pull of deltoid; F_G = effective pull of gravity.

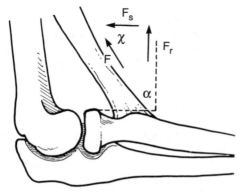

Figure 2.4 Example of how a muscle can provide a joint-retaining element while acting upon that joint. α = angle of tendinous insertion; F = force of contraction; $F_r = F_{\sin\alpha}$—rotatory component; $F_s = F_{\cos\alpha}$—stabilizing component.

mal motion or in a designed exercise program, is to increase the angle of application. From the above equations, this would increase the rotatory force, F_r. However, as the muscle length shortens by contraction, the tension on the muscle decreases proportionately and rapidly. This outweighs the advantage of increasing the angle of application (5, p. 69).

In some cases, the body design is such that the course of the tendon of insertion is deflected, thus negating the shortening tendency of the contracted involved muscle. The deflection of the quadriceps tendon by the patella prevents the quadriceps muscle from shortening appreciably, thereby preventing the tension decline that accompanies such shortening. This only works when a tendon is lifted off the bone, without a change in the plane of pull, like a pulley does and like the quadriceps tendon does. The pulley, another simple machine, provides one with a mechanical advantage in performing a task. This enables a greater load to be handled in any particular manner than would be allowed otherwise. If the plane of pull is changed, usually by injury to some retaining element(s), the action is impeded or made less efficient. Obviously, pain may result, as well. The heads of the gastrocnemius and the hamstrings are similarly deflected by the posterior protrusion of the femoral condyles during the plantar flexion of the foot and the flexion of the knee, respectively. Another type of deviation during motion occurs when the action of a deep tendon enhances the angle of a more superficial one, thus amplifying the action of the latter. This occurs with the tendons of the flexor digitorum superficialis and the flexor digitorum profundus, which traverses through the former at one point of its travel. Other examples of this process are the tendon deflection due to the action of the connective tissues in the volar carpal tunnel, and the analogous action in the tarsal tunnel.

There are very few muscles with large angles of application. The majority of muscles are arranged so that they are parallel to the lever arm axis, producing relatively large stabilizing components (5, p. 68). The pectoralis major is an exception, attaching itself at an almost 90° angle. The conclusion one might draw is that the maintenance of position, balance, and stabilization is really the primary function of muscles (5, p. 68). Joint stabilization is also enhanced by the action of the antagonist muscle. It is actually the net combined tonicity (as a vector sum) of both muscles (or groups) that stabilizes the joint. Some-

times, the antagonist action may even come from gravity (Fig. 2.5 **A** and **B**).

The arrangement of the stabilizer and the external load determines the type of lever action involved. Examples of each of the three classes of lever are:

First Order. Stand on foot and observe floor reaction on heel.

Second Order. Flex elbow against weight in hand.

Third Order. Rise on ball of foot and Achilles tendon increases tension against resistance of superincumbent body weight.

A muscle in contraction exerts a rotary effect on both ends, with the fixed end acting as the origin and the free end acting as the insertion. Usually, the two ends have vastly different masses, like the trunk versus the thigh, in the cases of the iliacus, or psoas, or iliopsoas. Since the angular acceleration is a function of the inertia, which is a function of the mass, the acceleration upon the trunk is proportionately smaller than that upon the thigh, assuming equal angles of application and equal applied forces. Angular acceleration, like linear acceleration, is inversely related to the mass.

Such a kinesiological evaluation of lever systems requires distinctive knowledge of musculotendinous origins and insertions, distance of insertions from their fulcrums (i.e., moments of force), angle of incidence of insertions, lengths of involved lever arms, and the position of operation of the levers. Another factor complicates the evaluation of these lever systems. It must be kept in mind that the motion of joints, which could be at angles to the specific planes of body motion described above, is not the same as the motion of muscles. However, it is the muscles that produce the joint motions. The difference is that the joint motion is a composite of all the muscular actions, as allowed by the joint's intrinsic retaining mechanisms. This means that, as we consider the joint motion, power, and work, we are again looking at the cosines of the angles of action of each of the muscular components that produce the action. Furthermore, certain muscles, as their respective joints go through their ranges of motion, actually reverse their force vectors as their lever arms change position far enough. A prime example of this is the adductor longus. It is a secondary flexor of the hip, but it becomes an extensor as hip flexion reaches 70°; the adductor magnus does the same thing at 50° (5, p. 74). This means, once again, that one cannot simply perform an exercise. It must be performed at the correct angles, through the correct ranges, and be begun at the correct starting point to obtain the desired result. One last complicating factor is the element of the number of joints that a particular muscle crosses, thereby affecting their motion. This factor makes calculations computer-complex and need not be algebraically considered at this time.

Neuromuscular Physiology

An understanding of the physiological aspects of rehabilitative medicine is required for the proper determination and application of therapeusis. Therefore, we have included this section on the physiological bases of normal and abnormal neuromuscular functioning. The psychophysiological aspects of neuromuscular training and rehabilitation will not be discussed.

Motor Unit

Depending upon the type of muscle, each motor neuron leaving the cord will stimulate a certain number of muscle fibers. All the fibers innervated by that motor nerve fiber, along with the nerve, are referred to as a motor unit. The number of muscle fibers supplied by a single nerve fiber is directly related to the movements expected to be involved. Generally, the more rapid and exacting the muscle reaction to stimulus, the fewer the number of muscle fibers in the unit, and the greater the number of efferent fibers to that muscle. In the control of delicate and precise motions, such as in the intrinsic musculature of the eye, the ratio of muscle fibers:nerve fibers would be no more than 10:1 (1, p. 307). In the gross and less complex motions of the larger muscles, such as the quadriceps the ratio may be 2000 to 3000:1 (1, p. 308). Other examples of ratios in the physiological motor unit are 342:1 (first dorsal interosseous muscle of the finger) and 1776:1 (medial gastrocnemius muscle) (1, p. 312). These fiber ratios vary from the figures in physiology texts, but one gets a good flavor for the concept using any of these sets of numbers, (2, p. 264; 3, p. 88). Adjacent motor fibers usually overlap by about 10 to 15 fibers, allowing

separate motor units to support each other's contractions. This phenomenon is most useful in the rehabilitation of nerve-damaged areas. Macro motor units (up to 10 times the normal number of muscle fibers) develop as healthy nerve fibers sprout new endings. This may decrease local control and fine tuning, but it allows muscles paralyzed by such entities as poliomyelitis to recover, after a fashion. It is an example of the so-called plasticity of the nervous system. The physiological motor unit (PMU) consists of the motor neuron, which stimulates the muscle, the fibers it innervates, and the axis of motion that is produced, all of which comprise the functional unit of the neuromuscular system. There are three categories of fibers in the PMU, determined by their speed and force of contraction and by their relative fatigability. The types are (a) fast twitch, high force and high fatigue; (b) fast twitch, moderate force, and fatigue resistant; and (c) slow twitch, low tension, and fatigue resistant. The faster the twitch the larger the motor neurons subserving them, because the larger neurons have faster conduction velocities. The slower twitch fibers are much more fatigue resistant. However, it should be remembered that some fast-twitch fibers can become more fatigue resistant with sufficient endurance training. Endurance training (discussed in detail below) refers to a specific program designed selectively to increase one's endurance. The slower fibers have a longer twitch contraction duration, can produce tonic contractions, and generally are redder in color due to increased myoglobin content. Although this myoglobin generalization is not always true, the slower muscles are mainly found distributed in limb extensors, serving postural functions (6, p. 293). The differences are seen in muscles such as the tonic soleus versus the fast phasic gastrocnemius. In a slow, maintained stretch the soleus can develop over 90% of its maximum possible tension, while the gastrocnemius develops only 10% of its maximum at the same time (6, p. 293). This indicates which muscle is injured, and later exercised, by the speed and duration of the stretch applied to it.

The terminal end of the axon of the motor neuron has many branches, needed to stimulate so many fibers. All of the myofibrils innervated by that axon have similar contractile and metabolic properties. There is some evidence of a trophic influence of the innervating fibers that may be capable of altering muscle characteristics (7, pp. 101–13, 8, pp. 258–9; 9, p. 71). In fact, Homewood presents evidence that all tissues may benefit from trophic neuronal influences (8, pp. 117–8). Furthermore, it is probable that the loss of some trophic substance secreted at the motor endplate by the nerve is responsible for changes in the muscle when denervation or severe nerve injury occurs (6, p. 178). It may be that specific nutritional factors added at the time of training may be necessary to take advantage of this capability. More study of this phenomenon is indicated. Depolarization of muscle fibers is probably not the only function of these nerves at the myoneural junction.

One of the basic neurophysiological principles involved here is the "all or nothing" principle, as espoused by Sherrington (5, p. 88). This means that the stimulus needs to be of sufficient magnitude to cause a contraction as the impulse reaches the neuromuscular junction. The force of contraction is varied in one of two ways. Either the number of functional motor units recruited is altered or the frequency of discharge is altered, the force of contraction being directly proportional to either of those variables. According to the load being moved, there is a blending of slow- and fast-twitch fibers, firing at specifically modulated rates to produce the speed and strength of contraction necessary for a given task. The heavier the load, the less options available, since the load of tension on the muscle fibers precludes such choices. The choice of fibers selected is also dependent upon the activity desired. It is the trainable ability of the human central nervous system to select fibers as best befits the maximum performance of a task, or set of tasks, that sets apart most people from highly skilled athletes, who have accomplished this to a great degree. How much of this is trainable and how much is genetic goes back to the age old polemic. However, that portion which is capable of training is that portion at which we aim. This ability also allows the doctor or therapist to rehabilitate a person with an injury or pathology. When a maximum effort is desired, synchronous firing of muscle fibers is necessary, with rapid recruitment of said fibers. When endurance activity is required, asynchronous firing is desirable so that there is a built-in recuperative period. This is important in the choice of exercises, as well as how the exercises are performed and under what conditions.

Neuromuscular Fatigue

In a strict physiological sense, fatigue is a tapering of the response to a stimulus, whether that stimulus is electrical, chemical or simply voluntary or involuntary effort (9, p. 42). There are several causes of neuromuscular fatigue. "Nutrient fatigue" results from a deficiency of muscle glycogen subsequent to submaximal exercise. A second type of fatigue, "anaerobic fatigue," occurs after short-term maximal exercise and is associated with the combination of an oxygen deficit, an increased serum and muscle concentration of lactic acid, and a lowering of the local pH (or corresponding increase of hydrogen ion concentration). It is also known that it takes sustained vigorous contractions greater than 10 sec in duration to deplete the myoglobin oxygen reserves, causing accumulated anaerobic metabolites, ischemia, and fatigue (2, p. 149). There are numerous potentially severe consequences of this second type of fatigue, which occurs under anaerobic conditions. Some of the changes occurring are an interference in the contractile mechanism, a depletion of high-energy phosphates, reduced activity of key enzymes, tubular system disturbances, and ionic imbalances (1, p. 314). Both nutrient and anaerobic fatigue are related to alterations in vascular flows (both supply and elimination). On the supply side, the tonic muscles have three times the size of vascular beds and flow rates as do phasic muscles, so they are less likely to go into "oxygen debt" (2, p. 149). However, on the elimination side, the tonic muscles have small or no recovery periods in which their myoglobin reserves can be recharged. Although this is not the only mechanism involved, it does suggest some therapeutic adjunct to the exercise program.

The last type of fatigue is called "neural fatigue." It occurs when the impulse fails to be transmitted across the myoneural junction. Other sources deny the possibility of neural fatigue, but common sense and recent publications indicate its validity (2,

p. 247). The precise mechanism of action is not known, but it can occur, for instance, after prolonged submaximal exercise, and further motor unit recruitment ensues. After a variable period of time, neural activity seems to decrease, suggesting neural fatigue as a factor. Although the authors are not aware of further specific research on this event, two types of mechanisms could explain this result. First, one could simply postulate a depletion of neurotransmitter substance or neural clearance substance, such as acetylcholine or acetylcholinesterase, respectively. This may or may not respond to increased blood flow, since the effect may not be simply due to lack of raw materials or accumulation of end products. Second, there is a well-known refractory period in neural stimulation and transmission of impulses. It may be that, with increased firing frequency or duration, the refractory period becomes either absolute or longer. It would seem that rest plays a more significant role in neural fatigue, in either case. The peripheral neuromuscular apparatus has a high threshold to fatigue; therefore, the fatigue is more likely to occur in the synapses of the central nervous system (9, pp. 42–3). Total rest and increased blood flow are not uniformly compatible, so some decisions need to be made regarding exercise design.

Steindler discusses three parameters of fatigue: biochemical, physiological, and physical relationships (5, pp. 87–90). There will be overlap with the above mentioned categories, but they are not identical windows through which to view fatigue. The biochemical type relates to the accumulation of lactic acid in the muscles, which may be 10 to 15 times greater than that in normal resting muscles (5, p. 87). This accretion is accelerated by the eventual "oxygen debt" that occurs as the oxygen intake either falls or the circulation is inadequate to handle the load. The lactic acid accrues initially at the motor endplates, but it rapidly diffuses throughout the muscle. If one had any question as to the origin of the muscle contraction impulse, this metabolic evidence would clarify it. One measure of the efficiency of the muscle is the ratio between the lactic acid removed for resynthesis in the liver and the lactic acid that is completely oxidized. This ratio is normally 5:1 (5, p. 88). It should be noted that it may take hours to dispose of the accumulated lactic acid from just a few minutes of violent exercise. Therefore, one can conclude that vigorous and severe exercising typically leads to a biochemical or anaerobic type fatigue in a relatively short period of time. This would lead one to question the validity of intense precompetition exercising.

Physiological fatigue relates to the neural stimulation of muscle fibers, usually in rotational or sequential fashion, during submaximal exercise. In this case, the fatigue factor is originally confined to a specific group of affected endplates. Fatigue begins to spread, eventually affecting the character and regularity of muscle discharges, as seen in electromyographic studies. The discharges eventually begin to resemble tremors as muscles become exhausted, finally resulting in a virtually flat amplitude graph, as the muscle appears paralyzed. From a physical standpoint, fatigue is the inefficiency in or inability to perform a task. Locomotor function diminishes and becomes less precise, the pulse rate increases, the blood pressure rises (proportionate to the exertion), and the respiratory rate increases. The resultant increase is eventually out of proportion to the external resistance, just as the muscle tension had become so, physiologically. An interesting factor concerning fatigue seems to cross these arbitrary lines of demarcation, to some degree. As noted previously, any fatigue factors that result from hypoxia or an accumulation of metabolites can be cured, to a certain extent, by an increase in blood flow. However, there exists the mechanical problem of maintaining such increased blood flow through a contracted muscular area, since the rise of intramuscular tension dampens the blood flow. Additionally, a great increase of blood flow, causing an increase in the extracellular fluid content, causes localized congestion, which is a factor in producing hypoxia. This becomes a problem for the lymphatic system, which is too often ignored clinically. Concern for and enhancement of the lymphatic drainage might well be a partial solution to these problems (discussed in the clinical sections). In any case, the solution has a point of diminishing returns. At this point, work becomes uneconomical and even counterproductive, a point well remembered by the doctor and the therapist. Finally, it has been shown that sympathetic stimulation seems to retard muscle fatigue, perhaps by an adrenergic effect (5, p. 90). This is a point well understood by coaches who motivate their athletes to perform well beyond what might be their normal limits, the so-called "giving 110%" cliche. The caveat here is that there are consequences of pushing someone beyond the point of fatigue, particularly someone who already has an injury or a compromise of function in some vital system. We have attempted to be acutely aware of such considerations in the design and implementation of exercise programs. Such concerns can only enhance the effectiveness while decreasing the risk, a factor that has become far more important in today's litigious environment.

Muscular Soreness and Stiffness

Soreness is of two basic types. There is a temporary soreness that begins with the exercise and may last for a few hours afterward. This soreness may be related to a temporary spasm of the muscle and is probably secondary to a localized hypoxia. This is the same kind of soreness that one experiences in angina pectoris and that is relieved by flushing the muscles with blood (therefore oxygen). This is why a shower or a steam bath may be just what the doctor ordered for this specific problem. Sometimes hot water and sometimes cold water is the better choice, depending upon whether the problem is not enough incoming blood (i.e., arterial) or not enough exiting blood (i.e., venous), respectively. There is no injury, per se, involved in this type of soreness. This may be the result of an improper warmup, excess environmental stress, anemic type blood conditions, or simply exercising too long. Any difficulty with proper respiratory function (both macro and micro) may induce this type of soreness, as well as the second type.

The soreness we must be more concerned about is the residual soreness, which usually begins some time after the exercise has ceased and may last for a few days. It is referred to as "delayed onset muscle soreness" (DOMS) and is apparently not related to significant elevations in lactic acid. (1, p. 392). Four main factors may be connected with DOMS (1, p. 392). Experimental stud-

ies have shown that eccentric contractions seem to cause far more muscle soreness than concentric or static contractions (1, p. 393). Although there is increased serum creatine kinase and serum myoglobin after all activities, one cannot seemingly differentiate the activity or degree of soreness based upon these chemistries (1, p. 393).

First, minute tears of individual muscle fibers have been hypothesized to be responsible for DOMS. It is known that eccentric contractions place a greater strain upon connective tissues and muscle fibers than concentric contractions do (see next section). Compare, for example, the difficulty running downhill (eccentric) versus running on flat ground (concentric). This is not all of the picture, since enzyme activity, which reflects tissue breakdown, does not show a one-to-one relationship with muscle soreness. Furthermore, if this is true, how do the fibers heal? In what period of time? What are the long-term effects of training on these tissues?

A second theory suggests that altered osmotic pressure causes fluid retention in surrounding tissues. The osmotic pressure is altered by accretions of metabolites in those tissues. This theory is also not adequate because concentric exercise produces five to seven times the metabolic stress of eccentric work (1, p. 395). The muscle spasm hypothesis also has much to speak for it, especially since symptomatic relief and a decreased EMG amplitude is created by appropriate static therapeutic stretching of the area (1, p. 395). Muscle spasms, or cramps, are involuntary, localized, painful contractions of muscle that may be protracted in duration but are often capable of being relieved by stretching (10, p. 439). Tonic myospasms are usually the result of ischemia, and any procedures, including stretching, that relieve the ischemia will usually have good results. We generally recommend static rather than dynamic stretching procedures, because they are less likely to initiate myotatic stretch reflexes (see end of this chapter), which could increase pain and spasm. Sometimes soreness was found in the absence of any relation to either myoglobinuria or EMG findings. Further testing revealed a significant increase in hydroxyproline 48 hours after exercise, which related to muscle soreness. This, and the fact that slow dynamic stretching as well as static stretching temporarily relieved the pain is the basis for the connective tissue damage theory.

Most of the time, a combination of factors is responsible for the symptoms. One needs to ask whether the long-term implication for serious muscle training is negative because of the tissue damage intrinsic to it. We believe that the benefits of training outweigh the harm, but there are proper ways to perform training activities. All of the answers are not yet known, but there is sufficient information available to design good rehabilitation programs.

Isometric Versus Isotonic Versus Isokinetic Exercises

Another model for the contraction of muscles is shown in Figure 2.6. The PECs are the structural muscle elements that are different from the contractile proteins, such as connective tissue sheaths and muscle proteins that basically provide scaffolding. The tendons essentially comprise the SECs, which are chiefly involved with the resistance to stretch. The CCs are the contractile fibrils in the muscles themselves. During a passive stretch of the muscle, they act as a passive viscous element and, like the PECs, provide little resistance to stretch. All of the above is the response to passive stretch. However, once the nerve stimulation has been received, the process becomes an active one, and the CCs become the main component involved. The CCs are able to convert electrochemical energy into mechanical energy, and the speed of contraction is an inverse function of the force opposing its shortening. This means,

in terms of exercise, that the potential velocity of contraction decreases as the load upon the muscle increases. This consideration will be further elucidated in the clinical section.

Muscle strength plays a role in all our concerns in this book. Muscle strength is the maximum force that a muscle can exert in a single maximum contraction (11, p. 3). A static contraction is one in which there is no associated joint movement, while a dynamic contraction is one in which there is associated joint movement. Static contractions are also isometric, while dynamic contractions can be isotonic or isokinetic.

In an isometric contraction, the CCs shorten, thus stretching the SECs. This contraction occurs without joint movement. Implicit in such motion is the fact that the force the muscle generates is equal to the force of resistance (or load). The myofibrils contract at maximum velocity initially, since there is no initial load. However, the stretching of the SECs gradually increases the tension and, therefore the load. Proportionately, the tension reduces the velocity of contraction. From this, it is also obvious that the isometric tension in a muscle is a function of the initial length of the muscle (2, p. 245). As the muscle length increases toward its resting length, the active tension increases. If the length is greater than the resting length, then the active tension gradually decreases to zero, because the actin and myosin filaments disengage due to the artificial elongation of the sarcomeres. At the same time, the passive tension increases from zero as the load pulls the muscle beyond its resting length. The quantity of elastic connective tissue (i.e., the passive component in the PECs) determines the actual form of the graph of muscle tension, since the active component (the CCs) always behaves the same in all muscles. This isometric contraction is utilized normally in maintaining posture versus gravity. This type of contraction is most effective during early stages of injuries (especially when joint motion is limited), when muscle strength is insufficient to utilize other procedures, and when other types of contractions may be contraindicated. To apply these concepts, it is necessary to differentiate and properly to diagnose the types of tissues and injuries so that appropriate exercises may be used.

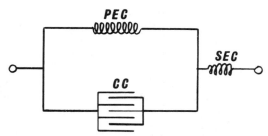

Figure 2.6 Electronic equivalent to muscle mechanics. *PEC* = parallel elastic components; *SEC* = series elastic components; *CC* = contractile components. (Reprinted with permission from Keele CA, Neil E: Samson Wright's Applied Physiology. 12th ed. New York:Oxford University Press, 1971.)

Isotonic contractions, on the other hand, do external work, as when one is pumping up a basketball or walking. However, walking, as do most complex motions, has isometric phases and actions as part of its process. The series of multiaxial, combined motions called walking, or gait, is accomplished by alternately moving agonists and antagonists, with the help of synergists, in a bilaterally symmetrical manner. The sequential fixing and releasing of joint areas is also necessary to accomplish this (see biomechanics texts for more information). Once the muscle contraction begins to overcome the load, if the force of contraction reaches a steady state, the load is moved, at a specific rate, and this is called isotonic contraction. In order for this load to be moved over a distance, the muscle must continue to shorten. However, one can perform an isotonic contraction in another manner as well. If one puts a constant load on a muscle and allows it slowly to overtake a contracted muscle, as that muscle gradually elongates we have the passive counterpart to an isotonic contraction, an isotonic stretch. Those who are familiar with exercise equipment such as Nautilus understand this principle.

The second part of each activity is a slower isotonic decontraction, where one resists only enough to slow down the relaxation curve. The first part of the exercise performed upon each of these machines is an isokinetic exercise, in which a particular load, which may be constant or variable over the range of motion, is moved relatively rapidly in an controlled angular acceleration over the portion of the joint's motion being exercised. The difference between isotonic and isokinetic is that, in the latter, the velocity and acceleration are controlled and, in the former, the load is controlled and held constant. Although isokinetic exercise sounds like the most attractive, particularly for athletes, its motion is only an approximation of the actions in those sports. The speed is relatively slow and constant, compared with the activity itself.

Isometric training has its own limitation as well. It is a very specific activity, such that strength improvement is usually demonstrated mainly in isometric contractions which approximate the training ones. (1, p. 379). If one is engaging in an activity, such as pitching a softball, that requires a specific motion, one needs to train specifically for that motion. The drawback is that such training is generally only applicable to that activity or an identical one. This means that, to train a muscle or group thoroughly, one must isometrically contract those fibers at a multitude of angles. This is usually inconvenient and time consuming. It is rare that all of the motion and power of a muscle or group is lost, except with severe injuries involving neurological deficit. In those cases, one must be that meticulous in training. However, it is very useful as a testing procedure to determine the angles (or range) of weakness, because such thoroughness is necessary when evaluating as well as when treating. Modern computer technology has enabled us quantitatively and qualitatively to analyze function over all of the ranges of motions of joints. Remember, the distance moved times the force exerted is the work produced.

Concentric Versus Eccentric

There is yet another way to describe types of muscle contractions. The first type is a *concentric* contraction, in which the muscle shortens as it develops tension and overcomes the resistance applied to it. This is typically the kind of contraction that is utilized in most sports activities, like weight lifting and hitting a baseball. The second type of contraction is called *eccentric*, in which the external resistance overcomes the power exerted by the muscle. This means that the muscle lengthens while it maintains an amount of tension upon it. This was called isotonic decontraction above. In weight lifting, as the weight is slowly lowered, this type of contraction is occurring. People engage in many activities that require them slowly to lower a load, just acting as a dampening force against gravity. This usually follows the concentric effort of lifting it in the first place. This combination has somewhat improperly been labeled as an isotonic exercise. The problem is that, while the load is constant, the tension is constantly changing, due to the equally constant change in angle of the lever arm and, therefore, length of the muscle. An interesting characteristic of eccentric contraction is that a muscle can produce more force in this manner than in a concentric manner, but with less effort. Therefore, it may be desirable to employ this mode of exercise, rather than a concentric or even isometric form, when there is considerable damage or weakness in a particular location (11, p. 3). This is another important consideration in the design of an exercise regimen, especially toward the beginning of such programs.

Progressive Resistive Exercise

A technique called progressive resistive exercise (PRE) forms the basis for most modern weight rehabilitative procedures. In each workout, the patient is instructed to perform three sets of 10 (for example) exercises, with a load that either increases or decreases per set. This is based upon the maximum load capacity. The idea in each of these sets is to produce fatigue in the muscles used. As the muscle strengthens, the load must gradually be increased. For example, one may begin with ⅓ or 40% maximum load, performed 10 times per set, abbreviated as ⅓ 10-RM or 0.4 10-RM. In the former case, this may graduate to ⅔ 10-RM and 10-RM, the last set being performed at maximum capacity.

Because there is a difference in the energy expenditure of an isometric versus an isotonic or isokinetic contraction, there is also a difference in their respective fatigue factors. In isometric contractions, where muscles do not change their length, no visible work is performed, but maximum tension is developed. The work produced here (since work must include some kind of motion, from a physics standpoint) is on the cellular and molecular level and involves electrochemical reactions. In isotonic contractions, there is a constantly decreasing tension, therefore the work (i.e., energy consumption) amounts to only one-third of its theoretical maximum. Contraction efficiency seems to increase as the contraction slows down, with 1.5 sec being the optimum contraction time (5, p. 91). In an isokinetic contraction, neither the load nor the muscle length may be constant. This means that the tension may not vary as much and the work accomplished may be closer to the theoretical maximum. In some ways, this type of exercise provides some of the benefits of both other types. Again,

speed of contraction is important, but there does not seem to be an agreement as to what speeds are best for what muscles and what intents. In performing either passive or active resistance rehabilitative exercises these facts are important to remember. If one performs isometric exercises and the external resistance keeps the muscle at its optimum length, then the muscle displays its optimum strength. However, if the external resistance is so strong as to overcome the muscle, the muscle will be forced into a passive stretch, thus changing its length from optimum and reducing its potential strength. The earliest signs of fatigue are a reduction of amplitude of the contraction wave and an imprecision of movements and increased effort necessary, on a macro level. It is wise to look for such signs, regardless of the type of exercise used.

Physical Properties of Muscle Tissues

The two main physical characteristics of muscle are its elasticity and its contractility. Tension, an external stressor upon the muscle, causes initial elongation and a reduction in the cross-sectional area of the muscle. The equation below shows the relationship between the various factors:

$$\Delta L = (F)(L)(E) / A,$$

where ΔL = elongation of muscle, L = original length of muscle, F = force applied (or tension), E = Young's modulus of elasticity (elasticity coefficient) (Actually this modulus has not been determined specifically for muscle fibers, so this is not a true Young modulus, but a constant of undetermined value. The Young's modulus is an imaginary constant that represents the ability of the body to elongate to twice its resting length without breaking—a feat not normally possible (5, p. 11)), and A = cross-sectional area of muscle. If we look at Hooke's law of spring motion

$$F = -kx$$

where F = force exerted, k = constant, according to material of spring, and x = distance spring travels, or elongation, we see a similar law, within which a linear relationship exists between the force exerted and the resultant displacement. The difference with muscles and body tissues is that the

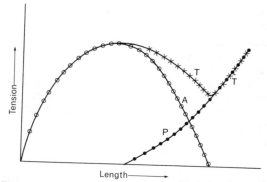

Figure 2.7 Relationship between tension and length in muscles. T = total tension; A = active tension; P = passive tension. (Reprinted with permission from Keele CA, Neil E: Samson Wright's Applied Physiology. 12th ed. New York:Oxford University Press, 1971.)

relationship is not really linear, but is hyperbolic (Fig 2.7) (5, p. 46). In a muscle, the elongation, a passive process, diminishes considerably after a certain point, though the tension may still increase a great deal. The unit resistance of the muscle to tearing is much less than that of its tendon (which is a much thinner structure still maintaining the same force as the larger muscle), and the fibers can normally be stretched to 1.6 times their original length without rupturing (5, p. 46).

It is important to consider elasticity for two main reasons. First, the tissue injured may or may not be of the elastic type. This means that the applied therapy needs to be altered to fit the injured tissue, as well as the type of injury. For instance, exercises can be done actively or passively, and different substructures are generally involved in each case. Second, one needs to consider whether to stretch or contract the involved structures and whether the agonist, antagonist, or other related muscles (such as synergists) need to be implicated in the treatment program.

The second main physical property of muscle is its contractility, an active process by which the muscle shortens in response to neural stimuli. The muscle more nearly approximates Hooke's law in its contracted state, where some elasticity also exists, than it does in other states. The absolute muscle power is found by the amount of tension necessary to stretch out a maximally contracted muscle to its original

length, over the cross-sectional area of that muscle. The maximum muscle strength, though, is found by applying a maximal innervation, under isometric conditions, to that muscle. If the muscle is allowed to shorten (i.e., isotonic conditions) then its tension decreases in proportion to its change of length, from 20 to 80% (5, p. 48). Remember that this muscle contraction occurs according to Sherrington's law on an "all or nothing basis," so the force of contraction is a function, neurologically, of the number of motor units "firing off" at a given moment in time. In isometric measurements of the *absolute* strength of the upper and lower extremities, the capacities in females were shown to average about 56% and 28%, respectively, less than in males depending upon the specific muscle tested (1, p. 376). Approximately the same results were obtained in dynamic measurements of absolute strength (1, p. 376). This is not true for all women and all men, but it must be kept in mind when designing and implementing exercise programs. Since our exercises are rarely performed near maximum capacity, this is significant only in finding the maximum as a limitation factor. It should be briefly mentioned that relaxation, the opposite action to contraction, is also an important facet. It is not merely the absence of contraction, for it is neurochemically an active process itself. Furthermore, it is necessary for an antagonist, or even a synergist, to relax so that an agonist can contract maximally.

Fiber Length

The fiber length in contracted versus relaxed states is dependent upon the elasticity and contractility of muscle. This is significant, in that the tension on the muscle represents the force, while the muscle length represents the distance over which the force operates. Without both factors, one cannot calculate the amount of work done, regardless of energy expended. Estimates of the actual ratios of contracted to relaxed fiber lengths vary, but we prefer Recklinghausen's estimate that the muscle only contracts to about 75% of its relaxed length (5, pp. 52–3). This is a conservative appraisal and will serve as a minimum guide for our purposes. The actual ratio will obviously depend upon the location, type, and action of the muscle and, probably, upon the nature of its specific fibers. On the other hand, a passive stretch could maximally add about 60% to the relaxed muscle length. All normal physiological motor activity should occur within this range of muscle lengths, or so-called amplitude of muscle action. Most muscles, however, display their maximum power or efficiency near their natural length, not at their extremes of motion or length. This is why muscles are more likely to be injured at other lengths; therefore, they may also need to be rehabilitated at those lengths. Muscles with a greater contraction length and less power are built for speed; muscles with a shorter contraction length have a larger index of efficiency and are built for strength.

$$E_m = \frac{1}{f(\Delta L)}$$

where E_m = muscle efficiency and ΔL = amplitude of contraction of muscle.

Often joints are supplied with pairs of muscles, so as to endow the joint with both capabilities. An example of this occurs in the knee joint. The medial hamstrings have a greater contractile length and provide speed, whereas the biceps has a shorter contraction and provides strength. This has obvious application for the surgeon who performs muscle or tendon transplants and similar implications for the doctor or therapist concerned with rehabilitative exercises.

Hypertrophy

As mentioned earlier, one of the later training effects that occurs with a strength program is a muscular property known as hypertrophy. This physiological adaptation to an increased load on the muscle is actually an increase in the size of the muscle fibers. One can have an increase in strength without hypertrophy of muscle fibers, probably by an increased efficiency of the neuromuscular mechanisms. Such hypertrophy does not occur much from weak, repetitive activities, but requires, instead, very vigorous muscle activity (to at least 75% of maximum tension) for only a few minutes per day [3, p. 91]. This is why isometric activity is so useful for developing strength. It is clear that muscle hypertrophy also requires a parallel increase in quantity and quality

of nutrients and metabolic processes, in general. For instance, the quantity of contractile protein is increased, but the quantity of mitochondria is not proportionately increased. This means that hypertrophy is useful for strength-related demands but may be detrimental for endurance training [1, p. 386]. Apparently, there is also a longitudinal splitting of the muscle cells, so that the number of fibers actually increases as well [1, p. 388]. However, this latter effect seems to contribute little to muscle hypertrophy. It also appears that the supporting connective tissues (i.e., the PECs) and the ligaments and tendons are amplified in some fashion by this process [1, p. 387]. This is actually a desired effect when there is ligamentous damage. For the record, the current data seem to indicate that women are not capable of achieving the same degree of muscle hypertrophy as men. This is theoretically due to the generally much higher level of testosterone in males. Despite the current interest in the use of anabolic steroids, this subject will not be discussed here. There are numerous pathological and pathophysiological situations in which muscle hypertrophy occurs as well. Some of these are discussed in the clinical chapters.

Physical Properties of Ligaments And Tendons

Although these soft tissue structures generally have a greater tensile strength than muscles, they are still subject to injury and need to be rehabilitated. This does point to the fact that muscle injuries are all too often misdiagnosed as damage to other adjacent soft tissues. Fascial tissues appear to have quite varying degrees of elasticity and tensile strength. However, their deformation is a function of both the quantity and duration of the applied external force, and it varies considerably with the individual and with the specific body area involved. The ligaments most exposed to tension stresses during their normal motion have the greatest percentage of elastic tissue within their makeup. A notable example of this is the ligamentum flavum, which is often seen thickened along the spine during certain medical imaging procedures [5, p. 55]. Such hypertrophy of elastic tissues within a ligamentous structure is probably a strong sign of the instability of that joint. If a ligament is continuously overstretched, it eventually loses its shape and size to some extent. Such events occur all too commonly in the deltoid ligament of the ankle, for example (due to chronic inversion sprains and foot pronation), and in the medial collateral ligament of the knee (due to the above mentioned events and others, such as genu valgus and chronic knee cartilage or patellar disorders).

The following is meant as a quick review. The places in the muscle where there are only white, fibrous, collagen tissue and no myofibrils are called tendons. In other words, tendons are muscles minus myofibrils. Tendons are found at the ends or middle (digastric or biventral muscles) of muscles. When there are two, three, four, or more muscle masses ending in a common tendon, the muscle is named bicipital, tricipital, quadricipital or multicipital, respectively (9, p. 48). These tendons serve as dampers, through their elastic structures, of the rough and digital motion of the muscles to produce smoother movements. The tendon behaves much as the fascia does, but tendinous ruptures usually occur either at the insertion to the bone or at the musculotendinous junction. The central artery of the tendon usually disappears sometime in the third decade of life, so early tendinous degenerative changes, leading to "spontaneous tendon ruptures," are not uncommon (5, p. 56). This degeneration occurs most commonly in the tendons of the extensor hallucis longus, tendoachilles, quadriceps, and rotator cuff muscles of the shoulder. This means that rehabilitative exercises performed for these areas must include a sufficient preliminary warmup structure to bathe these tendons in the circulatory overflow from adjacent structures. This tendinous degeneration also explains why avulsion type injuries are more common in younger individuals, while tendon tears are more typically seen in older persons.

Special Receptors

The afferent nervous system is composed of two categories of receptor nerve endings, *exteroceptors* and *interoceptors*. Exteroceptors include the cutaneous receptors for touch, pressure, pain, and temperature and the special sensors of the eyes, ears, nose, and taste sensation. Interoceptors include proprioceptors, visceroceptors (i.e., from the organs), and chemoceptors (i.e., carotid and aortic bodies). The proprioceptors, such as muscle spindle cells, Golgi tendon organs, joint receptors, and vestibular receptors, are the ones with which we are concerned here. These receptors inform the brain about changes in body positions and physical relationships. The vestibular receptors of the structures of the inner ear are not discussed in this text, but they are to be considered no less important.

Joint Receptors

Joint receptors are generally fairly large and fast-conducting nerve fibers (group IA mainly, with some group II in the capsule) that are located in the joint ligaments and, less so, in the joint capsule. They are divided into receptors that are slow adapting and mainly signal joint position, and others that are fast adapting and mainly signal joint movement. Conscious proprioception is solely provided by these joint receptors and their afferent pathways (2, p. 293).

Muscle Spindles

The muscle spindles are morphologically and functionally the most complexly organized proprioceptors and are found in muscles supplied by motor cranial nerves, as well as the locomotor apparatus (12, pp. 125–6). The muscle spindle is a fusiform structure, running in parallel to the myofibrils and attaching to their endomysium at both ends. The spindle nerve endings signal both the instantaneous length of the muscle and the velocity of contraction of the muscle. The former is called the *static response* and the latter the *dynamic response*, and each type is associated with a different neuroanatomical substrate (12, p. 130). Their primary function is to cause a muscle contraction reflexly in response to a muscle stretch. Perhaps it is injury to or pathophysiology of these structures that is responsible, in part, for serious myospasm and DOMS. It is, of course, the stimulation of the spindle cell afferent nerve which is testing the so-called H-reflex (10, p. 484). This cannot, however, be elicited in all muscles, and its relation to myospasm has not been well documented. Spindle cells are innervated by large, rapidly conducting group IA afferent fibers and end in annulospiral spindle endings. Even though the tendon is struck by the clinician's neurological hammer, it is the spindle cells that are responsible for the tendon reflexes being checked (2, p. 293). This is why calling this a deep tendon reflex is actually a misnomer. Like the density of motor nerve endings themselves, muscle spindles most densely populate those muscles in which finely differentiated movements occur (12, p. 126).

Myotatic Reflex

This apparatus is part of the two-neuron (or monosynaptic) reflex arc known as the myotatic reflex. Each spinal reflex arc is actually a mechanism consisting of five links: (a) the receptor, (b) the afferent conductor, (c) the "reflex center," (d) the efferent conductor. and (e) the effector (12, p. 132). We will focus on those spinal reflexes whose effectors are skeletal muscles. The first neuron is the afferent conductor fiber that

serves the spindle cell, transmitting the information to the central spinal locus, where it can be influenced by other inputs. This then synapses with the body of the efferent conductor motor neuron in the anterior horn. This second neuron's axon ends on the motor endplates of the same or related muscles. The receptor that begins this process is one of the receptors described above, and the effector is a muscle, gland, or vessel that reacts to the stimulus (Fig 2.8). This process is the mechanism by which the spindle cell controls the muscle length and, therefore, tone, and is known as a *stretch reflex*. One notes here that all motor reflexes, except this stretch reflex, involve multisynaptic arcs and, therefore, interneurons. That is why the stretch reflex is least susceptible to supraspinal influences (12, p. 201). It should also be noted that there are collateral fibers from the spindle cell afferent that send inhibitory messages to the antagonist muscle(s), thereby facilitating the stretch reflex. This is important when dealing with myospasm, which may

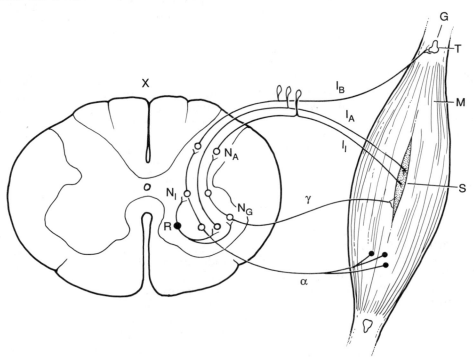

Figure 2.8. Schematic of basic neuromuscular control mechanisms. X = transverse section of spinal cord; M = muscle body; T = muscle tendon; G = GTO end organ receptor (in series with muscle fibers); S = spindle cell organ receptor (in parallel with muscle fibers): I_A = monosynaptic spindle cell afferent (primary); I_B = disynaptic GTO afferent; I_I = polysynaptic slower afferent; γ = gamma motor neuron; α = alpha motor neuron with flower spray endings; N_A = afferent nerve cell body; N_I = interneuron cell body; N_G = efferent nerve cell body; R = Renshaw (inhibitory) cell body.

DYNAMICS OF CLINICAL REHABILITATIVE EXERCISE

interfere with rehabilitative exercises, and gives us a rationale for a treatment approach. There is both a phasic and a tonic component to (or capability in) this reflex. The former occurs simultaneously with the actual stretch, and the latter occurs, after a short period of latency, during the period of constantly maintained stretch. Thus, this could also be considered one of the postural reflexes. Postural reflexes essentially attempt to maintain correct body posture by a constant alteration of musculoskeletal elements in response to external demands and intrinsic motions. Other postural reflexes include flexor, crossed extensor, and stretch flexor reflexes (3, p. 656; 12, p. 132).

Muscle Tone

Muscle tone refers to the partial state of tetanus (continuous partial muscle contraction) that occurs as a result of the asynchronous discharge of neuronal impulses to that muscle. It is more properly referred to as resting tone when referring to a muscle in a normal relaxed state. It is, of course, not really a resting tone, since it is busy maintaining the anatomical and functional relationships of the involved structures. This tone also varies according to the situation. For instance, it is lower during sleep than when awake, and it is higher when someone is poised for action but not yet moving. Various pathological or pathophysiological conditions cause this tone to vary and become greater (hypertonus) or less (hypotonus) than normal. Muscle tone is regulated by both myotatic and nonmyotatic influences, although the former clearly hold greatest sway (2, p. 294).

There is also evidence that there are separate α motor neurons specific to the tonic and phasic myofibrils within any given muscle, which innervate, respectively, the slow red myofibrils and the fast white myofibrils (2, pp. 294–5). The discharge of a tonic motor neuron is low threshold, long duration, and slow rate, whereas the discharge of a phasic motor neuron is high threshold and transient. Muscle tone is evaluated, without instrumentation, by palpation and by passive movement. Clinicians know that even though a muscle may not feel spastic, it may demonstrate increased resistance when put through a range of motion. The opposite situation

may also occur, but is not as likely. The explanation is fairly simple and accounts for most of the related phenomena. The tonic portion of the tone, or *reflex tone*, is used to maintain posture, and reflects the monitoring of length. This causes the contraction of red myofibrils, is generally a slow procedure, involving a time lag, and causes changes in the palpable resting muscle tone. To overcome the time lag problem, other neurofibers monitor velocity or change of position, respond more to passive motion testing, and produce phasic myocontractions, using basically the white myofibrils. Both types of γ neurons (which innervate the intrafusal fibers) and α neurons (which innervate the extrafusal fibers) are susceptible to extraspinal and supraspinal influences, such as mood (12, p. 137). This explains why a reflex or even a blood pressure may be increased in a doctor's office, especially during the early phases of treatment. Because many muscles have both types of fibers and, therefore, neurons, the type of training procedures used is important in most muscles and crucial in others. This information is significant in the design of exercise programs, in that the need for proper evaluation and diagnosis is further demonstrated. How patients perform the exercises determines how the neuromuscular system is affected and, therefore, what results may be expected. It is an oversimplification, but it may be said that one of the chief goals of rehabilitative therapies is to modify tone appropriately.

Golgi Tendon Organs

The Golgi tendon organs (GTOs) are located in the tendons of each of the muscles and are connected in series with the extrafusal fibers (as part of the SEC). They consist of a delicate connective tissue sac housing a spray ending of neurofibrils from a large myelinated nerve fiber, ending in the vicinity of the musculotendinous junction. Spindle cells are low-threshold stretch receptors. The GTOs are higher threshold stretch receptors whose main function is to cause reflex inhibition of the contraction of their respective muscles and simultaneously facilitate the antagonists of these same muscles. It should be mentioned that Charles Scott Sherrington, a late 19th century experimental neurophysiologist, elucidated many of the concepts presented here, including the concept of reciprocal innervation and inhibition, from which many modern theories are derived, (9, p. 465). Reciprocal innervation is the process whereby the pair of muscles that work in opposition to each other is alternately excited and inhibited, depending upon the intent of the stimulation. The GTOs are innervated by large, fast-transmitting group IB afferent fibers; they detect mainly muscle tension, not length. Because of the nature of their function, the GTOs are part of the mechanism responsible for protecting the motion units from overload. GTOs act in a slightly slower fashion than spindle cells, because they operate through interneurons, known as Renshaw cells (in a bisynaptic or three-neuron arc) in the anterior horn (12, p. 138). There are also reputed to be generalized receptors called pacinian corpuscles, which are small elliptical bodies that appear laminate, like an onion, and lie near the GTOs. They are fast adapting and seem to respond mainly to changes in movement or pressure, not absolute values of them.

Engrams

An engram represents the neurological organization of a preprogrammed pattern of muscular activity (13, p. 404). The nature of an engram is that, once developed, each additional excitation causes exactly the same activity. This concept will be discussed further under the heading of facilitation. This appears to differ, in substance, if not in theory, from the "engram" as described by L. Ron Hubbard in his book, *Dianetics*. The engram referred to here represents the sensory memory of a sequence or pattern of motor movements devised for a specific purpose. Memory is the key word here. In fact, the engram has been likened to a magnetic tape that can be played back (6, pp. 587–94). The normal proprioceptive signal pathway is designed to produce cerebellar control over the coordination of activities of the area originating the signals. The maintenance of posture is an example of the proprioceptive system at work (i.e., the sensors, the posterior columns, the cerebellum, and the vestibular system, all acting through reflex mechanisms) (14, p. 96). However, certain patterns of learned motor behavior can be stored as sensory engrams

and performed while bypassing the above systems. The proprioceptors would send information directly to the sensory cortex instead. Then the data are compared with the engram stored therein, and the motor cortex is then activated to stimulate or inhibit those muscles in proper sequence, time, force, and duration, which would produce the required task(s). In this situation, the motor system acts as a servomechanism to provide error signals for the sensory cortex so that performance may be modified by the engram.

When the sensory engram relies on kinesthetic feedback, it is rapidly responding. However, if it needs to depend upon the visual system for feedback, its response time is significantly longer (3, p. 689). Anyone who has learned a new sport activity is acutely aware of this phenomenon. In fact, if one tries to watch and think one's way through the activity, during the action, one is more likely to flub it. As the engram becomes less of a conscious activity, speed, coordination, and precision increase in direct proportion to that unconsciousness. Itzhak Pearlman and his "magic fingers" on the violin are a particularly pleasing application of this principle. When the recognition of a key triggers such a skillful response, this is also referred to as initiation of an *automatized preprogrammed pattern (or skilled automatic performance)* (13, p. 405). It is well established that frequent repetition is one of the main determinants in this process. The relatively "simple" tasks of walking, talking, and jumping required years of constant rote neuromuscular activity, including much trial and error, to bring a child's coordination skills up to adult levels. Once the sensory engram has been created, a motor engram is produced within the motor cortex. One must remember that the motor system is always run from this area. Now the function of the sensory cortex has been reduced to monitoring the activity to make certain it follows the engram. If it does not, at some point, the sensory cortex immediately initiates the necessary steps to correct the movements to fit the motor template.

Programs of therapeutic exercises are recommended to be repeated as often as possible, since engrams do not become well developed until hundreds of thousands of repetitions have been performed (13, p. 410).

This is particularly significant when training for activities requiring higher degrees of coordination. Therefore, many of these exercises are also effective for handicapped people and stroke victims. Coordination is effectuated by the same central mechanisms as is proprioception. Impulses transmitted through the posterior column system reach consciousness, while those passing through the cerebellum do not directly reach consciousness (12, p. 96). Therefore, part of the aim of our exercises is to reach the unconscious processes and mechanisms by conscious and deliberate activities. One must be careful, however, that exercises are done with precision. If extraneous motions accompany the desired motions, they will become part of that engram and the end product may be other than the preferred one. It should be mentioned that training includes promotion of the inhibition process in the formation of engrams. A concern only with the excitation of muscles producing a specific result indicates a lack of understanding of the coordinated process occurring.

Further Concepts

Some other reflex mechanisms should be mentioned here, because some exercise procedures will require that they be intact and well functioning. Many other reflexes have been discovered in laboratory animals as a result of experimental neurosurgical techniques. We will not be discussing these entities or animal reflexes, such as the scratch reflex. Tone can also be described as the resistance of a muscle to its passive stretching, which has to do with the characteristics of the individual fibers as well as the neuronal input into them (10, p. 480). There are tonic neck reflexes in the ligaments of the cervical vertebral joints, especially in the atlanto-occipital joints (2, p. 297). These reflexes may be related to activities and reflexes stemming from the temporomandibular joint apparatus. The tonic labyrinthine reflexes originate from the semicircular canals in the inner ear and respond to specific positions of the head relative to the transverse plane. These reactions are innervated by the vestibular nerve and are, therefore, under supraspinal control. A chain of reactions, collectively labeled the righting reflexes, enables the body to achieve or maintain an essentially erect posture. Full functioning of the cerebellum is prerequisite for the execution of the intricate and delicate reactions involved in these reflexes. They function in its absence, but not well. Another concept, first espoused by Sherrington, is that the proprioceptive beds of the more cephalad segments are influential in the reflex tone of a greater somatic area than the beds of more caudad segments (8, p. 126). If the head is rotated to the right, the tone increases in the limbs on the right and decreases in the left limbs. If the head is flexed, flexor tonus increases in the arms and extensor tonus increases in the legs. Head extension has the reverse effect. This reflex reaction may be of use in enhancing the outcomes of specific exercises. All of this is subject to supraspinal influences, such as the vestibular complex, and may not be applicable in persons who have deficits in those areas. How these reflexes affect tone and muscle exercise efficiency is discussed in the design of clinical exercise programs.

Furthermore, it should be mentioned that the corpus callosum serves as a bridge between the two cerebral hemispheres, allowing what Brodal called "interhemispheric cross talk" to occur (12, p. 678). The significance here is that the exercise of, for example, a right-sided, uninjured structure may positively enhance the performance of a left-sided, injured structure that cannot be moved itself for some reason. This procedure has been called cross-training, and the process has been labeled a *crossed reflex* by Hellebrandt. A certain amount of success has been attributed to it, probably because of the corpus callosum (9, p. 466). It has also been observed that a hemiplegic who exercises the unaffected side can usually witness an equivalent action in the affected side (12, p. 215). This is termed symmetrical associated movements, and, apart from the explanation just offered, there does not seem to be an acceptable accounting for this phenomenon. Again, this presents both a method and a rationale for treatment of certain conditions and situations, including a person with a casted or immobilized limb.

It is also of interest to recognize that there is a longitudinal branching of the axons of motor neurons, and interneurons such as Renshaw cells, from one to four segments, cephalward or caudally (12, pp.

139–40). This means that a loss of function of the biceps, for instance, may theoretically be treated by influencing the neurological beds from about the first cervical through the second thoracic levels. There is embryological evidence that muscles derive from several consecutive segmental myotomes and are, therefore, supplied with efferent fibers from consecutive neuromeres (8, p. 125). Another fact of particular interest is that the fibers of a specific muscle may exhibit different functions, according to the muscle's position in space and with respect to the rest of the body. For instance, in a neutral position, the deltoid may induce abduction in the shoulder joint. But, when the joint is approximately at 90° of motion, the same fibers may induce adduction to a certain degree. In fact, the same vector forces that produce joint stabilization contribute to such adduction. This means that the initial and working positions of exercise are very important with respect to desired outcomes.

Summation

Two other basic concepts may have a bearing upon the design and implementation of exercise programs. Summation, or addition of muscle twitches, occurs in two main ways: increasing the number of motor units contracting at once, or by increasing the velocity of contraction of the individual units. These neurophysiological doctrines are called temporal summation and spatial summation (3, p. 69).

In spatial (or multiple motor unit) summation it is assumed that there is some kind of "spreading" of the neuronal influence beyond its direct target into adjacent areas. This means that presynaptic terminals from disparate loci can converge upon a single neuron and summate their discharges to initiate action potentials in a particular neuron. The term convergence implies that a single neuron is controlled by multiple neurons (3, p. 550). Divergence implies that excitation of a single input nerve fiber can stimulate multiple output fibers (3, p. 551). Divergence may not be as important for our work, but such spillover effects can help account for positive influences upon an immobilized area from an adjacent structure. It is also assumed that these discharges were all subthreshold, that

is, unable to initiate the action potential, or the summation process would not have been necessary. From another standpoint, this means that recruitment of nerve fibers has occurred, due to the nature of the stimulus, and a multiple fiber summation develops, with a stronger signal ensuing (3, p. 546). It should be noted that the smaller motor units are much more easily excited than the larger ones. This is because they are innervated by smaller nerve fibers, whose cell bodies in the cord normally have a higher level of excitability.

Temporal (or wave) summation refers to the rapid and successive discharges from a single presynaptic terminal summating to create that action potential. This can also be called frequency modulation since the strength of the resultant signal is proportional to the frequency of stimulating impulses (3, p. 547). Temporal summation also implies that the resultant contraction is of greater magnitude or different character than a single postsynaptic discharge would produce in that muscle. What happens is that, when the frequency of stimulation is large enough, the first muscle twitch has not completely finished when the second one occurs. This causes a gradually increasing force of contraction, proportionate to that frequency and up to some inherent maximum. At that point, the frequency is high enough to cause the successive contractions to fuse and become indistinguishable. This state is known as tetanization, and the frequency of its onset is called the critical frequency. Two main factors contribute to the phenomenon of tetanization. Muscle fibers are filled with sarcoplasm (a viscous fluid) and encased in fasciae and muscle sheaths, which possess a viscous resistance to change in length. Also, the activation process itself lasts for a finite period and successive pulses can occur with sufficient rapidity to fuse into a continuous state of activation. This is probably because the free calcium ions persist indefinitely in the myofibrils and maintain the contractions. Once the critical frequency has been reached, further stimulation only can increase the force of contraction by a small percentage. Normally, both types of summation will occur during muscle function. The motor unit will normally fire between 5 and several hundred times per second (3, p. 89). However, no matter how slowly and weakly the motor units fire, the muscle contraction still appears to be relatively smooth because the motor units tend to fire asynchronously. This means that one relaxes as another fires, and so forth, through the zone of stimulation.

The maximum strength of tetanic contraction of a muscle operating at a normal length is about 3 kg/cm^2 (42 lb/inch^2 (3, p. 89). Because a quadriceps muscle may have as much as 16 inch^2 of surface area over the muscle belly, as much as 600 to 700 lb of pressure may be applied to the patellar tendon. This would explain some of the injuries occurring to the tendon or in the vicinity of the osseous attachment of the tendon. This is all too common at the tibial tuberosity, the attachment of the patellar tendon, and, especially, the calcaneal attachment of the Achilles tendon. After a long period of rest, the strength of muscle contraction may only be half its maximal level. It will gradually increase, over a number of twitches, to that plateau, a phenomenon called the staircase effect or treppe. This is theorized to be due to a net influx of calcium ions into the sarcoplasm and a delay in their recapture. Also the change in the ratio of intracellular potassium and sodium may potentiate the release of calcium from the sarcoplasmic reticulum. These principles may have implication in the treatment of patients suffering from paresis or even paralysis. It may be that a summation type concept can be applied to an exercise regimen so that a response is either enhanced or elicited where it had not been previously.

Facilitation

Facilitation refers to the excitation of certain neurons causing an enhancement of their action. This means that the postsynaptic potential, even though it may be at a subthreshold level, can cause the action potential to be thereafter more easily stimulated by subsequent presynaptic discharges, or, in a word, facilitated. This can also be applied to the muscles working with and in opposition to a specific muscle we are interested in moving. There is a brief period of facilitation of muscles synergistic to the reflexly activated one and an inhibitory effect in the muscles which antagonize this motion (6, p. 289). It would be difficult to display a stretch reflex without this phenomenon. Furthermore, this reciprocal innervation concept can be applied to muscle pairs, one spastic and the other hypotonic, in exercising or treating to rebalance them. Goodheart (as espoused in his lectures and research manuals) used this concept and the knowledge of the special receptors to create a manual (origin and insertion) technique to stimulate or inhibit aberrant muscle actions. Another technique (discussed later), called *proprioceptive neuromuscular facilitation* (PNF), also relies upon several of these principles.

However, there is another meaning which has specific bearing upon the material in this text. A *facilitated pathway* refers to a somewhat specious neurological entity that can be produced by repeated stimulus of a specific neural track. A law of facilitation states that once an impulse has passed through a certain set of neurons, to the exclusion of others, it will tend to take the same course in the future; each time it traverses this path, the resistance in the path diminishes (15, p. 801). Although there does not appear to be an anatomical substrate for this concept, it seems that, once this has been established, the process and end result become easier to attain and maintain. This is essentially the formation of a neural habit. Analogous to the rote memorization of a scholastic subject with the unconscious ability to regurgitate facts is the unconscious reproduction of some neuromuscular activity by excitation of a neuronal pathway. This is useful in the learning and production of skilled maneuvers, such as walking or playing a musical instrument, and it is equally useful in the rehabilitation of certain lost or reduced muscular functions. However, it can be a liability in the pathophysiological arc of pain and dysfunction involved in a myofascial trigger point (16, pp. 14, 31–4). At times like this the principle appears to be counterproductive, but patience and persistence in the establishment of new neural pathways can break the "bad habits" and implant the new healthier ones. There is some neurological evidence that repeated transmission across synapses that are highly resistant to transmission due to disease and disuse slowly reduces the resistances (9, p. 466). It was the neurophysiologist Herman Kabat who discovered the principle and labeled it *facilitation*. This was no different from Pavlov's discovery that he could produce conditioned reflexes in dogs to salivate at the sound of a bell.

Conclusion

The regulation of posture depends upon the integrated activity of all these mechanisms, both tonically and phasically. While postural movements can be made voluntarily, this status is actually maintained by unconscious processes, once they have been learned. This is important because posture is the basis of all movement and all movements begin from and end in a posture (2, p. 298). It is reasonable for the clinician to evaluate posture grossly and in detail before beginning certain exercise programs, since postural muscles will be involved. In fact, much of the function of the muscles surrounding and intrinsic to each joint is involved in counteracting the continuous passive motions created in everyday life, by that which "jars, jolts and jams" our body. This is especially true in the spine, wherein is housed the all-important lower central nervous system. Once one understands the perpetually changing nature of these servomechanisms, it is easy to understand the fatigue they experience and the eventual postural distortions that are produced with age. Perhaps it is a malfunction of these servomechanisms on a neurological level that is responsible for idiopathic scoliosis, or even fatigue or stress fractures (17, pp. 265, 369). Having evaluated and noted the patient's posture before the program's inception, it is equally proper to reevaluate it afterward. This, along with strengthening muscles and improving function, can be considered a primary goal of rehabilitative treatments. The work of Feldenkrais and others demonstrates how faulty postural habit patterns affect the structure and function of bone, muscle, and connective tissues (18, p. 50). If this is not considered, therapies may be only partially effective, which may lead to a recrudescence of the original situations that were treated. The neurological activities described in this chapter focus down to a single point, the target anterior horn motor neuron (along the "final common pathway"). It is from this point that all postural determinants are affected, and it is the focus of the exercise regimens we propose.

References

1. McArdle ND, Katch FI, Katch VL: Exercise Physiology. 2nd ed. Philadelphia:Lea & Febiger, 1986.
2. Keele CA, Neil E: Samson Wright's Applied Physiology. 12th ed. London:Oxford University Press, 1971.
3. Guyton AC: Basic Human Physiology. Philadelphia:WB Saunders, 1971.
4. Feather N: The Physics of Mass, Length and Time. Edinburgh:Edinburgh University Press, 1962.
5. Steindler A: Kinesiology of the Human Body. 4th ed. Springfield, IL:Charles C Thomas, 1973.
6. Ochs S: Elements of Neurophysiology. New York: John Wiley & Sons, 1965.
7. Hix EL: The Trophic Function of Visceral Nerves. Physiological Basis Osteopathic Medicine. Post Graduate Institute of Osteopathic Medicine and Surgery, 1970.
8. Homewood, AE. The Neurodynamics of the Vertebral Subluxation. Chiropractic Publishers, Willowdale, Canada: 1968.
9. Basmajian JV, Wolf SL: Therapeutic Exercise. 5th ed. Baltimore:Williams & Wilkins, 1990.
10. Campbell EJ, Dickinson CJ., Slater JDH, eds: Clinical Physiology. 4th ed. Oxford, England:Blackwell Scientific Publications, 1974.
11. Torg JS, Vegso JJ, Torg E: Rehabilitation of Athletic Injuries. Chicago:Year Book Medical Publishers, 1987.
12. Brodal A: Neurological Anatomy: In Relation to Clinical Medicine. 3rd ed. New York:Oxford University Press. 1981.
13. Kottke FJ, Stillwell KG, Lehman JF: Krusen's Handbook of Physical Medicine and Rehabilitation. 3rd ed. Philadelphia:WB Saunders, 1982.
14. Alpers BJ, Mancall, EL: Clinical Neurology. 2nd ed. Philadelphia: FA Davis, 1980.
15. Dorland's Medical Dictionary. 24th ed. Philadelphia:WB Saunders, 1965.
16. Travell JG, Simons DG: Myofascial Pain and Dysfunction; The Trigger Point Manual. Baltimore: Williams & Wilkins, 1983.
17. Schmorl G, Junghanns H: The Human Spine in Health and Disease. Orlando: Grune & Stratton. 1971.
18. Feldenkrais, M. The Elusive Obvious. Cupertino: Meta Publications, 1981.

3

Pathology and Pathophysiology

The rehabilitative exercises described in this text are designed for the improvement and restoration of normal musculoskeletal function. Impaired musculoskeletal function accounts for the majority of maladies affecting the public today, accounting for conditions ranging from lower back pain to muscular strain and sprains. In a 1974 study, insurance companies concluded that there were more claims for lower back disabilities than for any other condition (1, p. 131). In a study that followed, Kraus and Raab reported on patients with lower back disorders who were placed on a specific regimen of rehabilitative exercises. Of 233 individuals with low back pain, 82% reported favorable results after exercises. To properly understand and evaluate the various conditions presented in this chapter, specific disease entities must be explained, so as to allow the physician to understand the rationale for the prescription of an exercise rehabilitative program.

Muscle Atrophy

Muscle hypertrophy (see also Chapter 2) is a normal response of muscle tissue to exercise. Atrophy, a reduction in the size of individual muscle fibers, is a normal reaction to disuse or immobilization of muscular tissue. Denervation of a muscle over an extended period of time may result in irreversible muscular atrophy. If a patient is confined to complete bed rest, a muscle will lose approximately 10 to 15% of its strength per week, or 1 to 3% of its strength per day (2, p. 455). If bed rest is continued unabated for a period of 3 to 5 weeks, muscle strength may be reduced by as much as 50%. Bed rest, or complete immobilization of a muscle, not only produces muscle atrophy and incomplete muscle contraction, but also compromises blood supply. As a result of this reduced blood supply, metabolic activity is reduced, and muscle endurance is subsequently impaired. The impairment of muscle endurance is believed to be related to decreased oxidative capacity and a lowered tolerance to lactic acid and oxygen deprivation. Certain muscles are more susceptible to atrophy than others. The quadriceps and back extensor muscles are particularly sensitive to atrophy.

In a patient who must be immobilized, muscle atrophy can be limited by encouraging the patient to maintain some normal activities or by prescribing exercises. If the patient contracts the affected muscles at 20 to 30% capacity for a few seconds each day, or 50% of normal contraction for 1 sec/day, muscle strength can be somewhat maintained and the amount of atrophy may be limited. Exercise training may also cause an increase in the number of muscle fibers, referred to as hyperplasia. Disuse atrophy appears to result in the reduction of type I muscle fibers.

Muscle Fiber Types

As discussed in Chapter 2, muscle fibers are classified into three basic groups: (*a*) type I, slow twitch fibers; (*b*) type IIA, fast oxidative-glycolytic fibers; and (*c*) type IIB, fast glycolytic fibers (1, p. 135). An awareness of the various muscle fiber groups is important to determine exercises that will be effective. Studies have shown that type II muscle fibers decrease in area with aging. Therefore, strength exercises will be of little value, and any change in muscle strength is likely to be the result of neural impulse (1, p. 137).

Neurological Aspects of Muscle Function

Skeletal muscles are innervated via the lower motor neurons, located in the ventral horn (Fig. 3.1). Voluntary movement of skeletal muscles is also dependent upon the upper motor neurons keeping the lower motor neurons at a point of readiness. There are two types of spinal reflexes: cutaneous and muscle reflexes. Cutaneous reflexes result in a motor response to a cutaneous stimulation; they are also known as withdrawal or flexor reflexes. Muscle reflexes, adjust the tone and reactivity of the skeletal muscles.

The muscle reflexes function through two types of receptors, muscle spindles and Golgi tendon organs (GTOs). Muscle spindles relate information concerning the amount of stretch and/or length of the individual muscle fibers. The GTOs relate information concerning the amount of tension on a tendon due to the passive stretch or contraction of the muscle. This information is distributed through the spinal cord, with input into the lower motor neurons for such local reflexes as the muscle stretch reflex.

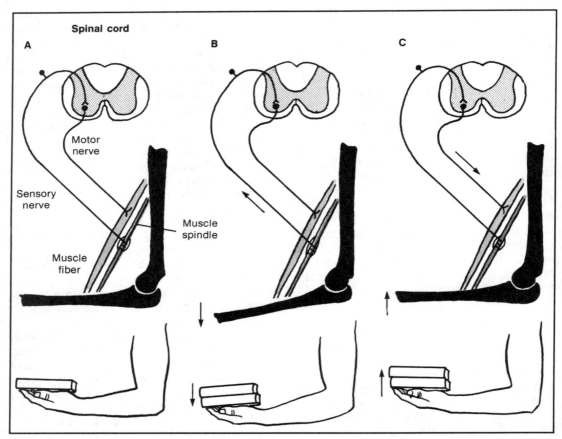

Figure 3.1 Schematic representation of stretch reflex. (Reprinted with permission from McArdle WD, Katch FI, Katch VL: Exercise Physiology. 2nd ed. Philadelphia:Lea & Febiger, 1986.)

Information on the immediate state of the muscles is also sent to the cerebellum, via synapses in the spinal cord. So that the cerebellum can coordinate voluntary movements directed by the cortex or adjust muscle tone from upper motor neurons in the brainstem. This is significant in certain upper motor neuron disorders (i.e., Parkinson's disease and polio) that result in neuromuscular dysfunction.

In upper motor neuron conditions, there is a loss of motor units, resulting in a loss of muscle tension feedback, which diminishes the capacity of the system to regulate force. As a result, rehabilitative exercises should be designed to allow for slow (tonic) muscle control, which is associated with low-threshold motor units (2, p. 176). In patients suffering from cerebral vascular accidents, there may be a reduction in the sensory threshold and an increased response to stimulus, resulting in an increase in tendon reflexes. The musculature of these patients is hyperflexive, and this must be taken into consideration when designing an exercise program. Since there is an interaction between the brain stem and other levels of the central nervous system, rehabilitative programs must focus on the patient's reflexive functioning as part of the redevelopment of voluntary movement.

The initial idea of movement occurs in the prefrontal (association) cortex, with the inception of a neural response. Delisa (2) reports of studies by Kornhuber et al. that show an 800-msec delay between the initial idea or readiness potential of motion and the subsequent voluntary movement. This is termed the readiness or *Bereitschafts* potential. This potential is a representation of the neural mobilization of the cortical areas, that are involved in the initiation, evaluation, and control of movements. Investigations by Freude and Ullsperger suggested the possibility that muscular fatigue may cause the Bereitschafts potential to increase. In another study, it was found that an increase in the Bereitschafts potential before complex muscular action indicates an increased activation of the supplementary motor area, prior to sequential muscular activity (3). Prefrontal lesions affect the ability to perceive motor action referred to as a general motor planning disorder. When one considers this delay, and the ones throughout the sensorimotor apparatus, the engram concept becomes that much more significant. To improve coordination and specific skills, the development of engrams is the only way more rapid movements can occur.

Neural impulses from the association cortex pass through to the basal ganglia (lateral cerebellum) before reaching the motor cortex. The thalamus appears to act as a relay center between the cerebellum and basal ganglia, with the premotor cortex. The premotor cortex receives input from the subcortical structures and the association cortex. It is the premotor cortex that seems to assist in the preparation of motor acts by the setting of postural tone and the timing of various motor sequences.

All the bits of information then are passed to the motor cortex, which is responsible for integrating this information and passing the signals down through the spinal cord. These signals are overseen by the intermediate cerebellum, which seems to be responsible for the control and monitoring of movement. With this many neural entities and sequences involved, there are far more reasons for abnormal motion then one normally considers. There are, however, a few distinctions that demand variations in the exercise program. If the premotor cortex is injured, postural exercises may need to be initiated early to improve muscle tone for later exercises. The cerebellum would best be benefited by exercises aimed at improving coordination. This is an oversimplification, but it serves as a starting point in developing a regimen (2, pp. 177–80; 4).

Clinical Entities

Sprains

A muscle sprain is a joint injury due to overstress. It is characterized by either partially torn or overstretched ligaments, joint capsules, or surrounding tissues. Sprains are further subdivided into three categories, based on the degree of injury (Fig. 3.2) (5, p. 79).

First Degree Sprain

In this degree of sprain there are only a few fibers that have been stretched or torn, with a minimal amount of hemorrhaging. Clinically there may be little or no loss of joint function and/or strength. Tenderness

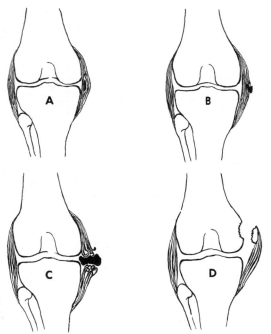

Figure 3.2 Various types of sprains. **A.** First degree (mild) sprain. **B.** Second degree (moderate) sprain. **C.** Third degree (severe) sprain. **D.** Sprain—fracture. (Reprinted with permission from O'Donoghue DH: Treatment of Injuries to Athletes. 3rd ed. Philadelphia:WB Saunders, 1976.)

may be elicited over the ligamentous tissues, with little or no edema present. In a first degree sprain, since there is no loss of function, treatment is directed toward reduction of symptoms. Rehabilitative exercises, therefore, are to maintain muscle tone. They can be initiated immediately, limited only by symptoms and patient tolerance.

Second Degree Sprain

This is a moderate sprain, with more ligamentous tissue tearing and increased symptomatology over a first degree sprain. There may be as much as 50% tearing of the ligamentous fibers, accompanied by noticeable plastic deformity of the ligament(s), with a subsequent functional loss of stability. Increased edema and internal hemorrhaging are present. However, separation of the fibers is minimal, and natural healing is still possible. If the amount of ligamentous tearing is severe, there may be permanent ligament scarring and subsequent permanent functional loss. With severe ligament tearing, it is necessary for the initial treatment

to be directed at keeping the torn ends of the ligament in close apposition to permit complete healing with minimal scarring. Rehabilitative exercises must be limited until the initial phase of healing is completed and the ligamentous tissue is whole again. The time for ligamentous tissue to heal is approximately the same as that for osseous tissue. Exercises are then initially prescribed to regain strength and endurance, beginning at a lower frequency, intensity, and duration. They should also be of a simple nature, i.e., planar, along the lines of strength of the joint.

Third Degree Sprain

This is a most severe condition, with complete tearing of the ligament. It is characterized by severe edema, hemorrhaging, and tenderness with complete loss of joint function. Because there is complete tearing of the ligament, immobilization is necessary to insure that the loose ends of the ligament are held in close apposition; and surgical intervention may be required. The ligament must heal completely before rehabilitative exercises are initiated. Therefore, rehabilitative exercises begin at a later date than in previous injury levels. If muscle action is attempted too early, further damage to the ligament may result, causing a permanent impairment. Initial exercises are to reestablish range of motion and muscle tone, then rehabilitative exercises follow to improve strength and endurance.

Strains

Strains are classified the same as sprains. However, strains are musculotendinous injuries. Whereas in sprains and dislocations one must limit joint motion to allow healing to occur, in strains it is necessary to limit musculotendinous motion for full healing to occur. This means that isometric contractions only are desirable early in the rehabilitative program and that loading must be minimized in the early phases of rehabilitation (5, pp. 62–70).

Fibrocartilage Injuries

Fibrocartilage injury, a condition usually associated with the spine, the temporomandibular joint, and the knee, is characterized by pain, which may be radiating, and loss of function in respective ranges of motion.

Spine

Within the spine, there is damage to the annular fibers of the anatomical motor unit. If the injury is severe, there may be a loss of integrity or malposition of the nucleus pulposus.

The intervertebral disc is attached in the anatomical motor unit to the superior and inferior endplates of the vertebrae. The intervertebral discs are connected to very thin layers of hyaline cartilage, which cover the superior and inferior endplates of the vertebrae. It is believed that this attachment to the vertebrae may be by means of Sharpey's fibers. As a result of this type of attachment, it appears that the diagnosis of a "slipped" disc is indeed a misnomer, as a slippage of the annulus would result in a tearing of the annular fibers, since the Sharpey's fibers are stronger than the annular fibers.

Disc injuries, where there is damage to the annular fibers, fall into three separate categories, based on the integrity of the nucleus pulposus. (a) A disc or annular bulge occurs when there is microtearing or separation of the annular fibers, allowing the nuclear material to extrude into the annulus. (b) A disc or annular protrusion occurs when the nucleus pulposus has been extruded into the periphery of the annulus, which produces a marked bulging of the annulus into the spinal canal or foraminal confines. (c) A prolapse or herniation is where a fragment of the nucleus pulposus has broken through the damaged annular fibers and separated from the rest of the nucleus, possibly migrating as a free segment into the spinal or nerve root canal.

Temporomandibular Joint

Temporomandibular joint cartilage injuries can be of an acute or chronic nature. They can be mild, with slight pain, to severe, with extreme limitation of jaw motion or even joint locking, severe shooting pains with various radiations, and a barrage of other symptoms, including head, neck, or ear pains. Although it is a postural joint, the weight bearing is generally minimal. Therefore, active or passive exercises, other than isometrics, do not impose significant loads, if the patient is not chewing. This joint is more delicately arranged then spinal joints, and exercises should be performed at a slower rate and with less than the full allowable motion.

Knee

Knee cartilages, especially the medial ones, are much more likely to become displaced physically. Therefore, one needs to be appropriately cautious in exercises not to move forcefully in the direction that causes such displacement.

Capsular Tears

Capsular tears are usually the result of an unexpected and abrupt joint motion, of a forceful magnitude, beyond the normal range of motion. Symptoms are similar to those of a third degree sprain and include edema, hemorrhage, and loss of joint motion. With respect to exercises, the same precautions should be observed as for a third degree sprain (5, pp. 80–1).

Dislocation

Dislocation, or luxation, is the result of the abnormal separation and displacement of opposing contiguous surfaces of a joint, secondary to trauma or a connective tissue disorder (Fig. 3.3). There is a loss of joint function that is directly proportional to the amount of luxation. There is a possibility of spontaneous reduction, where the opposing surfaces of the joint separate and then return to their normal position. The joint luxation, after the acute sprain, may be the result of either a slippage of the bone ends or an actual separation of those ends. A chronic dislocation, without evidence of new damage, is an indication of previous ligamentous damage. Luxation cannot occur without ligamentous damage. In an acute luxation, there is a fixed or unstable positioning of the joint elements, outside the normal ranges of motion. In a chronic luxation, the joint position may be normal, but there is a relatively high potential for an abnormal relationship to occur due to chronic joint instability. In the acute stage, there may not be plastic deformation of the ligamentous structures. In that case, the injuries may be virtually fully rehabilitated. The first phase of rehabilitation in all luxations aims at relaxation of the protective spasming and reduction in fear about moving the joint. The less the ligamentous damage and inflammatory response, the sooner strengthening is initiated to stabilize the joint.

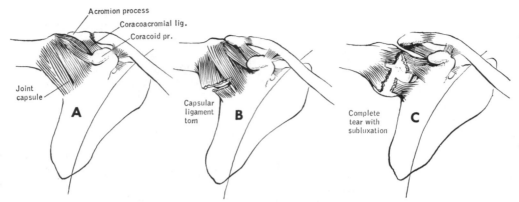

Figure 3.3 Complete dislocation with ligament damage. **A** to **C**. Successive stages in dislocation of the shoulder. (Reprinted with permission from O'Donoghue DH: Treatment of Injuries to Athletes. 3rd ed. Philadelphia: WB Saunders, 1976.)

Tenosynovitis

Tenosynovitis is an inflammation of the synovial tissue that surrounds a tendon. It may be caused by a strain, direct trauma, or infection. As a sequela of the inflammatory response, an increase of fibrin results in the production of adhesions between the tendon and its surrounding structures. As the condition progresses, the initial consequence may be a condition of adhesive tenosynovitis, followed by a constrictive tenosynovitis. In the majority of cases, the condition will subside with proper care, and normal function will return. However, depending on the severity of the condition and its location, permanent impairment may ensue.

In adhesive tenosynovitis, the tendon and its surrounding sheath stick to each other, preventing the normal sliding mechanism through which the tendon operates. In constrictive tenosynovitis, there is a thickening of the walls of the sheath due to chronic inflammatory responses, resulting in a narrowing of the lumen and subsequent loss of tendon movement within the sheath. If these conditions persist long enough, calcium deposits will be made in the irritated sheath, causing a calcific tenosynovitis. In adhesive or constrictive tenosynovitis a graduated passive, then active, exercise program will slowly increase the range of motion and reduce the inflammatory responses. However in calcific tenosynovitis, the same program may continually exacerbate damage to the tendons or the bursae and be counterproductive.

Bursitis

Bursitis is an inflammatory response within a bursa. The function of a bursa is to enable motion between contiguous body layers of soft tissues (5, p. 84) (Fig. 3.4). Continual trauma to the bursa produces synovial irritation, subsequent thickening of the synovium, and formation of excess fluid within the synovial cavity. Sometimes a calcific tendinitis will cause or exacerbate this problem. In the absence of calcified masses in the vicinity, bursitis will generally be rehabilitated in the same manner as tenosynovitis.

Synovial Hernia

Synovial hernia, or ganglion, is a result of a defect in the fibrous sheath of the joint or

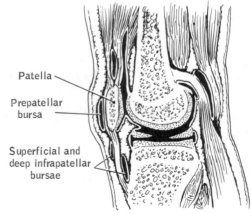

Figure 3.4 Patellar bursae. (Reprinted with permission from O'Donoghue DH: Treatment of Injuries to Athletes. 3rd ed. Philadelphia:WB Saunders, 1976.)

tendon, which allows the synovium and its contents to protrude through it. The condition is often the result of a mild strain. There may be pain, and the condition can be progressive. If this is the case, there may be some associated disuse atrophy. After correction, by surgical or nonsurgical means, rehabilitation consists mainly of improving the muscle tone and articular range of motion, followed by muscle strengthening exercises.

Stress Fractures

Stress fractures are initially difficult to diagnose and may be represented by negative radiographs. They appear as extremely tender areas over a trauma site. Later in their course, x-rays will reveal new callous formation, which may be the first indication of the stress fracture. Weight bearing bones are particularly susceptible to stress fractures. Generally, these fractures are small, well-aligned, and capable of full healing, provided further trauma to the site is avoided. This usually means avoiding protracted and strenuous weight bearing, but not avoiding all activity in the joint. Even in a non-weight bearing joint, continuous passive and active movements are instituted very early as the first phase of rehabilitation to prevent disuse atrophy. Subsequent rehabilitation, when the bones have knit sufficiently, includes strength and endurance exercises, as appropriate.

Fractures

Osseous fractures are of various forms, and treatment of the osseous damage is relatively routine. The physician immobilizes the bone and sometimes sets it if the ends are not in close apposition. However, it is important to realize that rarely is there an osseous fracture without concomitant soft tissue damage. Rehabilitation is necessary to restore soft tissue integrity, to reestablish strength, and to reeducate muscle. Rehabilitation is also necessary for surrounding muscular tissue that, as a result of the fracture treatment, has suffered from disuse atrophy. As with stress fractures, disuse atrophy is of particular importance, and it is necessary to properly evaluate the rehabilitative program to reestablish normal function (see chapter 4). The difference here is that immobilization is required for an extended period of time, making atrophy a more probable consequence.

Muscle Spasm

Muscle spasm may be the result of many common types of injuries. It may be caused by overstretching, direct or indirect trauma, increased contraction of muscle against a resistance, or the reaction of a muscular group to overcome another pathological process, such as discogenic disease. The agonist or antagonist muscle may be the primary problem in muscle spasm and/or cramping. If a primary muscle became weak, spasm may result in the corresponding antagonistic muscle. Therefore, it is necessary to examine and evaluate the spastic area properly with an orthopedic and neurological examination, to define the exact nature and etiology of the muscle spasm. In instances of nutritional or metabolic etiologies, the history and laboratory testing are more definitive procedures. In any case, muscle spasm is only a symptom. However, if it becomes chronic, it can become a second level primary disorder on its own merit. Once the cause is known, rehabilitation is first aimed at relaxation of the muscle spasm and possible strengthening of the antagonist musculature (5, pp. 106–8)

Contractures

When irreversible contractures occur, it is doubtful whether nonsurgical procedures can have a significant effect upon correction of the problem. Such contractures usually involve replacement of the normal elastic tissues with relatively inelastic tissues, such as bone, fibrotic tissues, and adhesive scars (6). In the case of ossific or calcific infiltration, mildly zealous stretching can cause further damage and inhibit the healing process. In fact, forcible stretching may cause fractures or hemorrhages within these solid blocks, causing the formation of more heterotopic bone (7). In other cases, there is a possibility of improvement. Therefore, a radiographic examination of joints we intend to stretch is often a prerequisite to treatment.

Peripheral Nerve Injury

Peripheral nerves, such as the ulnar nerve at the elbow, may be subject to direct trauma, thereby causing nerve contusions.

In this condition, there may be damage to some of the motor nerve fibers, resulting in paralysis of the associated musculature. It is imperative in such conditions that, after the nerve has healed, rehabilitative exercises for the muscles be considered. There are many causes of chronic pain, which include symptoms of a burning sensation, which courses a nerve pathway. Pain may be due to a hyperactive sympathetic nervous system. Causalgia is the result of a partial injury to a major nerve, with subsequent symptoms of an overactive sympathetic nervous system. Reflex sympathetic dystrophy is the result of a minor injury, or in some cases no apparent injury, with symptoms of an overactive sympathetic nervous system. Sudek's atrophy is another entity in this category. A common feature of all these disorders is a certain amount of osteopenia, along with muscle and inflammatory changes. Actually a more accurate name for all of them might be reflex autonomic dystonia (RAD), which describes all such problems at any stage of development. Symptoms may not correspond to normal dermatomal patterns or neural pathways. Pain may be caused by ischemia and/or any of the normal pathways for its reaction. It may be the result of neural compression, which can cause lower motor neuron lesions, in this case, due to nerve root impingement from numerous possible causes. Vertebral subluxation complexes, spinal canal stenosis, and entities causing encroachment in the vertebral foraminal confines are among the more common etiologies for neural compression syndromes.

Traction Injuries of Nerves

Traction stretch injuries to nerves may be produced when there is excessive joint motion. This motion must produce a centrifugal force vector parallel to the anatomical line of the neural axon. An example may be the overstretching of the peroneal nerve after the lateral ligaments of the knee are sprained by an excessive varus force applied to the knee joint. Again, it is imperative that rehabilitation be directed at the associated musculature as well as damaged nerves and ligaments. Regular evaluation of the strength of the muscles served by the hypertractioned nerve indicates which muscles are affected, to what degree, and what progress has been made. Care must be taken not to generate a significant force vector parallel to that which caused the injury. The early phases of rehabilitation concentrate on reestablishing the neuromuscular connection. Strength and endurance training come later, because a (partially) denervated muscle cannot be strengthened. It may take 6 weeks or more for phase one to be completed, due to the pattern of wallerian degeneration and regeneration (8).

References

1. Pollock ML, Wilmore JH, Fox SM III: Exercise in Health and Disease. Philadelphia:WB Saunders, 1984.
2. Delisa JA: Rehabilitation Medicine. Philadelphia: JB Lippincott, 1988.
3. Benecke R, Dick JP, Rothwell JC, Day BL, Marsden CD: Increase in the BP in simultaneous and sequential movements. Neurosci Lett 62(3):347–52, 1985.
4. Kottke FJ, Stillwell KG, Lehman JF: Krusen's Handbook of Physical Medicine and Rehabilitation. 3rd ed. Philadelphia:WB Saunders, 1982:248–51.
5. O'Donoghue DH: Treatment of Injuries to Athletes. 3rd ed. Philadelphia:WB Saunders, 1976.
6. Kisner C, Colby LA: Therapeutic Exercise: Foundations and Techniques. Philadelphia:FA Davis, 1987:119.
7. Basmajian JV, Wolf SL: Therapeutic Exercise. 5th ed. Baltimore:Williams & Wilkins, 1990:310.
8. Farber D: Neurorehabilitation. Philadelphia:WB Saunders, 1982:25.

4

Clinical Considerations for Rehabilitative Programs

The first step of any exercise program is to determine the needs of the patient. Are we rehabilitating toward a specific activity or set of activities? Has a precise impairment been determined, and are we aiming to improve upon this or merely to maintain the current disability level? Secondly, the patient's current capabilities must be ascertained. Any rehabilitation program must work within the patient's limitations; they must constantly be reevaluated and the program upgraded cybernetically to be as effective as possible.

Establishing Baseline

Whenever possible, one should first obtain a baseline set of values for the parameters being measured in the individual. It may not be possible to establish a true baseline since the person being rehabilitated is already injured and his capacities are already diminished to a certain extent. Therefore, for our purposes, a baseline is the current level of performance. The baseline information is combined with a carefully elicited history, a knowledge of normal populations, with respect to gender, age, and physical conditioning levels, and a physical examination of the patient. One needs also to be aware of any congenital anomalies or deficiencies that could limit the potential results. These data are usually elicited in the history-taking process, and the patient should be specifically questioned about them. An evaluation of all of this information allows one to prepare a realistic exercise program with realistic goals (Fig. 4.1).

Measurements

The establishment of a baseline is not always a simple process, although it is a fairly straightforward one. Depending upon the function and area to be rehabilitated, there are several parameters to consider. One can analyze range of motion (and/or flexibility), strength, endurance, respiratory capacities (and/or oxygen utilization), coordination, speed, and precision of motion. Range of motion is simply compared against acceptable norms for the variables of age, gender, and body type. There are several different sources for acceptable norms, many of which disagree. It is important to find one that you can live with and utilize it consistently. Our referenced norms are included in each chapter. We are currently researching better ways to standardize these values.

There are so many variables in strength that bilateral testing and comparison is imperative. This can be performed manually but one cannot obtain good quantitative data in this manner. We suggest either mechanical or electronic instrumentation to assist in this evaluation. Some of the better computerized units can provide dynamic and even real-time evaluations, with hard copy results that are specific in their find-

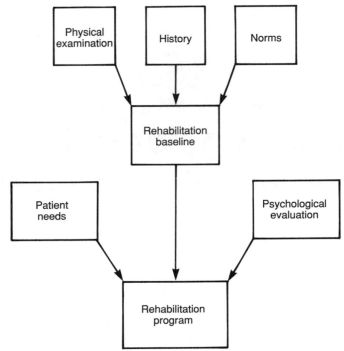

Figure 4.1 Program initiation flow chart.

ings. These systems are useful for designing programs but are not widely available at this time. It is also understood that any test that causes a great deal of pain or is not performable is not to be continued. It is recorded as "unable to perform."

Endurance and respiratory capacity have numerous specific charts that can be used as a basis for comparison, depending upon the specific tests used (1, pp. 184, 198, 359, 564; 2, pp. 496–7; 3, pp. 430–1). Endurance tests are generally tied in with cardiovascular functioning and should, therefore, not be performed by other than a physician if there is a known risk of cardiovascular incident occurring.

Tests of coordination, speed, and precision of movement are usually of a qualitative nature and require some experience with neurological methods and instruments. Speed may be tied in to endurance under certain conditions. These tests should also be performed bilaterally.

One last function to evaluate is skill level. This is probably more connected with athletic performance than other activities. Skill is usually a function of many of the functions mentioned above, along with balance and timing. It is difficult to evaluate

properly and requires a certain amount of experience by the examiner, relative to the skill being tested. It also may require some training of the performer, which brings other cognitive factors into play. Therefore, skill will not be considered a baseline component in this text.

Psychological Factors

Just as the physician and therapist must understand the goals and procedures involved, so too must the patient be actively involved. Along these lines, the attitude of the patient is sometimes critical in terms of the results which may be expected. Once the program has been determined, it is important that the patient be informed, in all necessary detail, about its content and its intent. The patient is much more likely to comply with the regimen if he understands it and is psychologically prepared to engage in it. A patient suffering from depression or who is unable to concentrate or motivate himself is going to have a difficult time with any program. This patient will need more support and reinforcement than the average patient. One may apply behavioral modification techniques to improve on compliance, when this is the case. Positive reinforcement is generally preferred. However, since patients usually have some pain, this negative factor may be exactly what motivates them. Remember to emphasize those conditions the patient needs to avoid absolutely to circumvent further injury. On the other hand, a well-motivated patient can be relied upon to perform home exercises and to observe necessary restrictions in order not to detract from the program. Patients' progress and success must be acknowledged in order to encourage their efforts. On the other hand, patients who do not comply with the program must be dealt with firmly, or they cannot be helped. It is the art of patient management in this science that can balance these attitudes to produce optimum results. All patients are not the same, and they must progress at their own rates. This is a trial-and-error process that requires clinical decision making and regular reevaluations to accommodate such individualities.

Program Reevaluation

It is absolutely necessary to reevaluate the program and its results regularly. Decisions as to how often and how thoroughly one reevaluates are based upon many of the factors described herein. If expectations are being met, then the program continues as presented originally. If results are not forthcoming or the patient regresses in some way, the program must be adjusted (Fig. 4.2). The program must have some initial projection as to how long it will be performed, as well as how much progress or rehabilitation is expected. Both the goals and the time elements that must be met in order to measure success. Although one must always approach the subject positively, there will be some failures or some patients who progress less than expected. For now, we will ignore this and concentrate on producing results.

In most cases, a trauma of some sort is responsible for the injury(s). When this is the circumstance, the patient may desire to be returned to preinjury status only, not to "complete health" or "wellness". This decision may also be mitigated by medicolegal circumstances and other parties. Real life exigencies must be accounted for in any practice. We categorize these as a factor in the development of pertinent goals. Once

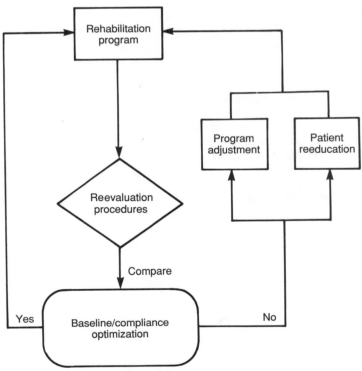

Figure 4.2 Program reevaluation flow chart.

those goals have been developed, the real work of this text begins.

Program Goals

Goals of a rehabilitative or therapeutic program fall under the following major categories: maintenance of disability (impairment) status, improvement of disability (impairment) status, return to preinjury status, retraining of new skills, and prevention of new or recurrent injuries. Of course, one needs to know the previous level of activity and skill in order accurately to assess the improvement. It may be of value to use mechanical and computerized functional capacity testing to evaluate skills and capacity levels. It is not the intent of this text to teach the use of such equipment, but they may be useful in determining needs, progress and even prognosis. By and large, we are concerned with rehabilitation of neuromusculoskeletal injuries and chronic conditions within these systems. Therefore, our goals and effects pertain to the application of exercise therapy to these systems. However, we do touch upon the respiratory and cardiovascular systems, to allow physicians to be involved in more complicated and more serious problems.

Goals must be realistic. This means that they must be achievable by the patient and biologically possible. Another suggestion is to involve all staff members in this process. Sometimes a patient may relate better to one staff member than another. It does not matter which staff member or what psychological strategy is necessary; if we achieve our goals we are successful and the patients benefit. Everyone who notices and mentions to the patient that progress has been made is part of the rehabilitation process.

Intent of Exercises

Within the framework of these goals, our exercises have specific intents, including the improvement, restoration, and/or maintenance of such parameters as strength, endurance, mobility and flexibility, coordination, respiratory functions, cardiovascular functions, relaxation, concentration, and specific skill levels. (Table 4.1). The lack of performance, according to established norms or one's professional opinion, in any of these parameters can be called impairment. Strictly speaking, im-

pairment is defined by the World Health Organization (WHO) as "any loss or abnormality of psychological, physical, or anatomical structure or function" (4, p. 254). Disability, on the other hand, is defined by WHO as "any restriction or lack (resulting from an impairment) of an ability to perform an activity in the manner or within the range considered normal for a human being" (4, p. 254). An extension of this concept is the notion of activities of daily living (ADL), those actions and behaviors which allow us to operate independently in the world. Inability to perform such activities is another way to rate a disability and to place a demand on a rehabilitative program. One may also measure the success of a program by regular reassessment of the ADL. This is a subjective process in which the patient completes forms describing activities performed. However, return to or improvement in ADL is truly a big portion of what we are trying to rehabilitate.

Table 4.1. Categories of Exercise, Motion, and Contraction

Attraction Type	Movement Type	Exercise Type
Isometric	Active	Balanced
Isotonic	Passive	Breathing
Concentric	Assistive	Complex
Eccentric	Resistive	Conditioning
Isokinetic		Coordination
		Endurance
		Aerobic
		Neuromuscular
		Lossening
		Minus training
		Mobilization
		Muscle reeducation
		Postural
		Progressive resistance
		DAPRE
		Manual
		Variable
		Proprioceptive neuromuscular facilitation
		Range of motion
		Relaxation
		Skill
		Strength
		Stretching
		Water

Means of Evaluation

The usual physician means of evaluation include a complete history or oral reevaluation, an inspection, and a physical examination. From a historical perspective, you will either be the treating physician or you will receive a packet of patient information from the treating physician. It is important to know and evaluate such factors as chronicity, exact location and pathophysiology involved, absolute and relative contraindications, and activities toward which rehabilitation is aimed. The physical components include vital signs, palpation (both static and dynamic), range of motion testing (active and passive), muscle strength testing, joint stability testing, and any necessary orthopedic and neurological tests. During the examination, it is important to note the exact points of motion at which pain is produced. This helps to define a parameter of the exercise known as range. Sometimes it helps to measure muscle size by circumferential tapes, along with the usual strength measurements. Joints often have accessory movements, such as traction and gliding, which are normal components of joint motion. These should be accounted for and should be present in normal amounts, or there is some amount of joint restriction.

Joint Play

A key factor to evaluate is "joint play." This is the normal range of involuntary movement that a specific joint can accomplish, which is beyond the normal active or passive range of motion (5, p. 28). This play occurs as the result of a partial loss of integrity of some of the elastic components of the joint's function.

The biomechanical cause of such loss of integrity is either multiple microtraumata or one or more macrotraumata. Microtraumatic events are very small and are usually not noted when they occur. They generally require frequent occurrence or long duration to be causal. In contrast, one is usually acutely aware of macrotraumatic events, and a single event can precipitate considerable disharmony and dysfunction. Congenital anatomical variations and certain disorders, usually of connective tissue, are also causative, but far less commonly. A partial summary of the mechanical situations categorized as microtraumata include postural imbalance, muscle imbalance at joint, overuse syndromes, repetitive tissue/joint shock, low-grade inflammations, and use of improper bedding or improper footgear. Some macrotraumatic situations include sprain/strain, work-related injury, athletic injury, recreational activity injury, slip-and-fall injury, whiplash type injuries, and injuries resulting from automobile accidents.

Documentation

A number of forms are needed to evaluate patient status and progress. One needs to give thoughtful consideration to parameters being monitored in order to create useful forms. Sample forms are not included here, but the information provided is sufficient to create such forms.

Therapeutic Intents

Strength

Strength has fascinated mankind throughout the ages, and high-technology equipment is available for its measurement. Strength can be measured and, therefore, developed in isometric, isotonic, and isokinetic modes. Absolute muscle strength relates to maximum tension per unit of cross-sectional area. This, of course, depends upon the type of muscle fibers, i.e., parallel, pennate, or radial. The cross-sectional area has to do with the plane that is perpendicular to the axis of the fibers. What is being measured in strength testing is a single maximal type contraction, developing maximal tension, whether static or dynamic. Improvement in muscular strength is determined less by total work done or power developed in the exercise than by the tension developed by the muscle during the exercise (6, p. 793). The development of strength is, however, often accomplished with far less than maximal contractions, repeated numerous times. The force output is also a function of the recruitment of the greatest number of fibers firing at once and the strength of their respective contractions.

Lower speeds of contraction seem to produce greater torque, probably due to the increased opportunity for recruitment, particularly of the slower twitch fibers (7, p. 97;

8, p. 352). In other words, as the load increases, the velocity or angular velocity decreases proportionately, and as the strength increases, the same load can be moved more quickly. Therefore, if isokinetic procedures are used, one should perform them toward the lower end of the torque/velocity curve to augment strength. Animal studies show increase in protein synthesis occurs within 8 hr following an increase in muscle load (5, p. 139). This loading can be accomplished by varying the number of repetitions or the amount of resistance. In any case, intake of proteinaceous substances within a couple of hours after such exercise allows for gastric clearance and the absorption of the necessary amino acids for the proteinogenesis. The performance of peak tension exercises every other day, to the point of complete peripheral fatigue, is the usual protocol for a strength regimen (5, p. 87; 9, pp. 87–90). It is evident that a daily regimen may lead to proteinolysis and be counterproductive. Therefore, one is advised to maintain an every-other-day program.

There are several guidelines for creating an exercise program that improves strength. The overload principle states that in order to increase strength, the load used during the exercise must exceed the metabolic capacity of the muscle (7, p. 11). This principle can be described as a process of applying a graduated load to a muscle by altering one of several parameters. Understand that this is not just another variant of the "no pain, no gain" axiom. In fact, we eschew that kind of process as potentially dangerous. The muscle must be exerted sufficiently for fatigue to set in, so that adaptive strength increases occur subsequently. One attempts to extend the limits of performance steadily and safely. This is why progressive resistive exercises (PRE) were studied and developed by DeLorme in 1945 (9, p. 34). There are numerous ways to load the muscle(s) to produce such exercises (see below). Additionally, the rate of improvement in strength is a function of the patient's compliance.

The strength increase occurs, probably, as a result of muscle hypertrophy. This is a biochemical process, especially involving increased protein content of the myofibrils. Therefore, prior to and during such activities, the patient's diet must have an adequate protein content. Because one desires to increase certain specific functions, it is necessary to consider joint position when that function is being performed. This is why we insist that position and form are as exacting as possible during exercises.

Endurance

Increasing endurance is another intent of exercise. This is a necessary commodity in order to perform repeated motor tasks or to sustain a motor activity over a period of time. The task may be of a static or dynamic nature. Depending upon the patient's needs, exercises are designed to follow that task aim. Endurance is a muscular phenomenon and is a function of the cardiac and pulmonary systems. The latter two categories will be discussed separately. Endurance can be mathematically defined as related to the total number of repetitions or the time necessary to produce fatigue. This tends to produce a hyperbolic endurance curve, plotting total number of contractions versus force or power of contraction (4, p. 437) (Fig. 4.3). The definition of endurance usually assumes that the intensity level of the activity is moderate, at most. In fact, Christensen states that one only applies the exercises at 50% intensity throughout the range of motion (5, p. 142). Therefore, in training for endurance, one never exerts full force for any significant period of time, but only insofar as strength training is simultaneously being applied.

Even without considering the other systems mentioned, endurance exercise is aerobic, in effect, because of its very nature. The constant repetitiveness or long duration of such endeavors surpasses anaerobic abilities. As a result, in muscles trained for endurance, there is an increased density of the capillary bed contained therein. This provides the greater amounts of oxygen necessary for aerobic activity and is why the cardiopulmonary system is intrinsic to muscular endurance.

There are several different types of endurance. Anaerobic endurance is measured under high-intensity (or isometric) conditions whereas aerobic endurance is measured under low-intensity (or dynamic) exercise conditions. Isometric, isotonic, and isokinetic endurance are measured under their respective conditions, maintaining

DYNAMICS OF CLINICAL REHABILITATIVE EXERCISE

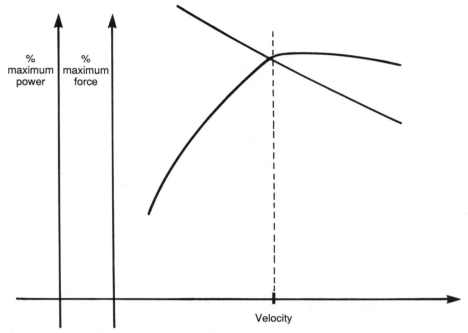

Figure 4.3 Relationship between speed of contraction and either force or power of contraction.

position or force, measuring repetitions with a specific weight, and repeating at a specific angular velocity without a loss of torque, respectively (8, pp. 362–3). At levels below 20% of the maximum voluntary contraction (MVC), there is a major reliance upon slow-twitch fibers, with increasing reliance upon fast-twitch fibers above this level (9, pp. 88–90). Force and endurance have inverse hyperbolic relationships. When force levels are less than 15% of maximum, endurance is maximal; when force levels approach maximum, endurance approaches zero, asymptotically (8, p. 351). This is true of intensity of work (as measured by average speed) versus the elapsed time in seconds (4, pp. 436–40) (Fig. 4.4). These relationships are very similar and demonstrate that only in a small segment of the curve, where the range of A on the ordinate and B on the abscissa intersect, are strength and endurance simultaneously trainable.

Fatigue

The physiological entity known as fatigue is a critical factor in all training. Fatigue is used to measure the end point of a specific set of exercises. If strength and endurance are the commodities, then decreased force or loss of form in repetition

will auger fatigue's onset. From a bionutritional point of view, depletion of ATP, creatine phosphate, then glycogen stores, in the absence of further incoming nutrients, signals the inception of fatigue (4, p. 440; 8, p. 352). An anaerobic exercise, like isomet-

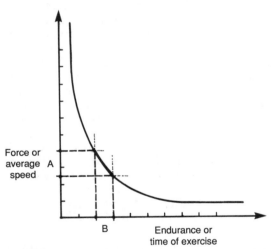

Figure 4.4 Relationship between force (or velocity) and endurance (or time of exercise). The zone marked off by *A* on the ordinate and *B* on the abscissa represents the range of parameters in which one may optimize all parameters, with minimal loss in any of them.

rics, reaches fatigue when anaerobic production ceases. Furthermore, static contractions greater than 60 to 70% of maximum cause interference with local circulation, which accelerates fatigue onset (8, p. 352). Lactic acid buildup is not a significant factor here, since its removal is actually faster at these levels than at lower intensities (8, p. 352). Exercise beyond or after this point is not only unproductive, but it is potentially harmful. Therefore, design of a program requires careful monitoring of fatigue so that we know exactly when it is produced. Trial and error is a necessary methodology to determine the point of fatigue.

Biological Task Equivalents

This brings to the fore the concept of biological equivalents of a task (9, p. 234). For example, if the biological end point is to induce fatigue, does it matter which type of exercise and which formats and factors are used? The answer is a resounding yes—and no. If we employ the techniques presented here, being mindful of the physiological constraints under which humans operate, we will see logically where we can cross-train (use different procedures for a congruent result) and where we cannot. Of course, a person trains best for a specific task by performing essentially that task, under controlled circumstances. Because of the increasing participation of fast-twitch fibers above 20% MVC, it can be said that there is a relative interchangeability of loads, between 30 and 100% of maximum, as long as the biological end point of fatigue is reached (9, p. 104). This is, of course, an approximation. We must emphasize that endurance implies the metabolic ability to supply the energy for the muscular activity involved. Sometimes, rather than cross-train or exchange activities, one can combine methods and produce what is known as "interval training." This means alternating aerobic and anaerobic activity (or stress and nonstress work), for example. It also provides a higher level of strength training than most endurance programs because the onset of fatigue is delayed. Some of the changes occurring in endurance training amount to actual physiological adaptations to specific conditions, such as an ability to function at altitude. One other very useful effect of endurance training is the resultant increase in the strength of ligaments and

tendons and the stabilizing of their attachment sites (8, pp. 361–3).

Mobility

The third intent of exercise is the improvement of mobility or flexibility. When the normal motion of body parts is restricted, adaptive shortening (tightness or contracture) of soft tissues and joints will occur (7, p. 13). Disease, trauma, and disuse (sometimes caused by immobilization treatments) can all cause such restrictions. It should be emphasized that there are actually two types of entities being discussed in this section. This follows along with the physiological breakdown (see Chapter 2) of tissues and/or functions into series and parallel elastic components. The parallel components are intrinsic to muscular function; therefore, muscular elements must be used to stretch such components, implying that active exercise is more important for this component. Series element involvement is likely to respond to either active or passive exercises, so mobilization maneuvers by the therapist are likely to be effective in this situation. There is the additional question as to whether muscle spasm is involved in the pathophysiological process. Failure to deal appropriately with spasm will reduce the effectiveness of other procedures.

Norms

One cannot discuss flexibility without introducing the concept of range of motion. This is generally the parameter by which one judges whether a person is normally or abnormally mobile. Hypo- and hyperflexibility are terms about which there is little agreement. We use the numbers for normal as presented in the American Medical Association's Impairment Guide, wherever available. Even with these numbers one must exercise clinical judgment and common sense to interpret proper norms for individual patients. Women are generally a little more flexible than men. In fact, barring other factors, such as specific exercise programs, boys tend to reach peak flexibility around age 10 and girls around age 12 (9, p. 459). Some activities, like swimming, produce longer and more flexible muscles, whereas others, where strength is paramount, may tend to reduce flexibility, but not usually below the norm for that particular age. Even these generalizations are not always true. There is also an important difference in active versus passive motions, in that the tissues that produce active motion are the same ones that limit it. Passive motions, on the other hand, are diminished only by restrictions intrinsic to the involved joints. It has been shown that elastic tissue is more resilient during joint excursion than is collagenous tissue (9, p. 459). Also, one must remember that flexibility in one joint does not necessarily imply flexibility in other joints.

Contracture

Soft tissue inflexibility occurs due to lack of mobility either in muscle, connective tissue, or skin. Muscles have elastic properties that, if not properly utilized, can lose some function and result in contracture. Contractures may be actively stretched but may require passive methods, such as stimulating spindle cells or Golgi tendon organs manually (Fig. 4.5), to produce a less painful result. Sometimes a spastic muscle needs to be more vigorously stretched or to have a faradic or tetanizing current applied for a period of time. This is usually contraindicated when inflammation exists. Even when one does choose to stretch more intensely it is advised to hold for a short while at the point of maximal stretch, and do not allow or perform jerking or bobbing motions at that point. This may induce con-

traction by stretch reflexes and be counterproductive. If there is inflammation, we use cold packs to assist with the exercising (10). In the absence of inflammation, we lean strongly toward the use of heat applied to the muscle area. Exuberant stretching techniques may also be contraindicated whenever there is a condition, such as osteoporosis, which may predispose the bone in the affected joints to fracture. It may be more desirable to stimulate antagonistic muscles than to inhibit the action of agonists, or to work the contralateral muscles in either stimulatory or inhibitory modes. Once again, this is a clinical decision based upon factors such as patient pain tolerance, degree and duration of contractures, presence of an immobilizing device, and specificity and degree of tissue injury.

Effects of Immobilization

Immobilizing devices, such as splints, casts, and slings, are applied for variable periods of time. The more effective the immobilization and the longer the duration, the greater the sequelae to the immobilized area. Animal experiments suggest that there is a decreased protein synthesis within 6 hr after a limb is immobilized (5, p. 139). This is part of the reason for the muscle and bone atrophy that occurs in immobilized areas. There is also a decreased impulse pattern in the motorneurons innervating the muscles of an immobilized limb. Remembering the trophic function of the nerves, one has yet another explanation for the negative consequences of immobilization techniques. The more mobile the joint is to begin with, the worse the sequelae may be. For example, a fractured finger in a splint for 3 weeks may present a far greater recovery problem than a knee dislocation casted for 6 weeks. This is not to say that immobilization should never be done, but one needs to be fully aware of its potential consequences. Once this awareness is present, immobilization can be more thoughtfully performed and rehabilitation can begin as soon as tissues and healing permit.

Tissue Elasticity

While skin is also somewhat elastic, it has no neurological organs to assist in the stretch. The elastic properties of the skin are shown in pregnant women and in fast-losing dieters, who may have "stretch

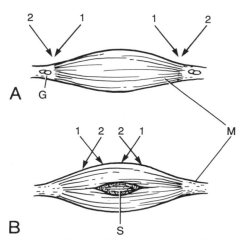

Figure 4.5 Origin/insertion and spindle cell manual muscle techniques. *M* = muscle; *G* = Golgi tendon organs; *S* = spindle cell organs. Force direction *1* causes muscle relaxation in each technique. Force direction *2* causes muscle contraction in each technique.

marks." By the same token, skin can be immobilized for a period of time and become relatively contracted. Other connective tissues may or may not have elastic tissues within them. To the extent that they do not, they are basically inert and simply follow the other tissues in their vicinity. However, the formation of scars, in the absence of adequate localized motion, can wreak havoc due to strictures passing through the connective tissue and affecting everything within their reach, even nerves and blood vessels. Passive mobilization is usually adequate to prevent such pervasive cicatrization (7, p. 14).

Joint Flexibility

Joint flexibility basically refers to mobility of the immediate structures in and around the joint capsule, the capsule itself, the retaining ligaments, cartilaginous surfaces or endplates, and the bony interfaces. Restrictions here can more likely be absolute, that is, of an osseous or calcific nature, in which joint motion is anatomically prohibited. This is usually permanent in the osseous case, such as an arthritic type spur. In that case, the intent is simply to maintain what mobility already exists. Overexercise can worsen this condition as quickly as no exercise will. The greater the inflammation, the more gently and slowly should one move the joint, sometimes only in a passive manner (4, p. 398). Joint mobilization techniques and chiropractic adjustments may be the only procedures, in certain cases, that can produce results. Tractioning and small-amplitude motions that abet joint play are often favored in such situations. During periods of immobilization, some form of limited motion will help to maintain joint flexibility (11, p. 409). This may include mild electrostimulation homolaterally and crossover training procedures. (See Table 4.2 for a summary of effects of immobilization upon body tissues and conditioning)

Warm-up Exercises

Warm-up exercises are designed to improve flexibility somewhat for a variably short period of time, depending upon the person and the exercising. Warm-ups are mainly thought of in connection with the beginning of an athletic endeavor, but they should be an intrinsic part of all rehabilitative exercise programs as well. In fact, in the more severe injuries, they may be the sum total of exercise for those local areas, in the initial stages. There are two types of warm-ups, general and specific. The first type is generalized body movement, such as calisthenics, that can be done by anyone. Specific warm-ups are the specific movements that rehearse the skills needed for the subsequent performance. There are six possible mechanisms by which warm-ups should improve performance, all related to increased blood flow and increased muscle and core temperatures (i.e., "warm-up"): (a) speed of contraction and relaxation of muscles increases; (b) lowered intramuscular viscous resistance increases mechanical efficiency; (c) hemoglobin releases oxygen more readily at higher temperatures, thus facilitating oxygen utilization; (d) the same oxygen effect is true for myoglobin; (e) nerve transmission and muscle metabolism

Table 4.2. Reconditioning and Prevention of Deconditioning

Immobilization Effect	Exercise Suggested	Intended Result
Cardiovascular		
Reduced venous flow	Dorsiflexion, plantar flexion, ankle circumduction	Simulates muscle pump, reduces blood pooling
Reduced orthostatic capacity	Active contraction of lower leg muscles prior to stand	Increase blood pressure reduces pooling
Reduced work capacity	Exercises performed frequently throughout day	Builds endurance
Musculoskeletal		
Bone	Isometric or isotonic longitudinal exercises	Increases longitudinal bone stress
Muscle	Isometric exercises, particularly	Maintains strength, mass, and joint stability
Joint	Range of motion, especially flexion/extension	Keeps connective tissue lattice open

are facilitated (possibly motor unit recruitment, as well); and, (f) hyperemia occurs through the active tissues (1, p. 412).

After age 25, there is a gradual and continuous loss of flexibility in all major joints, barring any serious attempts to improve mobility (9, p. 460). Therefore, there needs to be increased warm-up time and decreased intensity, with age, unless proven otherwise. It is also known that edema and a loss of circulation promote the formation of dense fibrotic tissues within an injured area (4, p. 392). Therefore, exercises that promote the entrance and exit of circulatory fluids are likely to encourage return of normal flexibility. Warm-up exercises should last about 20 to 30% of the entire training time, with a gradually increasing intensity (12, p. 300). When competition is to follow, warm-up time may be increased significantly. Furthermore, if warm-up is precedent to a rapid athletic event, such as a sprint, the warm-up time could be many times longer than the event itself. However, one is advised to be mindful of potential fatiguing or loss of energy stores. Additionally, the event or training should follow the warm-up closely so as not to lose the benefits mentioned above. Passive warm-ups, using massage or physiotherapeutic means, are generally to be considered as supplementary to active warm-ups. Of course, for someone suffering from paralysis, active warm-ups may not be possible, at least temporarily. It should also be mentioned that the counterirritative hyperthermic salves and lotions, currently in popular usage, probably only heat at surface levels. Therefore, if one relies upon them for proper warm-up, prior to competition, one may be unpleasantly surprised by injury during that event.

Warm-down Period

Those who are familiar with the aftereffects of rigorous training or competition are aware of the necessity for a warm-down period. The familiar victory lap after a competition is not just to bolster the ego of the victor; it provides him/her with the beginning of a warm-down effort. This allows for a more gradual cooling of the body and an increased level of oxygenation during the recovery period. Another reason to warm-down is that inactive postures following vigorous exercising allow large amounts of blood to pool in the lower extremities, thus reducing venous return to the heart, possibly resulting in syncope or worse (9, p. 454). The warm-down period should generally be within the 10- to 20-min range. In addition to the typical lower level activities that can be considered warm-down techniques, there is the category of relaxation techniques. This category includes saunas, steam baths, whirlpool bathes, and varieties of massage. A proper warm-down can help to prevent potential muscle and joint soreness.

One last point about joint flexibility should be mentioned. We usually consider limited joint mobility and reduced range of motion. However, sometimes excess mobility and range of motion need to be corrected. This hypermobility usually has a traumatic origin, but it can be inherited, such as in Ehlers-Danlos syndrome. Often, hypermobility is the result of an excess of motion generated in a joint whose adjacent joint(s) is hypomobile (Fig. 4.6). This is a normal physiological response to an abnormal biokinetic environment. Obviously, exercises intending to increase joint motion would be generally contraindicated in this situation. It is more important to strengthen the joint to be able to withstand day-to-day efforts, and still maintain enough flexibility. It is usually necessary to mobilize the fixated (hypomobile) area to create any real and long-lasting solution.

Relaxation

Relaxation refers to a conscious effort to reduce muscular tension. Actually, this refers to a psychogenic factor involved not only with the rehabilitative process, per se, but with the later performance by that person. We spoke earlier, in general principles, about properly "framing" the minds of both the therapist and the patient for best results. This production of positive motivation is essential; but, even with it, one can have a considerable amount of anxiety about one's condition or its prognosis. This anxiety translates into a hyperactivity in the central nervous system, which can refer to any and all bodily systems. The neuromuscular system responds with prolonged inappropriate contractions, which can be monitored by palpation or sophisticated electromyographic techniques. Monitoring can be a form of biofeedback, in which the patient is autogenically trained to alter his

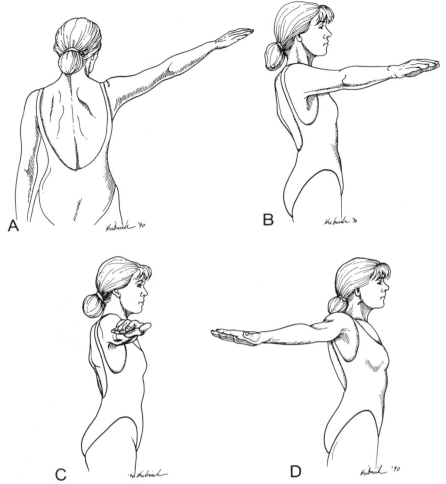

Figure 4.6 Joint movements progressing from simple planar to complex three-dimensional modes.

responses. Proprioceptive awareness can be taught by having the patient selectively contract and relax certain muscles and move their respective joints (4, p. 424). In fact, in addition to the typical headaches and muscular pains, most people suffering from chronic pulmonary disorders experience substantial tension in the associated musculature (7, p. 14). This is discussed further under "Respiratory Function."

Other than applying external agents, there are two main avenues for relaxation production. One can utilize the body's own reflex mechanisms, such as reciprocal innervation, whereby the contraction of the antagonist reflexly inhibits contraction of the agonist, that was in spasm. This requires a working knowledge of which muscles antagonize others. Also, the relaxation

of a muscle is proportional to its quantity of contraction. This means that a muscle which is held in contraction to a certain degree will thereafter relax to the same degree. Bringing this to conscious control and gradually decreasing contraction and increasing relaxation (progressive relaxation) is a process taught by Jacobson, and one that anyone can learn (4, p. 425). This is an example of the second avenue for relaxation, that is, conscious control of unconscious behavior. This is also exhibited in such techniques as transcendental or other types of meditation, in which one consciously focuses on either a body function (such as respiration) or an ideation. Actually, some meditation techniques involve defocusing, or making the mind blank, a difficult state to achieve. Also, an environment that is conducive to the activity or training described must be provided for the patient. This may include such considerations as a darkened room, an absence of noise or very controlled sounds, and a comfortable piece of furniture for the patient to use. Relaxation procedures are all teachable and can usually be performed, with little or no difficulty, by the patient at home and alone. They tend to enhance the effects of all other procedures as well.

Coordination

This is one of the more complicated neuromuscular functions, requiring constant feedback and cybernetic correction. Coordination is the ability to use the right muscles at the right times and with the correct intensity. By definition, coordination implies the use and interaction of multimuscular patterns. Many of the same neural pathways that regulate postural components and proprioceptive mechanisms are intimately involved in coordination efforts. Without coordination, one could not experience a normal gait or feed oneself. There are times when an emphasis on strength formation causes incoordinate movements, thus patterning a later problem (9, p. 355). This may be avoided by proceeding slowly with great attention to form and timing of exercises. As everyone who has worked with athletes knows, it is more difficult to untrain and retrain from a bad habit position then it is to train correctly from the outset. Coordination problems are rarely disorders of the lower motor neuron. They usually involve descending and efferent pathways. One tries to train both strong and weak muscles to work in concert, thus minimizing the incidence of late contractures (9, p. 355). This points out one of the most significant features of rehabilitative exercise. It should be started as early as possible, per area and condition, thereby acting in a prophylactic manner as well as a corrective one. If significant pain or muscle spasm is produced by the exercises, one is advised to discontinue them until such reactions no longer occur.

It is not clear what part of coordination is hereditary, what part is autonomic or unconscious engrams, and what part is voluntarily controlled. Only the genetic portion is probably uncontrollable. It should be mentioned that volition can stimulate and modify an engram as to its duration, but the engram is not alterable by direct conscious control (4, p. 405). However, the production of valid new engrams, by well-controlled repetitious activities, is one of the specific aims of coordination training. When an incorrect muscle or motion is added to an exercise, the therapist must immediately direct the patient's attention to this and reeducate the patient to avoid such future occurrences. Only after proper coordinated motion is achieved at a certain intensity and frequency level can one augment the strength program. In this alternating fashion, one gradually increases both strength and coordination, without sacrificing either. Sometimes strength is so diminished as to not allow motion of the joint versus gravity, a one rating. If this is the case, mild strength training must precede or coexist with coordination training.

Sometimes it is more important to work on the synergists or teach the patient how to let go (i.e., inhibit) of the antagonists. Relaxation techniques may be useful for the latter task. A specific knowledge of the anatomy and physiology can allow one to design more precise exercise patterns. Muscles of the same or adjacent joints that maintain the joint's position are used synchronously with the agonist (or prime mover) and they are called stabilizers (4, p. 404). In athletic competition it is often the stabilizers that are initially injured, sometimes in a minor fashion. Their lack of joint support may then cause other muscles to be injured, perhaps more severely, by performing unaccustomed actions or being overused. This sometimes occurs in baseball pitchers and may cause a work-related injury in a plumber or carpenter, for instance. Just as substituted gait patterns are always less efficient, substituted volitional muscle actions are also at a mechanical disadvantage (11, p. 563). One can discover when this substitution has occurred by examining the specific muscles involved. Various neurological tests determine balance, proprioception, and ability to perform coordinated activities. Furthermore, one can evaluate gait or motion of a limb visually, by various photographic means, with computer enhancement, and by various other technology, such as creative uses of infrared devices.

There are three general principles to follow in the development of neuromuscular coordination. First is constant repetition of a relatively few motor activities. It is important not to overload the nervous system with too many different motor functions at one time. One can envision the process of learning to play Beethoven's Fifth Symphony a bar or two at a time, gradually adding sections to learn each movement. The second principle advises us to use all sensory cues (visual, tactile, and proprioceptive) to enhance perception and motor performance. While the patient is performing the exercise, judicious placement of a mirror, and any other feedback available, is advised for the patient's benefit. In a patient whose proprioceptive reflexes are damaged, visual reflexes can, to a certain extent, replace them in the reeducation of coordination (4, p. 578). A corollary to this principle is that psychological reinforcement is equally important to the final result. The last principle is that one gradually accelerates the rate of the performance of the activities, as the engram becomes formed. Once again, one may recall the first notes played on the piano, guitar or French horn, and how the tempo was gradually increased as one "felt the rhythm" of the piece and learned to perform its content.

Respiratory Function

The aim of all exercises under this category is to improve ventilation. This means removing more carbon dioxide or increasing the oxygenation of the blood and tissues. Ventilation is a function of the lungs and bronchial tissues, the diaphragm, the thoracic cage (and its supportive structures), the abdominal wall, and the accessory musculature. Endurance, cardiovascular function, and relaxation are enhanced by a positive improvement in oxygen transfer. There is also an energetic benefit in that aerobic exercise is more energy efficient and, therefore, increases exercise tolerance proportionately. This is most important in athletic training. Table 4.3 lists the major respiratory disorders with which we need be concerned. Anyone with chronic obstructive pulmonary disease will benefit at much lower levels of performance and will be more likely to be helped overall.

As with relaxation procedures, a quiet area for interaction is best during the training. The patient also needs to be made comfortable, in loosened and nonrestrictive clothing. The supine position, with the head and upper trunk elevated about 45° is an appropriate starting posture (7, p. 537). In the beginning, sitting or standing postures may be too taxing and may be counterproductive. As with other body systems, observation of the patient's normal breathing pattern is vital to establish a baseline. The main categories of abnormal breathing are dyspnea, tachypnea, hyperventilation, orthopnea, Cheyne-Stokes, apnea, and hypoventilation. Dyspnea implies a shortness of breath or a labored breathing. Tachypnea describes rapid, shallow breathing; the tidal volume is decreased but the rate is increased. Hyperventilation is rapid respiration with an increased tidal volume. Apnea implies an absence of breathing, at least for an abnormal period of time. Cheyne-Stokes breathing is a situation where there is a cyclic increase and decrease in tidal vol-

Table 4.3. Characteristics of Respiratory Disorders

	Restrictive	Obstructive
Cause	Muscle weakness, inefficiency, or increasing stiffness of elastic components	Increased resistance to air flow through the tracheobronchial tree
Joint involvement	Possible	No
Respiratory phase most involved	Inspiratory	Expiratory
Vital capacity	Reduced	Reduced
Forced air capacity (% in 1 sec)	85% or more	<85%
Maximal breathing capacity	Normal or slightly reduced	Reduced
Diffusing capacity	Can be reduced	Not relevant
Total lung size (capacity)	Reduced	Normal or increased

ume, the latter being punctuated by a period of apnea. This often is the result of a head injury. In orthopnea, breathing is difficult in the supine position. Hypoventilation is often the result of an obstructive or a restrictive pulmonary disorder. When the lungs are unable to remove enough carbon dioxide, the alveolar concentration of CO_2 rises, which tends to produce respiratory acidosis.

This text is mainly concerned with exercising to assist people who are suffering with dyspnea and orthopnea. Hypoventilation often needs mechanical assistance in the form of an intermittent positive pressure breathing (IPPB) apparatus (4, p. 777). We are interested in tachypnea or hyperventilation only in connection with cardiovascular disorders (discussed below). Patients with pulmonary or cardiovascular problems are usually under ongoing medical care at the time breathing exercises are being used. Most exercises included here involve conscious retraining of normal breathing patterns.

Attention must be paid to the primary and accessory muscles that produce respiration. The major muscles to consider are the diaphragm, the intercostals, and the abdominal muscles. The main accessory muscles are the scalenus muscles, the levator scapulae, and the sternocleidomastoid. The diaphragm is by far the most complex of these muscles, and even has fibers interdigitating with the fascia of the psoas and the quadratus lumborum. Contraction of the diaphragm causes it to move inferiorly and decrease intrathoracic pressure, thereby causing inspiration. It is only mildly active during normal expiration but plays a crucial role in vomiting and defecating, as do abdominal muscles. It has been determined that the external intercostals act for inspiratory motion and the internal intercostals act predominantly in expiration, but have some minor inspiratory action (9, p. 567). The abdominal muscles mainly assist in expiration, but have little action in any but high levels of ventilation. The accessory muscles assist inspiration by elevating the superior thorax, thus further decreasing intrathoracic pressures. In breaths of maximum volume, the rib circumference increases by 8 cm, the anteroposterior dimension by 3 cm, and the lateral diameter by 1.5 cm, normally (9, p. 568). Changes in these measurements (which vary according to age, gender, condition, and other factors) are a means to determine the amount of restriction and to measure one's progress.

Eventually you will instruct the patient in the performance of their breathing exercises in as many positions, at rest and in activity, in which they are capable. Patients with respiratory difficulties are among the most difficult to rehabilitate and, at the same time, among the most rewarding. Their problems usually affect every aspect of their life, to some extent, and can be so ubiquitous as to literally drain them of most of their energy in just "staying alive." Therefore, each little step is an arduous task and yet can be very rewarding. Patients need to participate in goal setting because their self-esteem and their health, are dependent upon steady progression. Additionally, subjective improvement shows a decreased heart rate during exercise, and even severely restricted patients can increase exercise levels and oxygen uptakes by 20% (9, (p. 575).

Some advise that one should never allow a patient to force expiration (7, p. 537). The reasons for this are 2-fold. First, forced expiration increases airway turbulence. This can lead to bronchospasm or even increased airway obstruction. Second, the changes in intrathoracic pressure brought to bear in order to force such expiration may lead to a simultaneous collapse of the bronchial passages. This would obviously be contraindicated in a patient with an obstructive disorder. This latter is also true with respect to increasing the power of accessory muscles in order to aid respiratory efforts. Until a patient is more accomplished in breath retraining, it is not advisable to allow him/her a prolonged expiration. The subsequent inspiration is liable to be a gasp, may even scare the patient, and would tend to cause an irregular respiratory rhythm. This can be overcome in most people with practice and good technique, at least to a great degree.

Part of the technique, of course, is a relaxation process. By the same token, hyperinflation of the lung is equally undesirable in that it does not permit sufficient oxygenation with the next inspiration. Clearly, this is a problem of balance. In the beginning the patient is advised not to initiate inspiration with the accessory muscles or even the upper chest. This is not conducive to relaxation and thus may be counterproductive in the early and even middle stages of training, since it may produce hyperventilation. However, increased diaphragmatic excursion with reduced thoracic movements can reduce the neural input from muscle and joint receptors, thereby reducing the sensation of breathlessness (9, p. 576). This sensation potentially initiates a panic reaction, which produces a positive feedback loop, unless conscious control of breathing is assumed. Since alveolar and arterial partial gas pressures of O_2 and CO_2 are two important measures of ventilatory function, it is easy to see that exercises which alter content of inspired and expired air are highly desirable. This content is altered by changing the breathing patterns in the manners described above. It should be obvious, at this point, that relaxation and respiratory activities can and often should be performed at the same time. One last item to mention here is that the production and maintenance of proper posture are vital to efficient ventilation.

Cardiovascular Function

Two levels of cardiovascular problems must be rehabilitated. In the more severe problems, or in the immediate and acute phase of such problems, most activity is minimized. Exercise must be carefully selected and performed at the lowest energy levels, so as not to cause oxygen depletion or risk further cardiovascular injury. In more chronic or partially healed conditions, the exercise parameters can be augmented. There are several aims to this type of rehabilitation, depending upon the type and stage of the healing process. With respect to the heart itself, one may aim at compensatory hypertrophy, increased efficiency of electrostimulatory mechanisms, improved coronary circulation (increased collateralization), and better controlled and normalized cardiac rhythms.

Fitness

One could also talk about a level of cardiovascular functioning called fitness, which results in heightened energy reserves for optimum performance and well being (7, p. 590). What fitness means to a person is a function of their lifestyle. The more they can accomplish within their own normal living patterns, the higher their level of fitness is deemed to be. Actually, the more all of the therapeutic intents are furthered, the higher the level of overall fitness achieved. In terms of sports fitness, the exercise program is unrelated to the specific skills involved in the sports (9, p. 454). This has much to do with conditioning, which is an augmentation of the energy capacity of the muscle through an exercise program (7, p. 591). Fitness also depends upon gender, age, genetics, pathophysiology, and level of activity. One cannot have fitness without also having endurance. A conditioning program causes a cardiovascular and neuromuscular adaptation in the body such that the person's endurance is augmented. This is why cardiopulmonary training is intimately tied in with endurance training; the intents are interdependent, rather than independent. In this text neuromuscular (and even psychological) endurance is separated from cardiovascular endurance.

While all endurance is intrinsically related to the ability to transport and utilize oxygen, cardiovascular fitness has to do with specific avenues to accomplish this: the oxygen-carrying capacity of the blood, cardiac function, heart rate, and stroke volume. Exercises that can amplify such abilities are referred to as "aerobic." Exercises with little aerobic power are of little rehabilitative assistance to the heart and lungs. Endurance is measured as a person's maximum aerobic power, VO_2, and expressed in the following equation (7, p. 591):

$$VO_2 = rv(pO_2)$$

where r = the heart rate (beats/minute), v = the stroke volume (milliliters), and pO_2 = the arteriovenous oxygen partial pressure differential.

The pressure differential reflects the oxygen capacity of the skeletal muscle. This, in turn, is determined by such factors as the perfusion of the muscle and the enzymatic and mitochondrial content of the muscle. Perfusion is a consequence of cardiac function. While exercise can improve cardiac function, poor cardiac function can certainly limit exercise. Balance and moderation are usually the solution. Monitoring the above variables is a way to determine fitness level and ability to continue exercising at any particular level. Of these, heart rate is the most convenient and most accurate method. One could monitor pulmonary functions by respiratory rates, rhythms, and volumes as well, all which would reflect the patient's endurance. It may be wise to first obtain results from exercise stress testing before engaging in therapeutic exercises in anyone who has a history of cardiopulmonary disorders. Such tests would, of course, only be done under strict medical supervision, especially in a patient already needing rehabilitation. One other factor concerning cardiovascular stress is that it is considerably greater in water, especially as its temperature rises. The warmer the water becomes, with 34°C being the average starting temperature, the greater the peripheral arterial circulation. This, naturally, places a greater strain upon the heart, in proportion to the increased cardiac output needed to supply the periphery. Additionally, the hydrostatic pressure on the chest causes the heart to have to work harder than it would under the same circumstances on land. Therefore, it is recommended that underwater treatments generally be limited to about 20 min (12, p. 158).

Exercise Parameters

The parameters of any exercise are the variable factors by which the exercise can be modified to suit the individual and his or her specific needs at a given point in time. These parameters include intensity, frequency, rate, duration, and spatial and temporal configurations. First, one determines the goals and intents of the exercise program. Then one determines the locations to which the exercise is to be applied. Lastly, one calculates the boundary conditions for the set of parameters for the employed exercises. For example, exercise A will be performed on muscle X in order to rehabilitate it and its related joints to their preinjury status. It will be performed, in increasing levels of intensity and frequency, for the first 4 weeks over the entire range of motion to assist restoration of flexibility. Exercise B will be performed on this muscle from week 2 through week 6, at increasing intensity levels (i.e., loads), over the middle third of the range of motion in order to restore strength to the muscle and joints. This is a shortened and generalized version of a full rehabilitation plan.

Intensity

The intensity refers to either the external load on the muscle or the internal load assumed. This is the single most important factor in determining whether a conditioning effect is achieved (7, p. 597). In an isometric exercise, for instance, one can resist with maximum attainable force or any portion thereof, while maintaining balance with the external load imposed. To be able to determine what percentage of maximum the current load is, we had to establish a baseline and test for same. Obviously, the maximum will improve as the muscle and joint improve. Exercises for strength building generally require a much higher intensity than those for flexibility or endurance. However, an isometric contraction performed at about 40% of maximum, held for about 6 to 10 sec and performed three to five times daily, is sufficient to cause muscle hypertrophy (12, p. 97). If such exercising is begun within 3 to 4 days after immobilizing an injured extremity, loss of muscular strength can be greatly avoided (12, p. 97).

Duration

Whereas isometric exercises are performed at a low frequency (one contraction, three to five times per day) and a high duration (6 to 10 sec/contraction), isotonic and isokinetic exercise is just the opposite. Duration also refers to the length of time the phase of the exercise program is in force. For instance, how many weeks will an activity continue before it is discontinued or reevaluated? Although the duration of a single contraction is small (only a fraction of a second up to about 2 sec) in an isotonic program, the exercising lasts longer since many more contractions occur. Isotonic and isokinetic exercises can have some aerobic and endurance type benefits, if one programs them in that manner. They also can be used, in part, to teach skills and coordination, both of which are unavailable in isometric programs.

Rate

Rate refers to the speed at which an exercise is performed. This does not pertain to the isometric format and only vaguely pertains to the isotonic format. But it intimately relates to the isokinetic format, which is, therefore, better for training for specific skills where rate is a factor of performance.

Temporal Configuration

The integration of these exercises, in proper time sequence and proper amount, is referred to as temporal configuration. When do we add a greater load or change the frequency or duration of the exercise? These questions may not be able to be answered accurately until the patient is already involved in the program. When the patient is reevaluated, the temporal parameters can be set or reset.

Spatial Configuration

Spatial configuration refers to the Cartesian system discussed in Chapter 1. It has been suggested that one begin a program with one- and two-dimensional exercises (12, p. 101). Then, when a three-dimensional program can be instituted, one can work more intensively on increasing elasticity and add specific skill tasks to the program (12, p. 101). Generally, we begin with linear and planar motions, i.e., simple movements. As the joint unit begins to show improvement, we can add the third dimension, as movements become more complex and involve multiple interrelated structures (Fig. 4.6). Even in a simple exercise, the spatial configuration is paramount in producing "good form." Let us say we are going to perform an isotonic contraction of the biceps. Our data indicate that the muscle exhibits weakness between 70 and 120° of planar contraction, so the exercise may be structured to meet this spatial requirement. This is a simple example, and the problem may be in a synergist or co-contractor.

An interesting phenomenon, called coupling, occurs in human motions and is most easily seen in spinal movements. Coupling relates to synergistic and co-contractor actions, and is defined as a summary motion in which rotation or translation of a body about or along one axis is consistently and simultaneously associated with similar motion(s) about or along another axis (13, p. 63). For example, rotation (transverse or xz plane motion) is typically coupled with lateral flexion through most regions of the spine. The actual shapes and geometry of the facet joints are among the factors controlling three-dimensional motion at a specific level; this provides an anatomical substrate for such motions. It is easy to see how such concepts are related to the differences between simple and complex motions.

Exercise Categories

There are only a few different types of contractions of which the body is capable. Similarly, there are only a few different types of movement. Each classification is discussed below (Table 4.1).

Passive exercises refer to movements that are performed for the patient while the patient attempts to relax the related area. These can be produced by manual or mechanical means. They are preferred when other exercises are painful or are contraindicated. Passive exercises are usually less difficult to perform than other movement types when muscles or tendons are injured, and are, therefore, usually superior in augmenting flexibility. Many types of physical therapy, such as faradic current, also produce passive movements of muscles and joints. Alternately, a passive exercise can be performed with the assistance of gravity. An example of this is a squat, which is not produced by action of the hamstrings. This might be deemed an active exercise with a passive effect (14, p. 36). Active exercises are those that are performed by the patient alone, once he/she has been taught them.

Assisted exercises are performed by the patient with the therapist's assistance. They are particularly useful in the early stages of rehabilitation to guide the patient through the proper form of the exercises. They are also especially useful when teaching and conducting breathing exercises (14, p. 34). The aim of assistive exercises is always to reduce the amount of assistance, both in time and intensity, to zero, at the same time as motion and force are incremented.

In resistive exercises an external load is applied against the intended motion(s). These loads can be manual, mechanical, and variable. Resistive exercises are chiefly utilized to increase strength and endurance. When joint injuries are rehabilitated, especially postsurgically, it is probably prudent to avoid the extremes of the ranges of motion, especially with resistive exercises.

Balanced Exercises

These exercises have essentially three purposes; (a) they help to counteract the unilateral stresses that occur in certain activities; (b) they help to correct bilateral muscle injury or weakness; and (c) they assist in correcting and maintaining normal postural components. When there is a great unilateral weakness in a particular muscle or joint one is inclined to rehabilitate it unilaterally. This may work for a while, but it tends to create more unbalance and actually build in a neurological preference for that laterality in the form of an aberrant engram. Furthermore, balanced exercises act in a preventive mode by normalizing actions.

These exercises (and "Loosening," below) tend to resemble what may have previously been called calisthenics. It is recommended to begin all balanced exercises in the supine position (12, p. 308). It is also a good idea to perform them on a firm surface which is also well padded. They are for relaxation, warm-up, warm-down, and flexibility. As in progressive relaxation techniques, one begins at one end of the body, preferably the head, and works one's way through the whole body. The movements are performed slowly and regularly, and consist of an alternate series of up to 10 repetitions, each followed by an equal period of rest. During each session, one should complete the entire set of motions bilaterally, in all three planes of each body part exercised. The exercises begin with simple one- and two-dimensional movements and gradually include the complex three-dimensional movements that were discussed above. The primary purpose of this type of exercise is to mobilize the spinal column in a uniform manner to free it for all other activities. This is especially true in activities that require great strength, such as weight lifting or loading trucks at a dock. For people who are normally quite mobile, such as dancers or younger people, the final position of the exercise may be held for up to 7 sec to help with stabilization in otherwise hypermobile areas (12, p. 316). The body positions can be modified so that the exercises maximize results while minimizing adverse consequences. For example, a person with an increased lumbar lordosis, or whose activities accentuate this, might flex the knees in exercising so as to lessen the stress to the lumbar area and facilitate normal motion and posture.

Breathing

These exercises are usually important for the following functions: pulmonary, cardiovascular, endurance, and relaxation. Patients who need such exercises due to chronic or acute pulmonic disorders often experience coughing and the need to or the actual expectoration of phlegm. Such congestion often impedes the exercise. Therefore, in the absence of mechanical respiratory aids, one must be able to apply such techniques as postural drainage, cupping and various massage procedures to ease such congestion, so that breathing exercises can be continued. Postural drainage is contraindicated in the presence of severe pulmonary or cardiac conditions, hemoptysis, or recent neurosurgery (7, p. 554). Teaching the patient to cough more effectively is an asset at such times. Sometimes just changing the patient to a more erect position is sufficient. Specifically, one should sit or lean forward, with the neck slightly flexed, and review with and demonstrate to the patient the anatomy and mechanism of the cough. At times it will be helpful to stretch trunk and cervical muscles and joints, particularly the rib cage, prior to performing breathing exercises.

Conditioning

This refers to doing all which one can to promote the betterment of the health of all bodily systems, including the mental aspects. Implicit in this definition is that one is making the body better fit to survive, and even thrive, in the face of increasing stressors placed upon it. The physical fitness implied herein enhances performance, reduces chances of injury, and enhances recovery. A general and specific adaptation occurs in the body, as a result of conditioning, which is reflected as augmented endurance. Adaptation, of course, occurs over longer periods of time, and the greater efficiency that comes with it means the person will fatigue at a later time (7, p. 592).

Also implicit in conditioning, as with most intents of exercise, is that increased levels of demand are required to increase the final product. In fact, there is a rather specific protocol for cardiovascular fitness, as defined by Cooper (9, p. 453). The heart rate (i.e., pulse) must reach at least 70% of its maximum and the training effect does not begin until about 5 min after one starts the exercise period. Less vigorous exercising requires more time, and the result is ultimately dependent upon the oxygen consumption. Therefore, the more fit the individual is at the outset, the more vigorous the exercise needs to be.

Furthermore, we know that deconditioning occurs fairly rapidly in someone who is relatively or completely inactive. Among the results of deconditioning are increased resting heart rate; decreasing stroke volume; negative nitrogen and protein balance; reduced enzymes and energy stores; decreased vital capacity; decreased oxygen utilization and, therefore, aerobic work capacity; decreased circulating blood volume; decreased plasma and red blood cell count; decreased lean body mass; an increased urinary calcium excretion, which can lead to osteopenia; decreased muscle oxidative enzymes; and a loss of some proprioception and even neuromuscular responses (7, pp. 592–3; 10, p. 583). Therefore, it can be inferred that conditioning reverses all the above mentioned. Furthermore, it also causes cardiac hypertrophy, reduces body fat content, and reduces blood pressure during rest and exercise (10, p. 579).

Coordination

When coordination is lacking, it may be necessary first to teach the action of a specific muscle or muscles and later to integrate their action(s) (4, p. 406). This is the basis for formation of engrams. Of course, for this to occur, there needs to be a viable lower motor neuron pathway and intact proprioceptive pathways and receptors. There also needs to be a pain-free arc of motion for coordinate activity to take place. The therapist must also be cognizant of substitution efforts which can replace the limited abilities of an injured joint unit. When this is detected, sometimes only by electromyography, retraining is in order. Often, this is only possible by decreasing the intensity of effort and/or the rate of motion, or by assisted movements. Sometimes, one can teach with judicious application of tendon reflexes, but this is difficult when educating smaller muscles and finer

movements. When volitional attitude is inadequate to promote necessary motion, one may resort to some reflex facilitation procedure (see "Proprioceptive Neuromuscular Facilitation," for example).

Additionally, one could neurologically sensitize the tendon reflex by stimulation of the skin over the insertions or belly of the intended muscle (4, p. 408). This supradermal stimulation also brings conscious attention and proprioception to bear just prior to the volitional attempt. The stimulation can be any kinesthetic action or physical agent one desires to apply. This kinesthetic stimulation can be used to explain what is supposed to be felt, so that the patient's conscious mind can be involved in the process. In teaching control over these processes, especially the more complicated ones, we always begin with simple and low-resistance movements. In order for the patient to sense the motion of the prime mover, the resistance needs to be small; otherwise, some amount of recruitment, with contraction, is almost inevitable. This isolation in the feeling of the paretic prime mover is essential if normal coordinate function is to result. The body, all too readily, will substitute and utilize the synergists whenever necessary, thereby obscuring the injured part. This, at least partly, is responsible for many of the greater injuries in the first place. A smaller injury occurs, which causes an alteration in normal function and motion, thereby placing the remaining structures at a mechanical disadvantage in the performance of a task. This results in a much more severe injury, perhaps to a different structure, which, when treated successfully, still may leave the original lesion unattended. This happens frequently, for instance, in a baseball pitcher who has a minor hip injury, which then causes an alteration in his delivery, resulting occasionally in almost career-ending shoulder injuries. In any case, if the original lesion in the hip were not rehabilitated, the shoulder injury would be destined to recur.

Generally, there is a four-step approach, as described in Krusen, to the retraining of neuromuscular control (4, pp. 408–9). First, the motion is passively performed for the patient, along with supradermal stimulation, while the patient is instructed to think through the activity. Even this may produce a spillover effect, neurologically, with an amount of co-contraction. If it does, the patient is diverted somewhat, or told to reduce concentration a little. When this can be accomplished, the patient is asked to provide a minimal amount of active contraction. As the patient becomes effective in isolating the required component(s), he/she is then allowed to gradually increase active participation, while the therapist gradually reduces the passive constituent. Eventually, as the engram becomes formed, the therapist withdraws all passive elements and strength training is added.

For any of this to occur, the activity must first be analyzed to determine its basic components (unit motor tasks) so that we know what to focus on at any given time. Krusen calls this desynthesis, and its importance is directly proportional to the complexity of the involved task (4, p. 409). Patience is probably more crucial in this type of rehabilitation than in any other kind, because form and formation of proper engrams are very exacting. As soon as fatigue begins to set in the exercise must be discontinued. Therefore, frequent rest periods between small sets of repetitions are necessary to prevent accumulated fatigue. For a frame of reference, producing an engram for a specific industrial task required some three million correct repetitions, in a young adult with normal dexterity, in order to develop maximum speed and skill (4, p. 410). It is more or less for other tasks, depending upon their complexity and the extent of the injury. To demonstrate what this means, 1000 repetitions/day for three years equal one million repetitions. This assumes that all were done correctly. It should be mentioned that specific units of activity may have impact upon other tasks as well. However, they must be integrated into the engram for that task as well. As each subtask of an activity is perfected, it can be added to the chain of events, like another link. The conscious mind can only successfully select the engrams and the time sequence in which they will be utilized. Any other added variables will cause a tremendous proportionate increase in effort, and will eventually result in errors eventually. We urge you to work only within the boundaries in which success can be maintained and not to give up too early.

This is all the more important in physically disadvantaged people. For instance, if we train only two or three times for 10 min/day and allow incorrect activity to intervene between sessions, little will be achieved. Thousands of *correct repetitions* are needed to create a proper engram.

Loosening

These exercises were so labeled by Doris Eitner and consist of a series of alternating stretching and relaxing motions. The rapid reciprocating action could also be described as a series of shaking motions, which should be rhythmically integrated into the regimen (12, p. 128). When this is performed in a passive manner, it is useful for spastic muscular lesions (except those with upper motor neuron lesions and a tendency to clonus) and muscle contractures. The variables here include the magnitude and frequency of the shaking and the spatial and temporal configurations. Alternate tractioning and compressing of a joint also fits into this category, and is useful in increasing the joint play. The position of the body is important, especially if one is using the process as part of a relaxation program. These exercises are also useful in improving flexibility because the reduction of myospasms is usually integral to any program to increase mobility of a joint. One needs to be careful, especially if performing in a vigorous manner, since more than one joint may be moved and specificity can be lost. Such shaking is contraindicated in the presence of severe ligamentous or capsular damage. The more severe the damage, the slower and smaller the amplitude of oscillation should be.

Shaking is effective as a preventive measure, particularly in athletes prior to competition, and is often done actively by the athlete. Active loosening does not require the assistance of a second party to perform, but it needs to be carefully learned under professional supervision. An example of this is the twisting motion one might use to warm up for golf. This should be done slowly at first, then later increased in rate. Most of the time we advise against "jerky" motions, but finishing this "swing" with a "bounce" is akin to the way the motion is actually performed. Therefore, it can be done in such situations. Sometimes the use of weights, allowing joints to swing freely in gravity after elevation, or music can make the exercises more functional. If these exercises are done in a swinging manner, it is helpful to visualize a pendulum and imitate its rhythmic oscillations. This is also one of the uses of such devices as Indian clubs. One usually performs the exercise without the weight first, then with the added load.

The shaking type of active loosening is particularly useful just before one performs especially detailed and highly coordinated work, or after having completed it. It can also be used after exercising, such as jogging or other endurance or strength exercises, to facilitate the recovery period. Physiological experiments have shown that for two muscles of equal strength, the performance of the loosest muscle will always be superior (12, p. 134). Runners, chiefly sprinters, know this principle well and can always be seen warming up with this process prior to competition. Needless to say, the area immediately proximal to the shaking needs to be fixed (i.e., stabilized) in order to control the shaking. This means that this joint must have integrity and its muscles must be strong enough to support such holding. Additionally, some supporting structures may have to be provided in order to perform some of the motions, particularly those in the standing position involving the legs. Jumping rope is also an example of this type activity, but its rather high impact effect precludes its usage in even moderately injured persons. Some people have developed a type of jump rope, called a heavy rope, that is weighted, and would be inappropriate for this activity because it loads the joints too much. It is more useful as an endurance or strengthening activity.

Minus Training

This is called minus training because it involves exercising while there is a partial relief of body weight, or minus some of the postural load that one normally carries. Such exercises can be performed while the patient is in some sort of harness or support, perched upon a device (such as an exercycle), or immersed in water. One can graduate the minus training by gradually allowing more of the body weight to be supported normally. An example of this in water is to steadily lower the water level

through which one exercises, on a day-by-day basis or as rapidly as the healing process permits.

Muscle Reeducation

As the name implies, these exercises retrain individual function(s) in muscles. They also apply to augmentation of coordination in muscles recovering from injuries that leave them paretic or paralyzed or in tendon transplants. These exercises are already included in other sections under different names.

Postural

Intimately tied in with coordination and proprioception is the subject of balance. Balance has to do with the maintenance of equilibrium within the gravity field, in any position, when at rest or during activity. This is normally a constant process of reequilibration involving a specific set of servomechanisms that work through the final common pathway of the lower motor neurons. The majority of this activity is accomplished in the unconscious mode, unless a sudden physical force creates an imbalanced position. This force can be throwing a football, running into something or someone at work, or slipping on an oil slick in the garage. Once again, the formation of engrams is about the best method to improve both posture and balance. Because posture often appears to be relatively static, improvement in muscle strength may be of great assistance in the improvement of posture. Once the desired posture is established and it is determined which structures are failing to maintain it, flexibility and strengthening activities can be applied as needed. Balance engram formations begin after one carefully rules out neurological lesions in a related system. Gait training may come under this category as well, since it relates to both posture and balance. Such exercises as gait training and cross-crawl maneuvers (Fig. 4.7) can help to improve neurological integration of data and, therefore, augment virtually any exercise regimen. Gait is only proper when it is regulated by specific postural muscles; substituted gait patterns are always less efficient (15, p. 563). This is another reason why engram formation is desirable in this training mode. For screening purposes, it is recom-

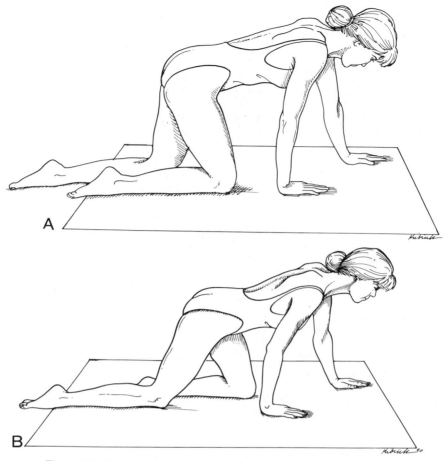

Figure 4.7 Basic postures for neurological gait training exercises.

mended to examine and treat the following muscles: gluteus medius, iliopsoas, vastus medialis, obliquus, and posterior tibialis. In testing, always look for substitution of muscles.

Progressive Resistance (PRE)

In this type of exercise, a mechanically applied load is gradually increased over time. PREs were originally designed to increase strength, but have been found to augment endurance and power as well. The De-Lorme axiom can be applied here. It states that high-power (resistance) and low-repetition exercises build strength, while low-power and high-repetition exercises build endurance (4, p. 450). It is believed that this axiom is true near the extremes but less so in the middle ranges. PREs are divided into load-resisting and load-assisting types of exercise. In the first type, the body part is moved actively against a certain resistance. In the second type, a load is used to assist motion of a muscle too weak to move even against gravity. This is one step removed from the assistive exercises that are performed by the therapist. The load in this case can also be administered, as per De-Lorme, by a system of pulleys and weights, to counterbalance the weight of the body part being moved (7, p. 96).

The repetition maximum (RM) is the greatest amount of load a muscle can move through the range of motion for a specific number of times (7, p. 96). The repetition minimum (Rm; our abbreviation) is the least load required to move a body part against gravity for a specific number of times (7, p. 96). The former is part of the description for resistive exercises, while the latter is descriptive of assistive type exercises. The RM is a baseline quantity from which progress can be charted. Normally, most programs demand from 6 to 10 repetitions, or reps (denoted 6RM, for example), at each load level. When 10RM can be easily exceeded at one load level, the load is appropriately incremented and one precedes at 6RM to perform the next sets of gradually increasing numbers of repetitions. With assistive exercises, the object is continuously to decrease the Rm so that the patient eventually requires no assistance. Then one switches to repetition maximum exercises. Each set of exercises is usually repeated a number of times, called bouts, with intervening rest periods. The exercise frequency is usually from three to five times per week, with the proviso that adequate recovery time from fatigue is allotted. The duration of an exercise program, in order to significantly increase strength, should be at least 6 weeks (7, p. 97). As mentioned previously, when the velocity of contraction increases the maximum tension developed decreases during concentric contractions. However, for eccentric contractions, the velocity versus tension relationship is reversed (7, p. 97). This may be a protective neuromuscular mechanism so that the muscle is less likely to be injured when excessive loads are encountered.

These resistive exercises can be performed using any mode of contraction described previously. When the isokinetic mode is used, strength gains occur over time, but only at speeds equal to or slower than that of the exercise (7, p. 97). Therefore, it is a good idea to perform such exercises at speeds that match or exceed the intended final activities. Since most activities consist of combined types of contractions, it is probably a good idea similarly to mix the types of contractions in the exercises. Isotonic contractions are generally done one of two ways, the DeLorme technique or the Oxford technique. In each, one first determines what the 10RM is. Then, in the former, one might begin with 10 reps of one-half of the 10RM, then proceed to 10 reps of three-fourths and the full 10RM. There would be a brief rest period between each bout of the session. In the Oxford technique, one proceeds exactly in the opposite direction. In the DeLorme technique, there is almost a built-in warm-up period,

whereas the Oxford technique affords a built-in resistance to the effects of fatigue.

The isometric procedure we prefer is known as brief repetitive isometric exercise (BRIME). In this technique, 5 to 10 brief, maximal isometric contractions are performed 5 days/week. It is also recommended that isometric training be repeated from three to five times daily for optimum results (12, p. 97). PREs may be performed for 12 to 15 times before increasing the load (9, p. 456). After the 15 reps have been easily performed, one adds an amount of weight so that only 8 to 10 reps can now be performed, even with some difficulty. Of course, the higher the repetitions the longer the exercise period, which can adversely affect both patient and therapist. Another process is to shorten the time required to perform the repetitions. An example would be to perform 10RM in 6 sec as opposed to 10 sec, requiring more power (9, p. 200). Also, exercises may be performed more frequently when the loads are small. It has been shown that PREs, when properly performed, improve flexibility as well as strength.

Another modification of this type exercise is the DAPRE (daily adjustable progressive resistance exercise) technique (10, pp. 413–5). The idea behind this process is that one has a means to determine the optimal time to increase the resistance and the optimal amount of extra load to add. If one is able to apply the DAPRE technique successfully, one will probably shorten the period and improve the efficacy of rehabilitation. There are four sets of exercises performed in this procedure, for each muscle group. In the third set, the patient is instructed to perform as many reps as possible at the predetermined maximum load. We use the number of reps in the third set to adjust the load for the fourth set. Then, the maximal reps from the fourth set is similarly used to determine the next day's load. From five to seven reps is the median amount. If more reps are able to be performed, the load is proportionately too light, if the patient cannot perform that many, the load is proportionately too heavy. In the first two sets, form is emphasized, and the patient is taught to perform the exercise within 3 to 4 sec, pausing at each extreme of motion, so that positive and negative work is performed. The exercise is performed, set after set, on alternate sides, beginning with the injured side. Of course, the weight varies according to pertinent factors on each side. This technique can be modified for an isometric contraction, when the isotonic one would be contraindicated. The contraction is held for 6 sec, and there is a 4-sec rest between contractions. In the third and fourth sets, the reps continue until the limb cannot hold the weight for the full 6 sec.

Proprioceptive Neuromuscular Facilitation (PNF)

This theory was first developed by Dr. Hermann Kabat of the United States during 1946 to 1951. These exercises can be performed isometrically or isotonically and usually have elements of both in them. In fact, static and dynamic contractions are alternately involved. In addition, the three planes of motion may be employed at any time, as exercises include multiplanar actions. When muscles contract in proper sequence, any stressed muscle group will overcome its load with maximum efficiency (12, p. 107). There are three modes of this exercise, slow turning, slow turning—holding, and rhythmic stabilization. In the first mode, an isometric, static contraction of the antagonist is followed by an isotonic, dynamic contraction of the agonist. For example, to strengthen a weak hamstring, we first isometrically contract the quadriceps, then isotonically contract the hamstrings. In the second mode, an isotonic, dynamic contraction of both the antagonist and the agonist precedes an isometric, static contraction of both muscles. In the last mode, an isometric, static contraction of the antagonist is followed by an isometric, static contraction of the agonist, which can be increased to a co-contraction, that is, multiple contraction of the antagonist. This is, as yet, an incomplete theory and its implementation is as individual and different as the therapists who apply it.

If one observes any movement in slow motion, linear or simple planar motion is rarely seen. Most activities require motions that spiral, twist, and bounce along with the simple translation or rotation that apparently takes place. If one considers the origin, insertion, and action of most muscles one can see the anatomical correlates to these functions. When PNF is performed, the spatial configuration is made nearly to approximate the activity for which the training is taking place. When done properly, this type of exercise is also excellent for skill training and coordination, as well as increased flexibility, because PNF works into the formation of engrams. Secondly, the stimulation of correct proprioceptive pathways helps the nervous system itself, by promoting neuromuscular reactions. It is obvious how important the law of reciprocal innervation is in these exercises. This type of exercise is also useful in correcting the chronic effects of the recurrent microtraumata of everyday life or the minitraumata of athletic competition. These complex motions utilize stronger muscles in order to stimulate and strengthen weaker ones (12, p. 115). Sometimes, as in bowling or carpentry, the activity is sufficiently one-sided that the exercise must be so also.

In all of this one must balance the relatively mobile PNF with other exercises aimed at strength building. A muscle in the pattern made too thick (or strong) may inhibit or exaggerate some of the motion. If, for instance, a tennis player injures his arm while serving, the triceps is a very important part of this motion. An overdeveloped triceps makes the motion incoordinate and an overdeveloped biceps (its antagonist) makes the motion more difficult. When using PNF for endurance training, many repetitions and low resistance are required; for strength training few repetitions and a high resistance are necessary (12, p. 121). Needless to say, injuries limit complex motions and, therefore, limit these exercises. However, it is still important to use the appropriate resistance, within the allowable range of motion. When an injury exists, it may be necessary to use only static exercises until healing permits dynamic motions. Patient positioning is also critical; one must be careful to fix and free up the appropriate areas so that the complex motion can take place in a precise manner. PNF can be used preventively as well as therapeutically. Under certain circumstances, one may wish to apply some form of concomitant physical therapy.

Relaxation

Relaxation has been discussed previously, mostly in connection with other types of exercise. One can discuss relaxation as a general condition or with respect to a specific part of the body. Such general techniques as progressive relaxation training, autogenic training, and biofeedback are beyond the scope of this text but are important parts of a rehabilitation program. They will be dealt with only in the section on respiratory exercises. Local relaxation procedures are similar to the above, but smaller in scope. Additionally, such modalities as massage and traction can be employed to produce a measure of relaxation. These exercises are prescribed for patients who exhibit persistent muscle guarding and hypertonic states. Relaxation is also critical for those whose energy level is so low that fatigue sets in relatively rapidly. Relaxation can help the patient recuperate more quickly, and can even reduce the response of the tonic neck reflexes. Anxiety produces a state of tension that increases central nervous system activity and the activity of many other systems (4, p. 424). This is directly reflected in the body's tension level, both generally and specifically. There is no limit to the frequency and duration of relaxation programs.

Skill

Skill exercises are those that train someone for specific activities, over and above the general need for coordination. They include the special activities that lead to increased preparation and performance by athletes and musicians. Some question the efficacy of traditional calisthenics in preparation for sporting event (12, p. 302). To some extent, we would have to be included in that group. Instead, more specific warm-ups and exercises are being used before such events. There is a principle which we will mention here but which has applicability in most of our exercises. This is known as the SAID principle, an acronym standing for "specific adaptations to imposed demands." To selectively improve strength in a single muscle or a specific set of muscles, one must contract it specifically against an imposed load. One must carefully identify each specific attribute and its components in order to train by this principle. While training for running through long-distance methods improves endurance, it also helps to train one for a marathon, for example.

Specific PREs or weight training will strengthen muscles rehabilitatively and will also prepare someone to perform those tasks skillfully. Skill training, like coordination training, involves the formation of engrams as gradually more complex maneuvers are executed and perfected by the patient. Of course, in order to perform tasks skillfully, one needs to acquire sufficient strength, coordination, and endurance.

Stretching

Not all flexibility exercises are stretching ones, but all stretching exercises are used to improve mobility. Stretching pertains to a conscious, controlled effort to elongate the elastic elements in the periarticular soft tissue structures. A minimum test of flexibility, suggested by Anderson, is fingers touching toes while the person is seated on the floor with the legs outstretched and the knees extended (15, p. 4). He also suggests sitting on the floor with the legs spread and touching one's forehead to the top of the fists, which are on the floor. Using these attitudes as guideposts, one can measure the patient's status and progress. Once again, relaxation is a definite prerequisite to effective stretching, showing the interrelationship between exercise forms.

Figure 4.8 shows the length relationships as one stretches a muscle further and further. In the early phase of the stretch, one only moves to position B for 20 to 30 sec, where there is minimal reflex counterac-

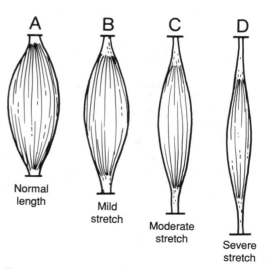

Figure 4.8 Relationship between amount of stretch and training benefit.

DYNAMICS OF CLINICAL REHABILITATIVE EXERCISE

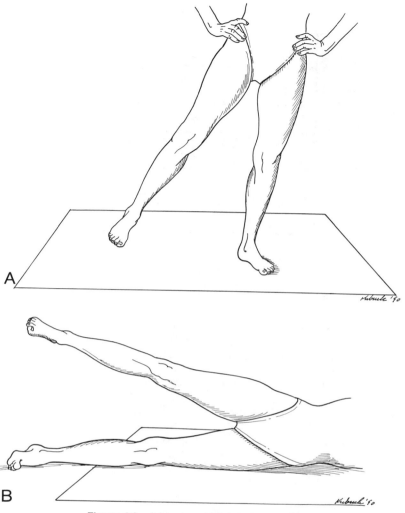

Figure 4.9 Adductor stretch in two positions.

tion to the stretch (15, p. 14). As one is ready, one proceeds to stretch further to position C, the developmental part of the stretch, for at least 30 sec more. In this phase, one should not actually feel pain, but will receive the maximum training benefit. It one moves into position D, the third phase stretch, one is likely to feel pain, and the training effect may be negative. There is obviously some subjectivity on the therapist's part, based upon experience, and some on the patient's part, based upon interpretation of pain. As useful training takes place, position C naturally lengthens; even position A may lengthen if there was initially some abnormal shortening (i.e., contracture) in that muscle.

There are some simple rules to follow in pursuing this type of training. One wants to evoke the feeling of stretching, but not the feeling of pain. Allow for individual differences in ranges of motion, and do not bounce to attempt to increase motion. There is a significant difference between stretching a muscle without regard to gravity and stretching while in the gravity field. In the former, one's position is such that the force of gravity does not influence the stretch in either way. In the latter, one is working against gravity, and thus must apply more force to stretch the subsequently loaded muscle. This is the difference between a hamstring or adductor stretch (Fig. 4.9) performed when one is

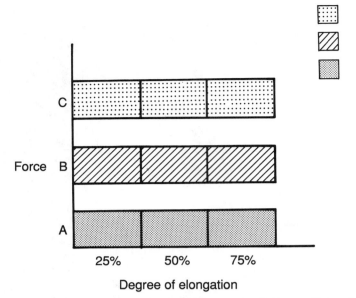

Figure 4.10 Progression of stretch routine. **A.** Done without gravity. **B.** Done with gravity. **C.** Done with light weight.

lying supine versus one performed in the standing position. The incumbent weight bearing of the latter position places a much greater stress upon the injured area. It should only be done after a certain amount of healing (to be determined by the therapist and patient) has already taken place. Whether one moves slowly, but repeatedly, through the motion or whether one fixes in one position of elongation is another variable to consider. Obviously, the greater the injury, the less motion is desirable. In fact, the amount of elongation is limited by the degree of injury. When the injury has healed to a greater degree, light weight may be used to assist in the stretching. Figure 4.10 demonstrates how one might progress through the stretching activities. When one

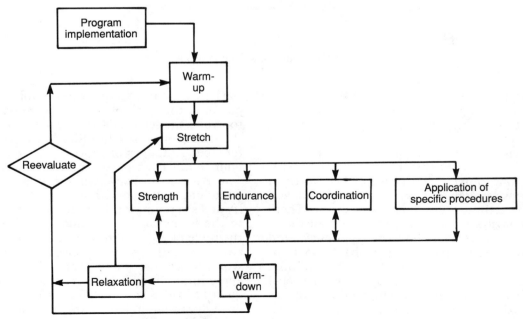

Figure 4.11 Flow Chart Model For Exercise Routines.

DYNAMICS OF CLINICAL REHABILITATIVE EXERCISE

can accomplish situation A at a minimum 75% proficiency, one proceeds to situation B, and so forth for situation C. It may take 2 weeks or more between changes, before one is safely capable of handling the higher level of force of the new stretch level. After healing this process may be applied in the course of a single session, with only minutes between the steps. Even an uninjured person will find a bilateral discrepancy in the feeling and/or results experienced. In order to heal properly, one should aim for as symmetrical a result as possible. Without symmetry of motion, all other exercises will be adversely affected.

As in all exercises, form is paramount. If the exercise is not performed correctly, either the wrong elements will be stretched or the correct ones will not be stretched. Concentration is important for all exercises. Learn to focus on technique, including time factors, can aid relaxation as well. Proper positioning is integral to good form. Just as proper stretching helps to warm up the areas involved, it would help the stretching if one warmed up first. Sometimes the application of some form of exogenous heat is sufficient, since stretching exercises are meant to be nontraumatic.

One needs to have patience in a rehabilitative program. One can do all that one can do, and no more. However, to do less is a disservice. Exercises must proceed in a logical and safe pattern to be effective. Figure 4.11 suggests a model for determining when certain phases are to be employed. Aquatic exercises were mentioned as an alternative, and they are discussed in Chapter 12.

References

1. McArdle ND, Katch FI, Katch VL: Exercise Physiology. 2nd ed. Philadelphia:Lea & Febiger, 1986.
2. Holvey DN: The Merck Manual. 12th ed. Rahway, New Jersey:Merck, 1972.
3. Pollock ML, Wilmore JH, Fox SM III: Exercise in Health and Disease. Philadelphia:WB Saunders, 1984.
4. Kottke FJ, Stillwell KG, Lehman JF: Krusen's Handbook of Physical Medicine and Rehabilitation. 3rd ed. Philadelphia:WB Saunders, 1982.
5. Christensen, KD: Clinical Chiropractic Biomechanics. 2nd. ed. Foot Levelers, Dubuke, IA, 1984.
6. O'Donoghue DH: Treatment of Injuries to Athletes. 3rd ed. Philadelphia:WB Saunders, 1976.
7. Kisner C, Colby LA: Therapeutic Exercise. Philadelphia:FA Davis, 1985.
8. Delisa JA: Rehabilitation Medicine. Philadelphia: JB Lippincott, 1988.
9. Basmajian JV, Wolf SL: Therapeutic Exercise. 5th ed. Baltimore:Williams & Wilkins, 1990.
10. Harvey JS: Clinics in Sports Medicine. Rehabilitation of the Injured Athlete. Philadelphia:WB Saunders, 1985, vol 4, no 3.
11. Micheli LJ: Clinics in Sports Medicine. Injuries in the Young Athlete. WB Saunders, 1988, vol 7, no 3.
12. Kuprian W, ed: Physical Therapy for Sports. Philadelphia:WB Saunders, 1982.
13. White AA, Panjabi MM: Clinical Biomechanics of the Spine. Philadelphia:JB Lippincott, 1978.
14. Cyriax J: Orthopaedic Medicine. 8th ed. London: Bailliere Tindell, 1982.
15. Anderson B. Stretching. Palmer Lake, CO, Stretching, Inc., 1978.

5

Program Design and Implementation

Readers are encouraged to design their own models based upon the data and principles provided here (including the information in Figs. 4.11 and 5.1). The exercise approach changes from the acute (inflammatory) to the subacute (healing) and the chronic (maturation and remodeling) stages. In this chapter, we will begin to explore some of the general and specific body conditions for which the exercises are intended. Throughout this discussion it should be understood that muscles move bones, nerves innervate muscles, and most of the soft tissue structures cross the joint lines described. Therefore, chronic disarticulation and chronic joint instability are considered as neuromuscular problems.

Laws of Muscle Action

As discussed in earlier chapters, there are two laws that define the operation of muscles. The law of approximation states that when a muscle contracts, it allows the origin and insertion of the muscle to come together. This is partially explained by the physiology of muscle spindles and Golgi tendon organs, and is the basis of the origin and insertion technique described elsewhere (1, pp. 20–1, 23). The law of detorsion states that during muscle contraction the origin and insertion of a muscle come together on the same plane, decreasing any spiraling of the muscle fibers. The laws of approximation and detorsion are seen in the

sternocleidomastoid muscle (2, p. 50). It also appears that during muscle contraction, if the synergistic muscle is not functioning properly, the amount of spiraling of the muscle fibers will be affected. Wolff's law of bone repair, which states that extra bone is deposited during the remodeling of bone at the stress sites and removed in areas where stress is not applied, may also apply to the failure of synergistic functioning of muscles. These principles, and the ones below, should be kept in mind when applying the exercises to patients.

Muscles never work independently, but rather in a group. This action is termed the mass action of muscles (2, p. 50). Mass action is best realized in postural mechanics, where if one muscle group acts independently of another group, proper posture is not possible. When establishing a program of rehabilitation, much more than the injured muscle must be taken into consideration. It is not uncommon to exercise every muscle group dependent upon, or precipitant into, the action of the injured muscle(s). This is why one refers to the open or closed kinetic chain of muscle reaction in, for instance, normal gait mechanics.

Muscle Fiber Types

As discussed in Chapter 2, muscle fibers are classified into three basic fiber groups, through muscle biopsy studies: (a) type 1, slow twitch fibers; (b) type 2A, fast oxida-

$$|\,\overline{\underset{\text{4–6 days}}{A}}\,| - |\,\overline{\underset{\text{10–17 days}}{S}}\,| - |\,\overline{\underset{\text{until full healing}}{C}}\,| \longrightarrow \text{time}$$

A = Acute stage: Possibly immobilize, with minimal rehabilitation. Use gentle motions only. Joint effusions and edema may minimize motion. Use active motions mainly. Do not force passive motion. There may be significant muscle guarding. Active motion is contraindicated at the site of active pathology. Pain occurs before tissue resistance.

S = Subacute stage: Increase mobilization. Exercise gently at first then slowly increase intensity. Tissue is still fragile. Pain is concomitant with tissue resistance.

C = Chronic stage: More vigorous motions may be used. Lengthen and strengthen as much as possible. Force passive motions to break adhesions. Pain is subsequent to tissue resistance.

Figure 5.1 Exercise time format.

tive-glycolytic fibers; and (c) type 2B, fast glycolytic fibers (3, p. 135). It is important to be aware of the various muscle fiber groups, to design exercises that will be effective. Studies have shown that type 2 muscle fibers decrease in area with aging. Therefore, strength exercises will be of little value, and any change in muscle strength is likely to be the result of neural impulse (3, p. 137). This again emphasizes that constant, repetitive activities, at lower force levels, will help to reinforce engrams.

Muscle Spasm

Muscle spasm may be the result of many common types of injuries. It may be the result of overstretching, direct or indirect trauma, increased contraction of muscle against a resistance, or the reaction of a muscular group to overcome another pathological process, such as discogenic disease. Muscle spasm and/or cramping may result from pathophysiology in the antagonist muscle. If a primary muscle becomes weak, reactionary spasm may result in the corresponding antagonistic muscle. It is necessary to examine and evaluate the spastic area with an orthopedic and neurological examination to define the exact nature and etiology of the muscle spasm. In instances of nutritional or metabolic etiologies, the history and laboratory testing are more definitive procedures. In any case, the muscle spasm is only a symptom. However, if it becomes chronic, it can become a second level primary disorder. Once the cause is known, the first rehabilitation exercises are aimed at relaxing the muscle spasm and possibly strengthening the antagonist musculature.

There are a number of situations in which we have found it extremely useful to utilize the Golgi tendon organ and spindle cell stimulation techniques (refer to Fig. 4.5) as described by Goodheart and others (1, pp. 20–1, 23). If a muscle spasm is unremitting and the muscle cannot be exercised sufficiently to accrue any benefit, these procedures may provide a partial and temporary neurological respite. Also, if it is very difficult to move into active or even assistive modes of exercise, one can usually produce a temporary boost in the muscle reactivity, so additional strengthening can occur. These techniques are not universal cures but they can help to break a positive feedback loop, thereby shortening rehabilitation time.

If myospasm limits motion and interferes with exercising, one may employ techniques of reciprocal inhibition and contract-relax inhibition to promote the motion (4, p. 271). Using proprioceptive neuromuscular facilitation to tolerance is a good procedure in most situations. If myospasm is a reflex response, a muscle guarding, rather than a protection of a damaged motor unit, for instance, one can force the action further by such methods. If the spasm is protecting injured tissues, this procedure may be contraindicated.

Stabilizing Areas

When joint instability is a key factor, it is necessary to strengthen the stabilizing elements before working on the injured areas. For example, when exercising the knee in a weight bearing fashion, one cannot afford to have weak ankles beneath the knee joints. The same is true for the joints contralateral to the injured joints. If one is fixating a shoulder to stabilize rehabilitating elbow motions, the shoulder needs to be strong enough to support whatever stress is applied to it from the distal activity. Therefore, when exercises are prescribed for the injured elbow, a weakened shoulder must also be exercised. If the stabilizing elements or joints are already at +5 (i.e., full strength), these exercises are not necessary. Stabilizing areas do not need to be exercised as part of a functional chain, even though they may be normal when tested independently. Sometimes it is necessary to stabilize joints with some sort of support, in order to prevent further injury. When exercising fingers distal to a casted wrist, removing the support would lessen the effect of the finger exercises and endanger the healing of the wrist. In this case, contralateral exercises, mild electromagnetic stimulation homolaterally, and mental stimulation of the involved area are recommended. Mental stimulation implies visualization of the involved areas and the intended actions.

Clothing

Specialized clothing, such as swimsuits, athletic supporters, and sports bras, may be needed. When exercising between 60 and 80°F., clothing should be loose fitting and light. Between 40 and 60°F. include a sweatshirt, and include sweatpants and/or thermal underwear when the temperature is below 40°F (3, p. 375). Shoes and socks should fit properly and provide enough support for the activities undertaken. Special shoes are necessary for jogging and running because of the excess stresses upon the pedal biomechanics. Wool and cotton socks are preferred because they "breathe" and are usually hypoallergenic. Some of the newer elastic materials may be preferable for patients with certain circulatory conditions.

Terminating Exercises

During the rehabilitation program, be careful to avoid further injury to the patient. Exercising should be stopped if the patient develops arrhythmias, palpitations, irregular heart rates, pain or pressure in the epicardium or arm or throat, vertigo or syncope, sudden incoordination, confusion or disorientation, cold sweats, pallor, cyanosis, or extreme rubor (3, p. 379). Those symptoms may indicate a precipitant cardiovascular incident.

Exercise Form

It is very important that the patient perform each exercise exactly as intended, that is, that the form be correct. Form is taught by careful explanation, demonstration, and pictures. Then, the therapist takes the patient slowly through each procedure, explaining exactly how and how often each motion is to be performed. When an exercise cannot be performed exactly as directed, the therapist modifies it in order to maintain the intent without causing further injury or pain. As the patient becomes more adept and heals more completely, the therapist remodifies the exercise so as to approach the ideal form. The positions of stabilization provided by the patient or therapist are just as important as the form of the exercise. If the correct areas are not isolated, the exercise will be ineffective or incorrect.

Patient Positioning

There are several conventional positions for starting exercises. Some exercises are better begun from variants of these positions; most can begin in one of these manners.

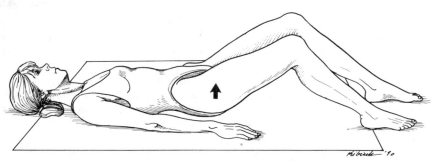

Figure 5.2 Supine standard position.

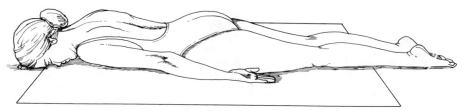

Figure 5.3 Prone standard position.

The supine standard position is shown in Figure 5.2. While lying supine the knees are flexed approximately 45°, the feet are flat on the ground, and the palms are down. This position removes a degree of stress from the hamstrings, low back, and shoulder areas.

The prone standard position is shown in Figure 5.3. Whenever possible it should be performed with the face directly down to relax the neck and shoulders and with the anterior legs resting on a pillow to relax the hamstrings.

The upright standard position is shown in Figure 5.4. It differs from anatomical position in the position of the hands, which are approximately how they naturally fall to the sides.

The sitting standard position is shown in Figure 5.5. Once again, the shoulders are relaxed by the arms falling directly to the sides and the feet are squarely placed upon the floor such that the knees are about at the height of the hips.

The side-lying standard position is shown in Figure 5.6. It is made easier by providing a pillow for the head. It can be done either with the bottom leg bent or straight, whichever is more suitable.

Conditioning versus Rehabilitative Exercises

Exercises are classified as conditioning or rehabilitative. The major difference be-

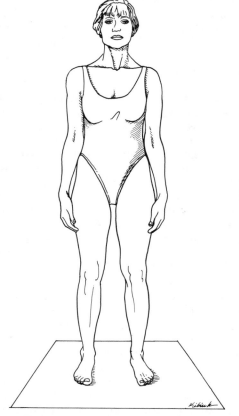

Figure 5.4 Upright standard position.

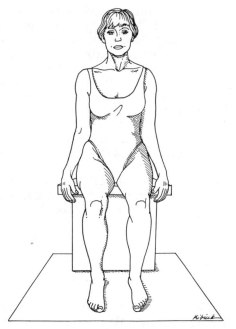

Figure 5.5 Sitting standard position.

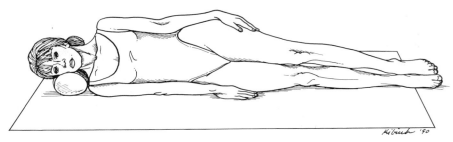

Figure 5.6 Side-lying standard position.

tween them is in their intensity. Conditioning exercises usually require a much greater intensity, especially in the early stages (2, p. 451). Additionally, in rehabilitative exercises, one must consider the patient's status and the kinetic hazards imposed by the exercises. Conditioning is primarily involved in producing the superior state of optimum fitness that is required for athletic activities. The essential intersection between these types of exercise is the category of skill exercises. Again, the difference is mainly reflected in the parameter of intensity.

Spinal Misalignment

The relationship between spinal misalignment and muscle imbalances is well established (5, p. 104–6). Whether the muscle imbalance precedes the spinal misalignment or the reverse is true, the end result is the same. It is clear that interrupting this positive feedback cycle at either end will favorably affect the patient. The approach, in this text, is to attempt directly to produce normal, balanced muscle actions. However, a misaligned spine will sometimes simply reinstate the imbalance. Therefore, spinal correction through manipulation or adjustment is likely to be needed as well. In no way do we denigrate the importance of either approach. The intent is to produce a beneficial therapeutic response in the patient by utilizing a series of exercises in a very specific manner. Although adjustments, physical therapy, injections, medications, or surgery may also be needed, they are not usually discussed. Conditions where surgical intervention is likely are excluded. We are more concerned with adding therapeutic exercises to the ar-

mamentarium of those who already utilize one or more of these other treatment modalities.

A 1983 national Gallup poll, conducted on behalf of Scholl, Inc., and the American Podiatry Association, uncovered a number of interesting facts (6). The most frequent sports-related injuries were of the knee (24%), followed by the foot (18%) and the low back (13%). Sixty-two per cent of those polled considered it normal for their feet to hurt. Furthermore, 75% of those surveyed admitted to being on their feet more than 4 hr/day. This is significant for those rehabilitating injuries of the spine and pelvis. Any time such rehabilitation is taking place it is vital that the lower extremities be fully evaluated for weakness, biomechanical faults, and stresses that would be transmitted upward. If they are not properly addressed during such a program, the spinal injuries will probably fail to respond or be reactivated shortly after treatment concludes. Those involved in regular running are particularly susceptible to such lower extremity difficulties. According to Bates et al., the most common problems of running athletes (in decreasing order) are knee pain (including chondromalacia patellae), posterior tibial syndrome (shin splints), achilles tendinitis, plantar fasciitis, stress fractures, and iliotibial band tract tendinitis (7). When these conditions occur, the resultant altered biomechanics eventually are reflected in aberrant spinal pathophysiology. Conversely, those who have spinal difficulties, ranging from vertebral subluxation complexes through compression fractures, exhibit altered gait patterns that will eventuate in one or more of the conditions listed. Only rest and immobilization will prevent such consequences, but immobilization produces its own sequelae. Rehabilitative exercises may well be better performed after the patient has been fitted and is wearing pedal orthotic devices.

Posture and Gait

Because posture is such an unconscious attitude of the body, one of the techniques for improving it is to make it a conscious process. In most of the exercises, the authors have endeavored to place all parts of the patient's body in space. Then each part is specifically moved, which is a good part of the reason for the precise mathematical definitions of space and motion that were employed. This raises the patient's consciousness of his own body, kinesthetically. Goodheart points out the highly pivotal role the upper cervical posterior musculature plays in the regulation of all muscular activities (8). He discussed the pioneering work of Alexander and Feldenkrais and how both inhibition and excitation of specific areas can be consciously controlled. We translate this into selective relaxation and strengthening, respectively, of those areas. This also suggests that cervical exercises may be beneficial for a large number of conditions, even those that seem unrelated to the cervical area.

When a person is reasonably flexible, one should emphasize good habits of alignment and development of proper kinesthetic sense to maintain position (9). Without such flexibility, it may not be possible to achieve a reasonably normal posture for a protracted period of time.

Posture may be defined as a biomechanical state of the body or as a functional relationship in which the body is supported, for example, static versus kinetic variations. In the latter case, what we are really dealing with is a series of chronologically ordered postures, much like the frames on a reel of film. In that case, we are more concerned with the relationship of the parts than the form of the whole. Any posture that is not determined solely by the gravity field is called an active state, since neuromuscular activity and precise control are required in order to produce and maintain it. The instantaneous postural state is a function (actually a vector sum) of all the forces acting upon the body and all the reactions of the body, both voluntary and involuntary, to those forces (10). When one considers the dimension of time, the analysis of this behavior actually requires differential and integral calculus. The vast majority of postural mechanisms and adjustments are performed either unconsciously or automatically. It is only in disorders of such mechanisms, such as Parkinsonism or drug-induced ataxias, that one becomes aware of those mechanisms at work. However, one must not label voluntary movement as simply a series of postures, since there are times when such movement can take place in the absence of true static postural support for the related body part. Other movements, such as emotional movements, movements of expression, and reflex movements (other than postural), may have no postural significance (10). Furthermore, some lesions of the basal ganglia will abolish many postural mechanisms, leaving voluntary movements intact (10). From an exercise standpoint, the performance of voluntary motions may not necessarily retrain or reactivate the normal postural mechanisms. Even strengthening the muscles needed by these mechanisms does not guarantee their service. One needs to establish the pathways for the mechanisms, recreate the engrams (exactly), and focus on the neuronal mechanisms while performing the exercise. This means performing exercises decomposed into their primary components, in an extremely deliberate manner, with attention to connecting sensory and motor constituents of the program. The usage of video equipment and mirrors, followed by visualization techniques, will help the patient learn to make unconscious processes conscious.

Several important large muscles engaged during the act of walking must be considered when rehabilitating disorders of the gait mechanism (11). The biceps femoris brings the body forward over the knee, the gluteus maximus completes extension of the hip, and the gastrocnemius gives a final lift by raising the foot lever on the distal end of the metatarsals. The rectus femoris and psoas major are lifting the other leg concurrently. Therefore, if a goal of the exercising is to improve posture, from a gravitational dynamic standpoint, improving the tone, strength and endurance of the above mentioned musculature is an imperative.

Warm-up and Warm-down

Pre- and post-exercise activity is as important as the actual exercise prescription and performance. During the warm-up phase, it is necessary to increase body temperature and circulation by initiating exercises of low resistance and velocity (12, p. 357). This prevents further damage to local tissue and produces a gradual increase in cardiovascular stress. During the cool-down phase it is necessary gradually to reduce the intensity and velocity of muscular activity, to lower the incidence of post-exercise syncope.

As in all exercises, form is paramount. If the exercise is performed incorrectly, either the wrong elements are stretched or the correct ones are not stretched. Concentration is important for all exercises, and should be stressed. Learning to focus on technique, including time factors, can help one to relax, as well. Proper positioning of the body parts is also integral to good form. Just as proper stretching helps to warm up the areas involved, it would help the stretching if one warmed up first. Sometimes the application of exogenous heat is sufficient, since stretching exercises are meant to be nontraumatic. Although various counterirritant type lotions and creams have been touted as being useful in this regard, their effect is superficial and relatively short-lived. They do not substitute adequately for warm-up procedures, particularly in an injured person, but they can be helpful.

There are exercises which might be called relaxed movement, which differ from loosening type exercises by virtue of their low level intensity and reliance upon the force of gravity for their main impetus. They are not usually performed passively, and they have essentially the same aims as loosening type exercises do. Their aims are as follows: (a) to prevent muscle shortening, that is, to counteract tendencies to develop contractures and adhesions; (b) to maintain suppleness of tissues; (c) to maintain freedom of movement of joints; (d) to hasten repair of injured structures; (e) to improve circulation; and (f) to maintain or improve proprioceptive sensations and reflex reactions.

Relaxed movements are always within the pain-free arc of motion and are performed in a pendulum-like manner. Figure 5.7 shows this type motion for the left shoulder. Relaxed movements can be performed passively, with a therapist's assistance, if the patient is unable to perform them actively. They are most useful for the early care of acute injuries, for postoperative patients, and for rehabilitation of neurological or cardiovascular disorders or incidents.

The warm-up should be performed slowly, gradually increasing the intensity so as to increase circulation and body temperature. The warm-down should be just as slow to prevent post exercise syncope due to blood pooling in the exercised extremity (12, p. 58). As this occurs, serum catecholamine content increases, which could lead to cardiac ischemia and dysrhythmias. This is of greater import to patients with cardiovascular derangements than to those without. But, if the patient has been in poor or fair condition for some time, syncope or vertigo would not be a totally unexpected reaction. Therefore, the more vigorous the exercise, the longer the warm-up and warm-down that are necessary. Be careful to allow sufficient warm-up without risking fatigue, which could be injurious. Figure 5.8 describes this relationship graphically. Perry recommends using 20 to 30%

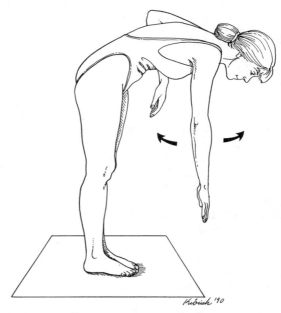

Figure 5.7 Example of a "relaxed movement" procedure.

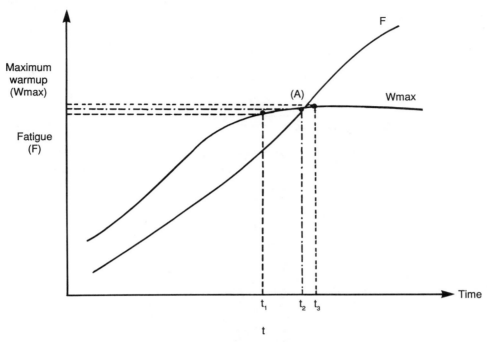

Figure 5.8 Relationship between warm-up times and incipient fatigue factors.

of the exercise time warming up and 10 to 20% of the time warming down (13). Warm-up exercises should involve antagonistic muscle groups (such as flexors and extensors, medial and lateral rotators, adductors and abductors, etc.) (14). This will help to prevent unexpected reactions when either is being exercised afterward.

Flexibility/Mobility

Mobility is the ability of articular structures to move with respect to each other. The greater the mobility, the more the joint approaches normal motion. If the joint's motion is excessive, the joint is hypermobile; if motion is limited, the joint is hypomobile. Flexibility is the ability of the soft tissues to move through their normal length, from shortest to longest positions. Hypoflexibility and hyperflexibility indicate limited and excessive flexibility, respectively.

Flexibility is most easily determined by a simple measurement of the range of motion of the involved joint and muscles.

The intensity and rapidity of a stretch determine the magnitude of the subsequent contraction. Thus, a brisk stretch, or even a

tap upon the tendon, will produce a greater facilitatory effect. On the other hand, a slow stretch is best for relaxing a given muscle (2, pp. 104–5). Therefore, the velocity of the stretch should be determined by the desired output of the muscle. This is part of the thoughtful design in which the doctor and therapist must engage the patient during each session.

There are some simple rules to follow in pursuing flexibility training. One wants to evoke the feeling of stretching but not the feeling of pain. Allow for individual differences in ranges of motion and do not bounce to attempt to increase motion. There is a significant difference between stretching a muscle without regard to gravity and stretching while in the gravity field. In the former, one's position is such that the force of gravity does not influence the stretch. In the latter, one is working against gravity, and thus must apply more force to stretch the subsequently loaded muscle. This is the difference between a hamstring stretch performed when one is lying supine versus one performed in the standing position (Figure 5.9). The incumbent weight bearing of the latter position places a much greater stress upon the injured area. It should only be done after a certain (to be

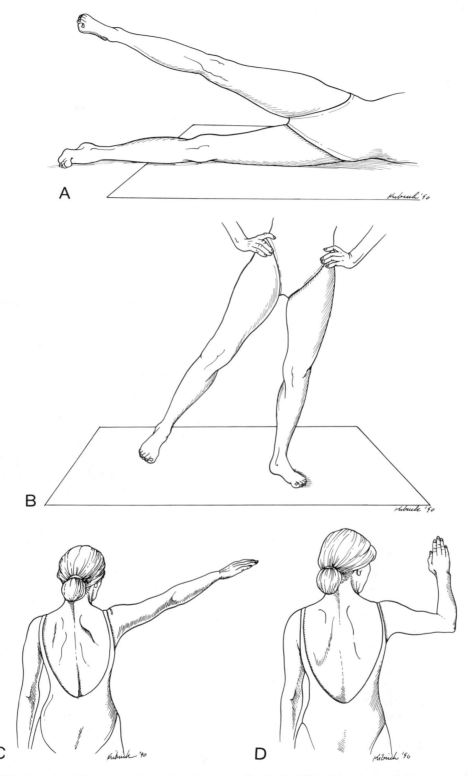

Figure 5.9 Example of how spatial configuration can affect both difficulty and potential benefit of exercise.

determined by the therapist and patient) amount of healing has already taken place.

Whether one moves slowly and repeatedly through the motion or fixes in one position of elongation is another variable to consider. Obviously, the greater the injury, the less motion is desirable. In fact, the amount of elongation is limited by the degree of injury. When more healing has occurred, some light weight may be used to assist in the stretching. Figure 5.11 demonstrates how one might progress through the stretching activities. Referring to the figure, when the first position can be accomplished at a minimum 75% proficiency, one proceeds to the second position, etc. It may take 2 weeks, or more, between changes, before one is safely capable of handling the higher level of force of the new stretch level. This process may also be applied, after healing, in the course of a single session, with just minutes between the steps. Even an uninjured person will find a bilateral discrepancy in the feeling and/or results one experiences. If one is to heal properly, one should aim for as symmetrical a result as possible. Without symmetry of motion, all other exercises are adversely affected.

Generally speaking, a tight joint should be less vigorously stretched than a tight muscle. Inflamed joints are more susceptible to injury than other tissues being treated in the area (15, p. 399).

A moderate prolonged stretch is more likely to cause a mild plastic change in the involved connective tissues. A short-term vigorous stretch is proportionately resisted and usually results only in elastic changes (15, p. 399). Elastic changes are reversible, whereas plastic changes indicate that a permanent deformation in the physical structure has occurred. Therefore, a vigorous, short-term stretch is really only useful to preload a muscle for a maximal contraction. This concept has more bearing upon strength training.

In early stages, and especially when moderate to severe muscle spasm is present, the cryostretch (or spray-and-stretch) technique might be reasonably applied prior to other exercises (16, p. 409). This involves the preliminary spraying of an aerosol substance, such as ethyl chloride or fluoromethane over the intended muscle area(s) just prior to stretching them.

When the parallel elastic component is injured, the active exercise mode is more important; however, series elastic components can be equally affected by passive exercise modes. This is another example of why it is important to differentiate the actual tissue site(s) of injury, not just the type of injury.

When poor posture is the cause of decreased flexibility, one should typically stretch the tight muscles of the hip flexors, the trunk flexors, the shoulder flexors, and the scapular protractors (4, p. 621).

When an agonist muscle is stretched, it is often helpful to strengthen its antagonist in order to maintain the longer position afterward (17, p. 40). For example, if an exercise is used to stretch the hamstring group, it would be wise to strengthen the quadriceps or psoas muscles, depending upon the specific function demanded of the hamstrings (refer to a table of agonists and antagonists).

Use extra caution when applying stretching, manipulation, or range of motion exercises to the fingers. If an extrinsic joint limits the motion locally, lengthen it over one joint only, while stabilizing the other joints (4, p. 134). Stretching a tendon across two joints could produce hypermobility in one of them. For example, when attempting to increase metacarpal motion, try to use the metacarpals, rather than the phalanges, as lever arms.

When stretching the hip into abduction, one is advised not to place the therapist's hand on the medial malleolar area unless there is considerable medial knee stability. This principle should generally be followed in all extremities, whether testing the muscle for strength or the joint for integrity, or exercising both in rehabilitation. Always be aware of the integrity of all intervening joints.

Within almost all of the exercises, there is an ability to utilize joint play somewhere within the range of motion in performing graded oscillation techniques (4, p. 159). Grade I uses small rhythmic oscillations at the beginning of the range. Grade II uses large-amplitude rhythmic oscillations within the range, but not at the extreme of motion. Grade III uses large rhythmic oscillations up to the limit of the available motion. Grade IV uses small-amplitude rhythmic oscillations at the limit of the available motion. When pain is the limiting factor, one usually uses grades I and II techniques. When stretching is the desired outcome, grades III and IV are utilized. This means that, when we stretch a hamstring or attempt to work a shoulder past a painful arc, any of these four approaches can be used, depending upon the attending circumstances. Such joint play techniques can also be used to help mobilize fixated spinal segments. It is recommended that treatments be initiated in the resting position for that joint, because this promotes maximum laxity of the capsule (4, p. 161).

Instruct the patient and incorporate into the program the important notion that joints distal to the injury must be actively mobilized, to the extent that they can be (4, p. 254). This is vital when a neurological insult is part of the clinical pathophysiology.

Lower loads, slower velocity, and longer duration produce longer lasting stretch effects, also assisting in endurance.

Isometric, Isotonic, and Isokinetic Training

In 1968, Perrine introduced isokinetic concepts. Isokinetic training allows maximum force production throughout the full range of motion, if the patient is sufficiently motivated (18). Another reason to utilize isokinetic training techniques is the ability to have variable speed rates over the motion ranges. The same procedures are used as for isotonic training, although one may mix fast- and slow-speed training, depending upon the nature of the injured tissues and the desired results.

Lower speeds of contraction produce greater torque, especially in slow-twitch fibers. As the load increases, the angular velocity decreases. Therefore, we recommend using isokinetic techniques at the lower end of the torque-velocity curve in order to increase strength. Strength is differentiated from power, which is a function of time and which requires incorporation of higher velocity techniques. For a frame of reference, 300°/sec is rapid, and 60°/sec is slow (3, p. 147).

Peak power is developed at about 50% of the maximum force (at the same velocity) (Fig. 5.10). This means that a middle velocity and force is a more useful overall (general) parameter and should probably be a part of most programs.

If muscular activities irritate musculoskeletal structures in which inflammatory processes are occurring, forceful muscular contractions are inhibited. This may provide insufficient stimulus to provide for muscle strengthening (15 p. 623). Isometric contractions may be more effective in such cases, but remember that the increased strength is mostly produced only in those positions trained. However, this is better than nothing. As the inflammatory phase subsides, one can progress to isotonic or isokinetic modes of activity.

Trunk mobility is defined in terms of trunk angle (i.e., range of motion) and trunk velocity of motion. Of the two, the change in velocity is the more sensitive as a rating of impairment (19). This can be plotted, if one has a device capable of measuring the parameters of the dynamic motion. This is useful in monitoring the progress of the rehabilitation program. In training for improvement in this realm, isokinetic exercises are advised because they are most sensitive to velocity changes.

Speed training is best accomplished by frequent repetitions of functional activities at increasingly faster intervals (20). The authors favor isokinetic techniques for speed training.

Aerobic Exercise

When training or rehabilitating athletes, an aerobic section is always included in the program. In rehabilitating a person whose demands are less strenuous, endurance exercises are included, but only in sufficient quantity to reconstitute what is normal for that patient.

Even though heart rates may significantly increase during weight training, aerobic training is still minimal (3 to 5%), regardless of the strength increase that may occur (21). The oxygen consumption is not high enough, due to the intermittent nature of the activity, to increase aerobic fitness. Therefore, when endurance training is sought, the third program (SF3; see "Summary of Exercise Parameters" below) is more desirable (Table 5.1), because it allows increased parameters on all counts.

The following five criteria must be met to define aerobic exercising (22). (a) The legs

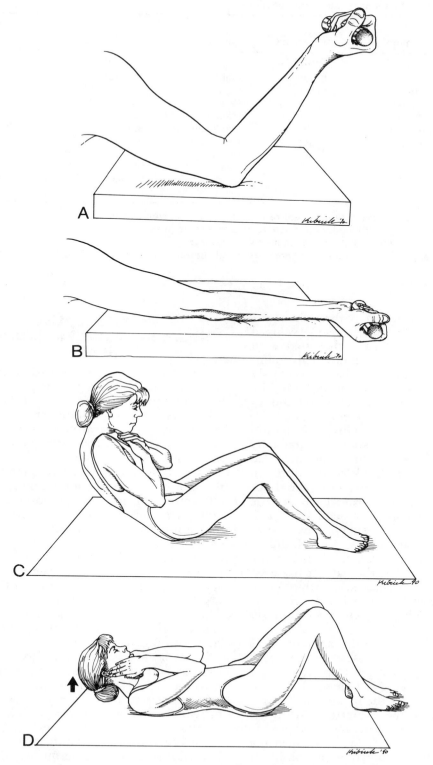

Figure 5.10 How spatial configuration alters the center of gravity and the length of the moment arm.

Table 5.1. Exercise Parameters: Standard Functions

Standard function	Frequency[a]	Duration[b]	Intensity[c]	Spatial Configuration	CE Ratio[d]
1	6–12/min	25–100 sec	Light	Full ROM[e]	1:1
2	½–1/sec	30 sec	Light	Full ROM	1:1
3	½–1/sec	30 sec	Light	Partial ROM	1:1
4	6–12/min	36–100 sec	Heavy	Full ROM	3:1
5	½–1/sec	20–40 sec	Medium	Full ROM	1:1
6	6–12/min	36–100 sec	Maximum	Static	3:1
7	½–1/sec	30 sec	Increment	Partial to full ROM	1:1
8	4/min	60 sec	Heavy	Static	3:1
9	6/min	40–80 sec	Heavy	Static	3:1
			Light	Partial	NA
10	10–15/min	40–80 sec	Light	Full ROM	NA

[a] Frequency refers to number of times exercise is performed in a given session.
[b] Duration refers to length of time for specific exercise in a given session.
[c] Intensity is characterized as light, medium, heavy, or maximal.
[d] CE ratio is the approximate proportion of time exercise is performed concentrically (C) and eccentrically (E), respectively.
[e] ROM = range of motion.

must be used continuously throughout the exercise period. The work load developed through the legs is greater than that with the arms and that level is more easily maintained. (b) The lungs must be continuously used, without straining or holding the breath. The goal of aerobic exercise is to saturate tissues with oxygen. (c) The exercises should be conducted for 15 to 20 minutes. (d) The pulse rate should be gradually increased to the submaximal rate intended and remain at that level for the duration of the exercise. (e) The exercises should be performed 3 to 5 days/week. There is little advantage to increasing frequency to 6 to 7 days/week (14). In fact, such increases may have detrimental effects. In helping to evaluate the safety of an aerobic program, one should note that the patient has a return to the resting heart rate within 6 min and a feeling of full recovery, without fatigue, within 1 hr after vigorous exercises (14).

In aerobic fitness training, a frequency of less than three exercise sessions per week will result in a loss of the adaptive changes that one had gained (22). One needs to exercise at 70 to 85% of the maximum attainable heart rate to be operating within the "target zone." Beginners are instructed to exercise at an intensity level that does not cause a shortness of breath which prohibits conversation (22) (refer also to "Cardiovascular Rehabilitation" below).

Proprioceptive Neuromuscular Facilitation (PNF)

A number of the exercises described in the following chapters lend themselves to being performed as PNFs. Format 9 (Table 5.1) is designed to accommodate such exercises. They are typically performed alternating an isometric contraction for 6 to 10 sec with a relatively small passive motion. This process is continued throughout the range of motion of the joint, and it is usually capable of improving motion immediately. To apply this type of exercise, the doctor must determine exactly which muscle must be contracted so that its antagonist can be stretched further. PNF may even be useful in the early treatment of highly spasmodic conditions, such as torticollis. PNF is not advisable if torn or severely damaged tissues are being stretched or contracted. An example of this process is shown in Figure 5.11.

It has been suggested that PNFs be utilized as part of the treatment regimen for myofascial pain syndrome (23). The authors believe it assists resolution of the condition in two distinct ways. It increases local circulation to increase waste removal, and it helps break positive pain feedback loops. PNF is useful for numerous conditions, usually only limited by the doctor/therapist's imagination.

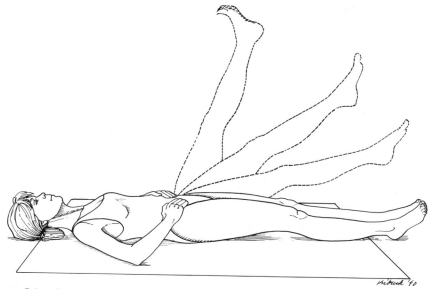

Figure 5.11 Example of proprioceptive neuromuscular facilitation for hamstring flexibility.

Eccentric versus Concentric Contractions

Part of the delay between the onset of neuroelectrical activity and recorded muscle tension may be the time required to stretch the series elastic component of the muscle. This delay is less during eccentric contraction than during concentric or isometric contractions (24). Of significance, partially contracted muscles can generate rapid forces more readily than relaxed or stretched muscles. This may explain, in part, the extra soreness and fatigue that accompany eccentric contractions, as opposed to other types.

The concept of concentric versus eccentric exercises was defined and explained in Chapter 3. The authors have taken a simple stand on how to apply them to an exercise program. The simplicity of it allows those who are relatively inexperienced in rehabilitative procedures to decide on their usage. Although eccentric exercises can maximize tension and force on a muscle (thereby, a joint), they also tend to produce undesirable delayed onset muscle soreness (DOMS). Therefore, virtually none of these exercises is designed exclusively as an eccentric exertion. However, as seen in the standard function chart (Table 5.1) there is eccentric ac-

tivity in virtually all exercises. This is untrue only if the patient is allowed to contract concentrically (in any action mode) then instructed to simply let go and "drop" the body part. This is very difficult to do. Our bodies are designed to let go gradually, and very few of us can relax any part that quickly, especially after a substantial contraction. Also, it is not desirable to produce such a contrasting reaction in a muscle, except under very controlled circumstances. That may be possible in an office, but not at home. The sudden relaxation, if it could be done, could cause an injurious reflex contraction or reaction in a synergist or antagonist. An example of slowing too rapidly occurs in the baseball player (who suffers a hamstring pull) while running to a base. There is also a difference between a "healthy" and highly trained professional athlete and an "unhealthy" patient, who may not be in very good condition. In Table 5.1, the concentric-eccentric ratio reflects the approximate time and effort exerted in those modes. When the ratio is 1:1, the patient takes approximately the same time and effort in raising the load, for example, as in lowering it. When the ratio is 3:1, the load is released fairly rapidly, and the eccentric portions may be either undesirable or unnecessary.

Modifying Contractions

Contractions may be labeled in rather vague terms, such as mild or moderate, and vary by patient, age, gender, and condition. Other specific modifications, such as those in a progressive resistance exercise, are discussed in the following sections.

It is suggested that the patient start movements for most strength exercises from a prestretched position. This means that a relaxed muscle is pulled into a position of increased tension just prior to the contraction. As discussed earlier, this allows for greater loads to be handled by using a greater mass of muscle.

The countermovement jump (CMJ) describes a forceful and relatively rapid prestretch movement that potentiates further activity. Prestretching enhances the average concentric force and average mechanical power by large percentages. This potentiation is directly proportional to the force at the end of prestretch, the prestretch speed, and the brevity of coupling time between the eccentric prestretch and the concentric contraction. This coupling time was a function of the angular displacement and the reaction force curves (25, 26).

One probably should revise the application of resistance or decrease the amount of resistance if the patient cannot complete the full range of motion, the site of application of resistance is painful, muscular tremors develop, or substitutions occur (4, p. 79).

Modifying Frequency

Some of the information in this section has a bearing on contraction modification. Often, the frequency and intensity are interactive, rather than independent, variables.

Eccentric work is not only associated with delayed muscle soreness, at its worst during the second day following exercise, but electromyographic parameters also take more than the 2-day recovery period of concentric exercise (27). Therefore, the frequency of exercise sessions is modified accordingly. If the patient performs essentially eccentric exercises, a minimum of 2 open days is allowed between sessions, rather than the single day between concentric exercising. When sessions are mixed, clinical judgment is necessary. Essentially concentric exercises rarely require greater than 1 day of rest between sessions. This may be a program variant observed and created from Table 5.2.

Frequency of exercise, presuming regularity, should be at least three to five times per week (3, p. 248) (Table 5.2). However, there are certain circumstances and certain kinds of exercise that should be performed daily, if reasonable results are to be obtained. Loosening, relaxing, stretching, and skill training usually require significant daily activity. However, with such a program patient compliance can be more difficult to secure. In fact, these types of exercises may be performed several times, briefly, over the course of each day, due to the number of proper repetitions required to form an engram. For some people who are sufficiently out of condition, old, or injured, low-level programs performed twice per day are desirable. One option is to require daily sessions, but alternate between light and moderate sessions, so that the body can adapt to the stressors. One of these options is often selected when weight reduction is a necessary component of the rehabilitative program, so that caloric expenditure can be maintained at a high enough level.

The 10 repetition maximum (10RM) load can be determined by the trial-and-error process of beginning with a small load and progressively increasing it. Of course, fatigue is a factor, and protracted trials are contraindicated, both for patient safety and

Table 5.2. Exercise Parameters: Frequency and Duration

Program Parameter	Bouts/session	Sessions/day	Days/week	Phase Duration	Intents
I	3	1	3	6 wk	General
II	3	2	3–5	4 wk	Strength, endurance
III	4	3	5–7	4 wk	Skill, endurance, mobility, stretch

for accuracy of information. There are a number of ways to design a progressive resistance program, based upon this reference point. According to DeLorme's protocol, the following formula is applied to each successive bout:

$$X \text{ contractions at } Y\% \text{ of 10RM}$$

X is typically between 10 and 12 repetitions. Y is a variably increasing percentage of the 10RM, which is characteristically incremented by a regular amount. For example, one might begin at 10% and increase in increments of 10%, up to 100%; or one might begin at 25% and increase in increments of 25%, up to 100%. The sum of these 10 or 4 bouts, respectively, would equal one session. The sessions take place from one to several times per day and usually from three times a week to daily. Usually there is a 2- to 4-min rest period between bouts. About once weekly, the patient is tested to determine whether the load can be incremented. Recall that in the Oxford method the load is decremented in the same manner as it is incremented above.

We do not generally recommend the brief maximal exercise format since it is wrought with danger for those not sufficiently versed in its usage. There is sometimes a fine line between therapeutic and injurious, and that requires delicate decision making from an expert point of view. Whether performed isometrically or isotonically, brief maximal exercises may well be too stressful to be accomplished without significant risk of further injury. These are normally more advanced exercises and should be performed either in later stages of rehabilitation or for athletes who wish to improve their performance, relative to strength. Much of this information on frequency also refers to temporal configuration. These parameters are inescapably related and they may be modified individually or simultaneously.

Modifying Spatial and Temporal Configuration

In the early stages, the position in which an exercise is performed may be critical. That is because the force of gravity is significant, compared to the load moved, initially. Sometimes, an exercise can be modified in this manner so that it can be used much longer during the exercise program. Referring to Figure 5.10, if a situp type maneuver is begun in the first position the patient will have an easier time performing the exercise because the length of the moment arm is less in this position, so less force is needed to overcome the resistance in moving the center of mass against the gravity field. Figure 4.9 shows the relative result of abducting the hip from a standing versus a side-lying position, over the same arc of motion. Since the distance over which the force vector acts is greater in the second position, the task is more difficult to perform in that position. Therefore, to alter the effective intensity of an exercise (or its impact on a particular muscle action), one could simply have the patient perform it from a different starting body position. Similarly, the instantaneous position of the body, with or without load, varies throughout time, i.e., the intensity perceived by the muscle(s) can be varied by the specific arc of motion utilized during the exercise, regardless of body position. When a muscle is injured or weak it is far more easily damaged. Therefore, it may be advisable to perform exercises only within the strongest portion of that arc, unless that is the specific location of the injury or where it manifests. Then one can gradually move through the weaker or more injured portions of the muscle range as the other portion strengthens to support it.

Another way that spatial configuration can be of assistance is shown in Figures 5.9 and 5.10. In this case, the fulcrum-weight distance is affected by the change in position of a joint distal to the affected muscle(s), by the same principle described above. In position B of Figure 5.10, the effort required is diminished, so the potential for injury is decreased. These types of parameter changes can only be accomplished after careful and exacting examinations prior to exercising. This relates to the spatial configuration parameter, and this is one of the main ways to determine how to vary it. It should be mentioned that these principles apply to passive and stretching type exercises as well as to other types.

We discussed the concept of beginning exercises with simple motions, either in anatomical planes of motion or into specific joint motions. Not only is this easiest on the joints and soft tissues, but it applies the exercises more specifically, allowing for better control over results. However, as the patient assumes a greater percentage of the range, the motions usually become more complex. Eventually, one can begin to perform patterns of motion, through multiple motion segments, which simulate or duplicate motions and activities later required. This, then, becomes much more than just range of motion exercise, also involving skill training. For example, to reach the full range of shoulder abduction, the humerus must also be rotated externally and the scapula upward (4, p. 25). Because some muscles cross and affect two joints and their motions, the way in which the joint motion is stabilized determines which effect will be enacted. The biceps brachia can cause flexion of the shoulder joint or flexion and supination of the elbow joint. The quadriceps muscle can act as a hip flexor or a knee extensor. In each of these examples, the more distal motion is the chief motion available, but the other motion must not be ignored. Sometimes stabilization is assisted by the patient's position at the time of exercising. For instance, a supine position may be useful to stabilize the shoulder or inhibit certain motions of the shoulder, such as extension while flexing, adducting, or abducting the joint. On the other hand, hip or shoulder extension is most easily isolated in the prone position, to eliminate the normal extraneous motions that would accompany extension. This is why many exercises for these areas take place in the prone position.

To achieve full dorsiflexion of the ankle, one needs to flex the knee joint as well (4, p. 40), because the tension on the fully extended, two-joint gastrocnemius inhibits such motion. Dorsiflexion with the knee extended emphasizes stretching of the gastrocnemius, whereas dorsiflexion with the knee flexed stretches mostly the soleus muscle (4, p. 143–4).

When muscle strength is rated at fair or better, exercises can be performed in an antigravity position. When the strength is rated less than fair, exercises should be performed in a gravity-eliminated position (4, p. 94). This configuration difference may need to have external mechanical support to be accomplished, rather than postural change.

An important characteristic of an exercise regimen is its rhythm. This refers to the relationship between the effort and rest cycles and the relationship between the separate exercises in each set or bout (2, p. 143). As the sessions progress, both the patterns and the timing become subconscious and almost effortless. Compliance with the program is usually directly proportional to the ability to establish and follow a comfortable rhythm.

As a general rule, perform all exercises in their full range of allowable motion, except for isometrics, which are static exercises. Exceptions to this rule are decided at the discretion of the treating physician. If the range of motion is possible but painful, the exercise may be contraindicated or at least require modification. If pain is caused by a calcific tendinitis or a healing fracture, motion should probably be restricted so as to avoid further injury. If pain is caused by adhesions or lack of conditioning, the exercise may be continued, but cautiously. Sometimes, a patient can passively be moved beyond a painful arc and the exercise can be continued throughout the rest of the range. This is important to know and to do, since this latter motion could otherwise be weakened or even lost. Sometimes the painful arc can be avoided by performing static exercises around the zone of pain. Sometimes an isokinetic exercise will be more effective when performed over a portion of the full range; and other times you may want to vary the speed over different portions of the normal range of motion. If performance over a particular portion of the range causes pain, it may be possible to eliminate the pain by reducing the speed of contraction. The authors also recommend performing isometric exercises at various aspects of the range of motion, so as to train a greater portion of the myofibrils over the range of motion. These are examples of how to control the range of motion (and all aspects of spatial configuration), but there are always exceptions to rules.

If there is to be only a single exercise period during the day, the recommended times are in the morning before breakfast, late in the afternoon before dinner, or at least 90 min after a meal. At other times, digestive processes could interfere with exercise, or the converse, reducing the potential result.

Summary of Exercise Parameters

The following general protocol is recommended for an exercise session, with appropriate modifications to fit individual circumstances. The first stage is the warm-up program, which is designed to increase local and general circulation. As mentioned earlier, this should occupy from 20–30% of the total training period. The older the person, the worse the state of conditioning, and the greater the injury, the longer this should be. If there is any doubt as to how to design this portion, imitate the same activities for which the patient is training, but at a much lower intensity and frequency than during the middle portion of the session. Circulation needs to be increased to the exact areas being rehabilitated, perhaps initially with the assistance of physiological therapeutic modalities.

The second stage generally involves stretching (i.e., flexibility exercising) to begin to involve the nervous system. The third stage is comprised of the rest of the specific exercise formats and categories designed to achieve the program intents. The exact order of exercises, and which intent is first to be sought are determined by the clinician on an individual basis. The only guideline here is that one needs to be most cautious with the exercise type with the highest magnitude of parameters, because it has the highest potential for reinjury or exacerbation. Therefore, it should be performed at the time the maximum warm-up curve intersects the lowest point on the fatigue curve with which it intersects (Fig 5.8). The warm-up is maximum just prior to the time that the body institutes its thermoregulatory mechanisms, mainly perspiration. This does not necessarily mean that the local physiological motor units are sufficiently warmed up to perform vigorous activity. Fatigue is more subjective. It is during this time span that the most vigorous exercise will have optimum effect.

The fourth stage is the warm-down period, which generally is slightly less than the warm-up time, but otherwise similar in content. Stretching and/or relaxing exercises may be appropriate during the warm-down.

As exercises progress, a set of controls is exerted upon the various parameters to graduate the program from its initial to its final stages. Progression of the program is based upon regular and frequent evaluation of the patient's progress and accomplishments. Then these results are compared with program objectives and modified with respect to patient feedback.

For pulmonary and cardiovascular purposes, an adequate program that stresses the various exercise components should be designed to last approximately 60 min, depending upon the desired outcome and the number of structures affected (3, p. 246). The four main components include a warm-up (10 min), a muscle conditioning (10 to 20 min), an aerobic portion (20 to 40 min), and a cool-down period (5 to 10 min) (3, p. 247). The times for each component vary depending on the patient, the condition being treated, and the intended activities. Besides actual time spent, energy cost may be a determinant for the duration of the session. This is most important in cardiorespiratory endurance or weight control programs. Usually, the patient should burn 900 to 2500 Kcal/week, or 300 to 500 Kcal/session (at three to five sessions/week) (3, p. 247). Of course, highly trained athletes, particularly in such fields as weight lifting and distance running, will burn considerably more Kilocalories per week. Of course, a 60-min session may be impractical or undesirable, and the duration may require modification.

Standard Functions

The standard functions and program parameters (the exercise formats) proposed in Tables 5.1 and 5.2 are examples established by the authors as a guideline for doctors and therapists. They can be used as presented or modified to suit the therapist's and the patient's needs, according to the physiological principles explained here. As the patient begins to heal and strengthen, the load (i.e., intensity) is usually increased first and the duration or frequency secondarily. Usually the secondary factors are only increased if they were underperformed from the outset. The parameters set down herein are not sacred, but they are effective and, if properly utilized, will produce steady patient progress with only minor risks of injury exacerbation.

The parameter of respiration is not included, because of its variability and its varying degrees of applicability. Some maneuvers, or parts of them, are better performed during inspiration, whereas others provide better results during expiration. Some of this effect is due to the specific motion which the part being exercised undergoes while the two phases of respiration take place, and some is due to the increased intraabdominal and intraspinal pressures and muscle tensions that occur during deep phases of respiration.

Standard function (SF) 1 (see Table 5.1) is designed to be performed slowly, usually with a built in hold at the extreme of motion. It is a useful format for isotonic exercises. A variant of this function is to lower very slowly and change the concentric to eccentric contraction ratio to 1:2, similar to the format used in Nautilus exercises. This variant should be used very cautiously, for the reasons stated above. SF 2 is designed for either isotonic or isokinetic contractions. According to the joint area being exercised, the speed may vary considerably, as evidenced in the frequency parameter. SF 3 may be used for isotonic or isokinetic action, in which the full range of motion is unnecessary, undesirable, or unattainable. SF 4 is a combination of dynamic stretching through the motion and an isometric contraction at the extreme of motion. The frequency may actually be considerably slowed according to the needs and abilities of the patient. Similarly, the isometric component may need to be gradually phased in from light, through medium, then to heavy (submaximal). Only in final phases of the rehabilitation, when the person is virtually fully recovered, are maximal contractions permitted. It is intended that the muscle be relaxed rapidly after the isometric component, thus the concentric to eccentric contraction ratio. When healing is nearly complete, the ratio may be changed to 1:1 to increase the work output and endurance aspects.

SF 5 is designed primarily as an isokinetic exercise, with the intensity, frequency, and spatial configuration being the most manipulated parameters. SF 6 is intended to be strictly an isometric format, with the load and spatial configuration being the principle parameters manipulated. This is usually performed multiple times, at multiple positions, over the range of motion. SF 7 is the format designed mainly for progressive resistance exercise programs; it has a few different variables built into it. SF 8 is designed to function essentially within the framework of slow postural exercises. These positions are held for relatively long periods of time, in an attempt to reinforce proper neural pathways. The intensity and duration here are strictly a function of the patients's ability to maintain good form. SF 9 is a proprioceptive neuromuscular facilitation format. As such, it is biphasic, with a heavy, active, isometric component followed by a very light, passive, stretching component. Also, like SF 6, there are multiple contractions. SF 10 is the format for a passive stretch maneuver. The isokinetic abilities of each function are often brought out by performing the exercise to a rhythmic cadence, so as to control the speed. The speed should ultimately be regulated to at least match the intended result. The program parameters are self-explanatory and can be altered to suit the patient and the conditions.

Regarding the program parameters, early stages of rehabilitation usually require a low work intensity so that one can exercise daily (27, p. 794). Then, as the intensity is increased, the workouts are generally reduced to the more typical three times per week. Beginners maintain this thrice weekly exercise schedule to allow for a rest and recuperation day between sessions. During an athlete's competitive season, exercises will probably be reduced to twice per week. The same is true for advanced trainees who work at higher intensity levels. This allows the person to engage more fully in the normal physical activity for which he is training.

Strength and Endurance

The usual strength protocol advised by the authors is performance of peak tension exercises every other day to the point of complete peripheral fatigue. This is the application of the overload principle, and conforms to the progressive resistance (PRE) exercise format of DeLorme.

In general, to enhance endurance, a more moderate intensity level is suggested, of less than or equal to 50% of maximum, performed aerobically.

To strength train the fast-twitch fibers,

one needs to train with an intensity greater than 20% of the maximum voluntary contraction (MVC). If the force levels are less than 15% MVC, then endurance training is maximal. This indicates the minimum levels necessary to increase strength effectively. This is why strength training is not possible in the early stages of rehabilitation for more severely injured parts.

Interval training consists of alternating aerobic and non-aerobic activities. Such exercising provides more strength training than most endurance programs and more endurance training than most strength programs. Endurance training is useful to strengthen ligaments and tendons and stabilizes their attachment sites on the bones.

The authors recommend the basic PRE protocol, as prescribed by DeLorme, as the starting point. After one determines the 10RM, each bout of each session is performed as follows: 10 repetitions at one-half of 10RM, 10 repetitions at three-fourths of 10RM, and 10 repetitions at full 10RM. The fractions can be varied and the number of intervals can vary. A patient should not be performing near the 10RM level until sufficient healing has taken place. Normally, three bouts of each series are performed during each session, but this varies and is under the doctor's control. One can increase the number of bouts and decrease the intervening rest periods as the patient becomes stronger and endurance increases.

The authors have combined the PRE concepts of DeLorme and Watkins with the Oxford technique for a different approach to strength training (3, p. 144). The result is gradually to increase resistance to maximum, set by set, then gradually to decrease resistance to minimum before finishing a workout. One can vary the frequency and number of sets as well. This has a built-in partial warm-down, as well as an endurance type training effect. This can be more effective and safer and can increase the endurance aspects of training. This does not mean that the standard protocols cannot or should not be utilized, but consider the possibility of combining processes.

Prestretching is always important in strength training because it engages a greater percentage of the muscle mass, thus allowing one to handle a greater weight. In any case, from 8 to 12 repetitions at maximum intensity is the recommended program. If the patient cannot perform 8, the load is too great; if he can perform more than 12, the load should be increased (2, p. 456). Because one is working to momentary muscular exhaustion for strength building, it is important to rest those muscles for about 48 hr after training. Also, it is better to work larger muscles first, so that fatigue is not a factor. This provides the greatest stimulus to growth (2, p. 456).

As a general rule, once the proper number of repetitions at a particular weight are accomplished easily, the weight can be increased by 5 to 10 lb for arm exercises and by 10 to 20 lb for leg exercises (3, p. 294). To emphasize strength training, the load and probably the number of sets would be toward the higher ends of the ranges.

It is important to know the angle of maximum strength for each joint in each degree of freedom. Since the maximum force able to be exerted by the joint varies with the angle of application of that force, an isotonic or isokinetic (i.e., dynamic) contraction would have a different effect at different angles of application (3, pp. 141–2). This refers to the parameter of spatial configuration. Therefore, according to the injury, one may skip the minimum strength portions of the range to avoid the need for recruitment and the potential for further injury. In a healing situation, one may apply a variable resistance over the range of motion to attempt to match the strength differentials in a given muscle. Such devices as the Nautilus, which employs eccentric cams within its system of movable levers and pulleys, may be used. However, this should not be confused with an isokinetic system, because velocity is not so easily fixable. It is not as difficult to apply these principles as one may think. It is easy to see how computerized testing can provide the necessary data, but even normal testing at multiple positions can provide enough information to begin a program.

In the moderately injured person, it is recommended to use isometrics at about 67% of maximum (but not less than 50%), which Hettinger and Muller originally found to increase strength (3, p. 144). It may be desirable to aim closer to 100% of the maximum force, but this is not without substantial potential risk. Exercises should be of about 6 to 10 sec duration, repeated 5 to 10 times daily. Specifically, the contraction needs to last long enough for full recruitment to take place within the muscle. Therefore, one needs only measure the time it takes to reach maximum contraction and hold for a few seconds.

Plyometric training involves a sudden loading of a muscle (such that it is forced to stretch), followed by a rebound contraction of that same muscle. The stretch loading increases the tension so that a maximal force production is more likely to occur (3, p. 146). This is like a combined eccentric-concentric maneuver that loads both the parallel elastic components and the series elastic components. However, it is not without some danger to those tissues and should not be performed until a much later time in the program. Its benefits have not been fully confirmed in the literature. This is not simply a prestretching procedure, but it is a loading procedure and has some attendant risk.

Circuit training was first introduced by Morgan and Adamson in 1953 in London. It is frequently used in health clubs and on sports fields (3, p. 147–9). It requires the person to proceed, at 15 sec intervals, through a series of 30-sec work stations, exercising at 40 to 60% of 1RM. The work and rest intervals can vary to match the individual. Then, after a suitable interval, another circuit follows, for as many as necessary. This type of training is most effective for strength, endurance, and flexibility training. It is somewhat less effective as a means of altering body composition (i.e., percentage of lean mass), and least effective in increasing maximum oxygen uptake, because of its relatively anaerobic nature.

The strength of a particular muscle is usually assessed by measuring the 1 repetition maximum (1RM) through a series of trials (3, p. 228). Weight is progressively added to a comfortable starting weight until the subsequent weight can be lifted only once correctly. This is not attempted until there is a significant improvement in muscle and joint integrity.

Endurance measurement is sometimes a tricky business. One needs to move a resistance a great number of times, but the difficulty is in determining just how much resistance is appropriate for each muscle in each individual. Two specific ideas were to take a percentage of body weight or a percentage of the 1RM and repeat the movements either rapidly within a short period of time, or as many times as possible. The first concept tests endurance as a function of the body as a whole, whereas the second tests endurance as a function of isolated muscle strength. It has been recommended, and the authors agree, that one use 70% of the maximum strength to test endurance (3, p. 230). Of course, this is reduced according to the amount of concurrent injury. Sit ups, push ups, and pull ups are typical tests of endurance. These tests can be modified to adjust for body type, gender, and age, both in form and in expectation. For instance, push ups are more easily performed in the bent-knee position. These are actually exercises, but they are also considered measures of accomplishment. Expectations may be determined by counting performances over a 30- or 60-sec period.

In terms of strength, and even endurance, brief isometric maximal exercises (BRIMES) are at least as effective as isotonic (PRE) exercises (2, p. 316). Therefore, the question exists as to which type exercise is best to perform under which conditions. An important concern with BRIMES, just as with any exercise that maximally stresses structures, is the enhanced potential for damage. Therefore, the authors reserve such activities for later stages of the programs and believe they are generally more suitable for conditioned athletes.

Specificity and Skill Training

Explosive training techniques (high velocity, low force) can be used selectively to train the production of fast force contractions by specific development of fast-twitch fibers, even though hypertrophy of the whole muscle is minimal (29). With reference to the specificity of training concept: working with heavy resistance causes a large increase in maximum strength with insignificant changes in time of isometric force production. On the other hand, explosive strength training, low loads with high contraction velocities, demonstrates exactly the opposite effects (30).

When training either slow-twitch fibers or for slow-twitch type activities, large angular displacements and slower speeds are in order. The exact opposite is true for fast-twitch fibers and more rapid activities. This is theorized to be due to the storage and longevity of elastic potential energy stored in the muscles and the cross-bridges. This again speaks for specificity of training (31).

When a patient is being retrained to perform actions requiring high degrees of coordination, a significant amount of constant and regular feedback is necessary. Be persistent in the training methods, pointing out and demonstrating exactly what is the desired action, as slowly as necessary to perform it correctly. Motions are very deliberate here, and isokinetic training is not initially as useful, even at the lower end of the velocity curve, since strength is not the main intent.

Although there is some contradictory evidence, the authors fully support the "specificity of movement" school of training (3, p. 147). Whenever possible, we promote training that fully simulates the movements that the patient intends to perform later, in all parameters of such motion. This does not sacrifice the need for the type of exercises proposed here, but indicates how to augment the program. The speed of the exercise ultimately should match that of the activity for which one is training, because the training will only support subsequent strength increases at speeds less than or equal to the training speed (4, p. 97).

Many activities require short bursts of rapid movement, which is often specialized and complex and usually of a maximal nature, surrounded by periods of submaximal activities and/or rest. The specificity of exercise principle requires exercises to duplicate such actions. For an injured shoulder, the exercise types and parameters are different for a weight lifter versus a tennis player, even when the same muscles are injured. Obviously, for the weight lifter, more power needs to be generated, and strengthening modes are give priority. The tennis player probably needs more flexibility and a greater arc of motion. Both activities require speed during the course of the activity, but in different parts of their different arcs of motion. Isokinetic exercise is usually best to develop speed in a specific portion of the arc of motion.

When an activity is too difficult, perform it at lower parameter levels, modify its form to suit the patient, or find an easier activity to substitute for it. One must be cautious, in modifying the form or substituting other forms, that the original intent is still being served. If the activity was being performed properly and the patient is no longer able to perform it, first ascertain why it can no longer be done. The patient may be tired due to any number of reasons, and this would be a transient phenomenon. However, there is always the possibility of reinjury, exacerbation, or underlying pathology. A dysglycemic metabolic condition or a simple infectious disorder can lower one's energy level and cause relative inability to perform usual tasks. It is always recommended that a doctor reevaluate any patient whose performance level falls without an obvious explanation. Even a reinjury requires reevaluation, for medical and medicolegal reasons. Even when skill training is a primary objective, adequate strength to perform a task is prerequisite to its accomplishment (2, p. 455).

Probably no exercise type needs more initial assistance and more patient persistence than skill and coordination maneuvers. Neuromuscular reeducation begins without external resistance. Then loading occurs slowly and only when competence has been ably demonstrated. For instance, the ability to contract the prime mover completely independent of other interactive muscles is a necessity. Several factors tend to increase incoordination. (a) If the patient needs to support himself against gravity, overcome a resistance greater than his available strength, or is simply weak, coordinated movements will be difficult. (b) A spillover effect from coordinated adjacent neuronal activity may cause incoordinate motion. (c) Excess emotional stimulus usually decreases coordination. (d) Pain potentiates a great increase in neuronal activity, which can have direct or neural spatial summation effects upon coordinate activity. (e) Fatigue causes incoordination, probably related to a reduced ability to inhibit excess neuronal stimuli. Therefore, to increase skill and coordination, one should avoid doing things that tend to produce these factors. When such factors do occur, the therapist must support the patient better, modify the exercise, or curtail the session.

In rehabilitating a muscular problem, it is sometimes difficult to isolate the actual weakness, even though a problem is clinically obvious. George Goodheart suggests that if the muscle is tested repeatedly, the weakness will often show after about four attempts. This may be necessary to discover the specific weakness in an antagonist or synergist.

Most doctors today think in terms of orthotics when a chronic foot problem is diagnosed, especially if it has an aberrant biomechanical origin. The authors would concur that this is a primary consideration. However, it would be just as wise to consider how to modify the pedal biomechanics or how to support the application of the orthotic for long-range benefits. Since the "average" foot collides with the ground about 10,000 times on an "average" day, it is easy to see how improper biomechanics can cause abnormal muscle action and how the reverse can occur just as easily (32). Each of the musculoskeletal motions connected with normal gait (and even standing posture) is associated with some similar (or compensatory) motion in the superincumbent joints. Pronation unlocks the foot for surface adaptation and shock absorption, whereas supination locks the foot so that it can act as a rigid lever during the act of propulsion. Weaknesses, injuries, or myospasms in the soft tissues that perform these acts (even up through the hip joints) need to be addressed for lasting relief to be possible. The closed kinetic chain of structures and events that occurs during gait movements can be implicated wholly or in part in any of a number of disorders, from the feet through the spine. Conversely, when correcting such disorders by exercising, any and all components of the kinetic chain may require treatment. For example, pronation difficulty in the right foot may require contralateral hip strengthening in order to be corrected.

Acute, Subacute, and Chronic Injuries

Exercises over the full range of motion of a joint may be impossible due to traumatically induced injuries. Injuries in which there is actual damage to the integrity of the joint structure demand special precautions at the extremes of ranges of motion. Early stages of rehabilitation for acute injuries of this nature preclude complete range of motion because of the high risk of further structural damage. Examples of such conditions are severe sprains, luxations, and capsular tears. Conditions in which there is marked inflammatory response, particularly edema, also curtail full joint movements, due to fluid dynamic pressures. In this case, encourage as much motion as possible to enhance removal of excess interstitial fluids. For patients with traumatic injuries and inflammation, follow the former guidelines, to avoid additional injury. For all disorders with an inflammatory component (especially in the acute phase), relaxation exercises are required first. In resistive exercises, loads should be small, repetitions high, and form maintained by not allowing much fatigue. If these guidelines are not observed, the strengthening portion will be counterproductive to the relaxation portion of the rehabilitation.

Treatment for acute pain tends to make chronic pain worse, and visa versa (33). Acute pain is usually accompanied by tissue damage, to a degree which depends upon the severity of injury. Typical treatment options include rest, medications, gentle manipulations, physical therapy, and surgery. Chronic pain requires exercise, perhaps psychological therapy or behavior modification, reduction in medications, and generally no surgery. The notable exception to this is chronic pain caused by cancer, for which surgery is a routine option.

In the early stages of moderate to severe injury rehabilitation, or with debilitated patients, it is often better to employ shorter and more frequent exercise periods during the course of the exercise day. The stage of injury recovery influences decisions about how to employ all the parameters of exercise.

Mode of Action

If one keeps in mind that passive exercises are essential to prevent contractures in joints and connective tissues, it is possible to utilize them even in severe joint injuries (2, p. 918). However, one would not utilize stretching procedures in the early stages of this type of acute injury because joint structures would be passively stretched as well, possibly worsening the injury. Joints can be put through their range of motion passively (PROM), in a partially assisted manner (AAROM), in an active manner (AROM), and in an active resisted mode (ARROM). An exercise regimen generally proceeds in the order of modes as listed above. DeLisa believes that strength is the key determinant in progressing through the modes of exercise (12, p. 356). That is, as the joint or muscle becomes stronger, the patient is able to exercise more actively. One needs also to consider the other aspects of the anatomical (AMU) or physiological (PMU) motor units with respect to their integrity and degree of tissue damage. The less the integrity and the greater the damage, the lower the mode of exercise allowed. After a patient has suffered a recent fracture or tendon repair, immobilization without immediate rehabilitative exercises is contraindicated. Specific range of motion exercises, if properly prescribed and performed, may be essential for the restoration of a preinjury status (12, p. 365). Range of motion exercises of a slow velocity and smooth motion, avoiding irregular motions so as not to stimulate the tendon reflex mechanism, are necessary to maintain articular ranges of motion.

In performing passive range of motion exercises, do not force the motion. If you do so, you will be performing a stretching technique, which may not be appropriate at that time. The object here is to maintain the scope of the current free range of motion, that which is available without forced motion or pain. If the plan is to provide active range of motion, assistance is only provided as necessary for smooth motion.

Because of the danger in spinal injuries, spinal motion is usually encouraged actively first, to determine the first level of limitations. The patient will generally know his/her own limitations and not permit them to be exceeded. Once this is reasonably well established, passive motions can be safely undertaken. However, in musculotendinous injuries, active motions may be more painful and injurious, so passive motions must precede others. This is both a differential guide and a therapeutic necessity.

Exercise Phases

Rehabilitative exercises can be divided into three distinct phases (34, p. 102). The first phase is the activity permitted during the time of immobilization. During this time, isometric and isotonic exercises of the contralateral side, careful homolateral exercises, and isometric or isotonic exercises of adjacent joints are permitted. Also, activities to promote and maintain a higher level of fitness are desirable on a limited basis. Simple motions are preferred through most of this phase. Generally, the production of pain is sufficient to cause the activity to be contraindicated.

The second phase, labeled the partial stress phase, occurs once movement is again permitted. Exercises on the healthy side can be pursued vigorously, as can fitness improvement that does not overstress the involved area. Exercise of the injured area proceeds from passive to assisted to active to resistive, as stress loads are gradually increased. Minus exercises (as discussed in Chapter 4) and water exercises are generally easier to accomplish and potentially less injurious, especially early in the program, (i.e., through phases one and two).

In the third (full stress) phase of activity one can eventually utilize maximum or submaximal stress loads on the injured area(s). One is more likely to be able to use complex three dimensional motions without fear of exacerbating the condition. Use of mechanical and electronic devices to augment the exercise parameters is encouraged, as necessary and as tolerated. Exercises designed for specific activities and the patient is pushed to his limits during this phase of the program.

Phase one activities include cross-over training, relaxation procedures, and controlled exercising of adjacent joint areas. This means that adjacent structures can be moved only when they do not interfere with the primary immobilization intent. Phase two activities include isometrics (at submaximal levels), carefully graduated isotonics, and exercises where the injured area is somewhat supported, as in water or mechanical sling devices. Stretching type activities may begin here or in phase one, but, as in all exercises, they are gradually increased in parameters as tolerance and ability permit. For a while, it may be necessary during each session to begin with assisted modes and finish with active or resistive modes. Coordination and skill training can be begun in phase two, but it is in phase three that these exercises are most effectively performed because the patient has already improved in strength and endurance and increased the range of useful motion considerably. At some point during phase three, maximum intensity can be reached and, thereafter, maintained. This is desirable, if the patient is to return to full preinjury status. In fact, it has been shown that intensive dynamic back extensor exercises, conducted over about a 3-month period, are more effective than other therapeutic regimens (35). Therefore, as soon as more intensive exercises can be tolerated, they should be implemented. What is true for the spine is highly likely to be true for less critical areas of the anatomy.

Exercise Qualifiers

There are some precautions that one should observe with respect to stretching exercises. Since one is never quite sure, at first, what a joint's allowable range of motion is, one should never passively force a joint into such motion. Since connective tissues lose tensile strength and elasticity after periods of immobilization, one should avoid vigorous stretching in the immediate post-immobilization period. A joint or muscle pain that lasts for more than 24 hr after stretching indicates that the force applied, the range pursued, and/or the speed of contraction was excessive (4, p. 145). Edematous tissues and weak muscles should be stretched mildly and cautiously, if at all, because such activity can worsen a patient's condition. When stretching areas that involve knitting fractures, it is imperative to stabilize the area between the fracture site and the joint being mobilized, to protect that healing bone. In fact, it is advisable to stabilize the body segments on either side of the mobilized joint in most stretching procedures (15, p. 399).

Generally speaking, a tight joint should be less vigorously stretched than a tight muscle. Inflamed joints are more susceptible to injury than other tissues being treated in the area (15, p. 399). A moderate prolonged stretch is more likely to cause a mild plastic change in the involved connective tissues. A short-term vigorous stretch will be proportionately resisted and usually results only in elastic changes (15, p. 399). Therefore, a vigorous, short term stretch is really only useful to preload a muscle for a maximal contraction. In early stages, and especially when moderate to severe muscle spasm is present the cryostretch (or spray-and-stretch) technique might be reasonably applied prior to other exercise formats (36, p. 409). This involves the preliminary spraying of an aerosol substance, such as ethyl chloride or fluoromethane, over the intended muscle area(s), in certain locations, just prior to stretching them. It is effective when pain is a limiting factor, especially when pain tolerance is low.

The only true contraindications to stretching techniques are hypermobility and inflammatory reactions (4, p. 157). This is somewhat distinct from joint mobilization or range of motion exercise, which may be lightly performed when those conditions are mild. A swollen joint should not be stretched since its capsule and soft tissues are already stretched by the joint effusion. Such techniques may only be applied in the vicinity of a hypermobile joint when the joint is properly stabilized to allow force to be transmitted across it without disturbing its intrinsic structures.

Generalized or localized osteoporotic conditions act as relative or absolute contraindications to certain types of exercises. Any exercises, like progressive resistance and weight bearing, that increase the osseous load may be risky, except at low intensities. Stretching must not be too forced or loaded either, since the tension the muscle can withstand may far exceed what the related bones can bear.

When irreversible contractures have taken place, it is doubtful that nonsurgical procedures would have a significant effect upon correction of this problem. Such contractures usually involve replacement of the normal elastic tissues with relatively inelastic tissues, such as bone, fibrotic tissues, and adhesive scars (4, p. 119). In the case of ossific or calcific infiltration, mildly zealous stretching can cause further damage and inhibit the healing process. In fact, forcible stretching may cause fractures or hemorrhages within these solid blocks, causing the formation of more heterotopic bone (2, p. 310). In other cases, there is a possibility for improvement. This is why a radiographic examination of joints we intend to stretch is often a prerequisite to treatment.

There is a relative (or absolute, depending

upon degree) contraindication to using heavier weights when the patient has hypertension, coronary artery disease, or certain other circulatory problems (3, pp. 275–6).

Avoid Valsalva maneuvers during exercise (have the patient exhale) to avoid abnormal stress on the cardiovascular system and the abdominal wall (4, p. 72), particularly in patients who have a medical history in those areas. This is an especially important consideration in isometric exercises or any movements against heavy resistance.

Avoid abruptly starting and stopping exercises because this can cause arrhythmias. The patient should avoid alcoholic beverages, because of impaired judgment, and steam bath type activities 30 min before and 60 min after exercising, due to increased cardiovascular loading (37).

It is usually contraindicated for patients with low back disabilities to perform such exercises as trunk raising and double straight leg raising until quite late in their programs (17, p. 42).

The sit-up position causes the highest intradiscal pressure, so consider the effects of a sit-up type exercise on a patient with disc problems. Isometric exercises, which increase both intra-abdominal and intradural pressures, are usually contraindicated in the acute stages of intervertebral disc syndromes. Absolutely contraindicated in patients with disc lesions is any motion that peripheralizes the symptoms (4, p. 460).

Resistance exercises are usually contraindicated when a muscle or a joint is inflamed or swollen, because the resistance can increase such a response (4, p. 76). It usually does not matter whether the inflammation is infectious or arthritic. However, the consequences of the former tend to be more serious, much sooner.

In active inflammatory conditions, such as rheumatoid arthritis, the patient fatigues easily and requires longer rest periods between bouts and sets (4, p. 238). Maximum resistive exercises are contraindicated during these periods, because there is always a compressive element perceived in the involved joints when strengthening exercises are implemented. Such conditions eventually have pathological changes that weaken the structures, both locally and systemically, and make the person more susceptible to damage from even moderate exer-

cises. Sometimes medications, such as corticosteroids, further weaken structures (e.g., demineralization of bone), causing even more damage. A thorough history can prevent mistakes from being made. Inflammatory conditions are not an absolute contraindication to rehabilitative exercises, but rather exemplify the factors to consider in setting the boundaries for exercises.

Special consideration needs to be given when facet arthrosis is known to be present. Usually, extension, especially coupled with rotation, is to be avoided, because it tends to narrow the already diminished foramina (4, p. 469).

A number of general precautions are necessary for postsurgical rehabilitation. Avoid specific motions and weight bearing predicaments consistent with the surgical procedure performed. There is normally a certain amount of local inflammation after surgery. Therefore, the normal precautions and contraindications concerning inflammatory reactions must be observed. Stretching and resistance exercises should not begin on surgically repaired muscles, tendons, and ligaments for about 6 weeks postoperatively (4, p. 244). If there is a continuation or increase of drainage, edema, or pain during or following exercise, the exercises should be modified downward or discontinued. Depending upon the duration of casting and the activities performed during casting, the newly freed area will usually be weak and atrophied. The area is very much in need of rehabilitation, but such a process must proceed quite slowly. There is usually some pain from stretching the contracted structures simply because of the swollen tissues. Whenever there has been a fracture, if there was concurrent soft tissue damage, an inelastic scar will form. When one attempts to stretch this tissue, either pain or decreased motion will result. If mobilization procedures are not utilized, the consequences may include a permanent loss of motion. Exercises that result in joint swelling lasting longer than 4 hr, require medication, cause a decrease in strength, or cause rapid fatigue have too high parameters or are being increased too rapidly (4, p. 236).

The presence of myositis ossificans is a contraindication to most dynamic exercising because the added trauma may further injure the muscle and increase the calcific deposition (15, p. 677). Once the calcific deposits have been essentially resolved one may begin activities, including an exercise program.

Due to the numerous altered hormonal concentrations during exercise, there are several other precautions and concepts to consider (38). For example, changes in insulin, glucagon, and epinephrine secretions are significant for a diabetic. Because fibrinolysis increases, there is a tendency toward bleeding and away from clotting. Certainly those with blood dyscrasias and liver dysfunctions need to know of this proclivity.

Additionally, there are a number of less severe orthopaedic repercussions which ought to be considered in the performance of rehabilitation programs. Such entities as blisters, muscle soreness, muscle cramps, and abnormal callus formation can hinder or retard the program's progress. Blisters and calluses are usually the result of ill-fitting footwear or an initial overuse, producing a constant abrasion of the feet and/or hands. This problem is easily solved by utilizing only properly fitted foot gear and by properly performing the exercise regimen. Muscle soreness is a function of the type of exercises performed, the state of conditioning of the patient, and the parameters of the exercises performed. These factors have all been discussed previously and are accounted for in all the attitudes we promote. If the warm-up and warm-down and exercise level are all appropriate, soreness will be minimized. Muscle cramps can have mechanical, biochemical, or pathological origins. The latter are beyond the scope of this text. Mechanical factors have to do with following the proper procedures, particularly warm-up and stretching, in the exercise protocols. Biochemical factors usually involve simple corrections in the intake and utilization of certain serum or cellular electrolytes, such as sodium, potassium, calcium, and magnesium. Imbalances or deficiencies in these biochemicals can be responsible for such involuntary spasms. This condition is usually correctable by providing adequate intake of minerals and fluids before and during the exercise, if necessary. Fatigue was discussed in detail in earlier sections of this book. Remember, tired muscles are much easier to injure. Also be cognizant of such environmental conditions as temperature, humidity, air pollution, and altitude and how they impact exercise physiology. Another factor of concern is patient motivation and concentration. It has been estimated that only 60 to 85% of those beginning an exercise program remain with it for at least 10 weeks. Therefore, the rate of success will be severely limited by the patient's ability and desire to continue with the program and follow it as closely as possible. Of course, compliance will be markedly increased by the attitudes and abilities of the therapist, as well as those of the patient.

Overuse Syndromes

More than two-thirds of injuries in recreational athletes have been reported to be due to overuse syndromes, i.e., they develop from repetitive trauma to muscle and bone (39). Therefore, it is important to know how to diagnose, treat, and, ultimately, prevent this entity. One of the key precautions here has to do with one of the main treatments for this type condition, rest. Prolonged rest, like immobilization, has untoward consequences, such as loss of muscle tone. The result of this is a proneness toward future reinjury. Thus, it is suggested that the patient return to normal function, within a normal environment, as soon as possible.

In any overuse syndromes, some rest must precede any exercise regimen. This is obvious from the descriptive name of the clinical entity. Exercise must be initiated very gradually; the aim is to rehabilitate with endurance exercises. Active motions, especially while weight bearing, are more easily and effectively accomplished in water, or utilizing some supportive structures, as in negative exercises.

Many injuries can reasonably fall within this category. Usually, they are problems in the lower (weight bearing) extremities. For example, patients presenting with lateral femoral epicondylar pain, without joint effusion, are often showing the results of an overuse syndrome (40). This is relatively common in distance runners and is usually only exacerbated by continuous running sports or sprinting. An adequate tensor fascia lata stretch, along with proper training and running techniques, can usually prevent such a syndrome. Once someone has been diagnosed with an overuse syndrome, the same stretching procedures are useful in treating it. One could normally examine for this by testing muscles, either manually or mechanically, with pain and weakness being positive findings.

"Shin splints," or anterior/posterior compartment syndromes, are another example of an overuse syndrome. "Tennis elbow" is a typical example of this in a non-weight-bearing limb. In shin splint conditions, one must differentiate between involvement in the anterior and the posterior compartments, correlating with the swing or stance phases of locomotion, respectively (41). Depending upon relative hypertonicity and weakness, muscles need to be stretched and strengthened, respectively. Anterior compartment muscles include tibialis anterior, extensor digitorum longus, extensor hallucis longus, and peroneus longus. Posterior muscles include tibialis posterior, flexor digitorum longus, flexor hallucis longus, flexor hallucis brevis, and adductor hallucis. The anterior muscles are normally somewhat weaker, making a dynamic balance a tricky business to achieve. Patients with these problems are often using inappropriate gear and improper technique or skill.

Running injuries may need either a flexible or rigid orthotic, at least temporarily, as part of the rehabilitation program (22). Sometimes, weight-bearing exercises performed while wearing orthotics are more effective in recreating balance. The orthotic helps to correct the weak arch resulting from excessive exercise or from immoderate obesity, often secondary to a pronated foot.

Sprains and Strains

As discussed in Chapter 3, there are three degrees of sprain or strain. They are classified according to the amount of injury sustained and the amount of function lost. No matter what joint is involved, the principles are the same. Furthermore, the rehabilitative process relates directly to this classification of the condition being treated. The less severe the injury the sooner one can begin to rehabilitate and the greater the intensity permitted. The more loss of function there is, the less the capability to rehabilitate. In the most severe injuries, active rehabilitation may be delayed in favor of immobilization and symptom abatement. If surgery is required, rehabilitative exercises begin postoperatively.

For a simple, mild to moderate sprain of the ankle (i.e., swelling is minimal and there is very little instability) initiate gentle active range of motion within 48 to 72 hr. As soon as patient tolerance allows work the range of motion passively and apply stretch activities. Isometric exercises are the usual third stage of activity, while there is still protective weight bearing (with a cane or crutches). Severe injuries may require 3 to 6 weeks of immobilization and even surgical repair before this kind of rehabilitation is possible (42). Rehabilitation for weight-bearing joints, although they are much stronger, must be approached cautiously, since they usually carry much greater loads.

Janse and Kissinger noted an important relationship between an inversion sprain and what they termed a tensor fascia lata syndrome (43, p. 5). Whether one is dealing with cause or effect here, the objective is always to balance muscles and restore normal function. This model is suggested for deciding how to rehabilitate any chronic injury. There is often an underlying or complicating neuromusculoskeletal factor in a chronic or repetitive injury. If one seeks that factor and proceeds to rehabilitate it, along with the primary injured site, chances are the result will be more complete and longer lasting. The authors suggest that you first investigate the immediate proximal joint and its surrounding structures. If this provides no new information, evaluate other structures that somehow balance this structure in overall body motion. An example of this is the compensation that occurs in the cervical or lumbar spine when the other is injured, misaligned, or stressed. If one area is injured, frequently secondary effects in the other need treatment.

Quoting from Ruth Jackson, M.D., "Sprains of the ligaments and capsules heal within six to eight weeks by the formation of scar tissue, which is less elastic and less functional than normal tissue. Varying degrees of residual alteration of their functional capacity is inevitable" (44, p. 21). This again points to the considerable need for the earliest possible rehabilitation. It is important to provide range of motion and stretching procedures as a first step. Not doing so may cause the propensity for residual dysfunction. When reviewing the case of an individual with chronic weakness and dysfunction in an ankle or wrist from a sprain (or series of sprains), one can see this underlying functional disability as causative. The more mild the injury, the sooner it heals and the more likely it will be to heal by first intention (that is, with minimal or no cicatrization). However, the more often it becomes reinjured and the more loading put upon it, the less likely it will heal at all. This latter fact is why apparently minor injuries can come back to haunt someone, even when the symptoms resolved within days or weeks of the initial injury. Manipulative procedures within the first 6 months can be the difference between proper healing and permanent loss of function (45, p. 101). The authors suggest range of motion and stretching exercises, as soon as immobilization is completed. The more serious the condition, the more passively exercises are begun. This assumes that the pain-free arc has been established, so as not to exacerbate the injury.

Although joint motion must be limited for sprains and dislocations to heal, in strains it is necessary to limit musculotendinous motion for full healing to occur. Therefore, isometric contractions only are desirable early in the rehabilitative program and loading must be minimized in the early phases of rehabilitation. Reparative function is directly related to the length of time injured and the extent of immobilization used. This is particularly true of these soft tissue injuries because they tend to be relatively ignored, as opposed to fractures and more visible wounds. Although mobility is usually a considered goal, flexibility is often forgotten.

The ankle and knee joints are most prone to ligamentous sprains (46, p. 6). Among the more serious injuries is the sprain or tear of the cruciate ligament(s) of the knee. Rehabilitation of cruciate ligaments of the knee often presents the clinician with unique and difficult problems. This ligament has spiraling fibers, rather than the straight linear fibers of most ligaments (47), which provide a greater than normal degree of effective contractility. However, these fibers are more likely to present a difficulty in surgical repair or in healing through normal pro-

cesses. If left alone and not rehabilitated, a cruciate ligament injury probably will cause an unstable knee, soon subject to reinjury. In early stages, it will need to be treated like any ligamentous tear or sprain. This ligament limits anterior slippage of the tibia under the femoral condyles, so such motion will have to be gradually trained. This requires both reeducation and strengthening. Balancing the muscle strength from front to back is also essential, with the hamstrings eventually producing about 80% of the strength of the quadriceps (47). Avoiding sudden accelerations or decelerations is paramount in the early and middle stages of treatment.

Without severe ligamentous tears, it is reasonable to expect at least 10 months of continuous rehabilitation before the structure approaches normal tensile strength (47). Even after that amount of time, it is unlikely that normal structure will be formed, so the function will only approximate its prior capability. Therefore, surrounding tissues must be strengthened above their previous levels in order to provide the initial state of conditioning and strength.

Whether cruciate ligaments are surgically repaired or conservatively treated, vigorous rehabilitation is ultimately necessary. It is likely that a severe ligamentous rupture, with or without avulsion of bone, will require surgical intervention prior to conservative management (47), but mild or moderate ligamentous damage may respond adequately to less drastic procedures. It may be necessary simultaneously to treat the area with cryotherapy, pressure bandaging, and elevation. Sometimes contrast baths are also employed. The key is that the fibrous tissue that repairs the ligament is laid down in a biomechanically suitable pattern, which maintains as much strength as possible, without producing limiting adhesions within the adnexa. Braces that limit motion may also be a necessary early adjunct to therapy, and therapy may be expected to continue for at least 10 months (47). It is most important in such injuries to rebalance muscles in rehabilitation programs, so that the hamstrings are approximately 80% of the strength of the quadriceps (47). In early stages, there is very little loading, and one mostly attempts to increase motion, within limits of stability.

One may only be able to utilize contralateral crossover training for a certain time. A little later, water exercises may be included, as strength and endurance exercising begins. Slowly, one adds loads, especially through the range of motion, either isometrically or isotonically.

Tendinitis and Bursitis

Restoration of pain-free movement is one of the most important goals of treatment for chronic tendinitis (48, 49), but is not always easily accomplished.

If these conditions persist long enough, calcium deposits are made in the irritated sheath, causing a calcific tenosynovitis. For tendinitis and bursitis, a graduated passive, then active, exercise program will slowly increase the range of motion and reduce the inflammatory responses. In a calcific tenosynovitis, however, that program may continually exacerbate the tendons or the bursae (see below) and be counterproductive. Physical therapy devices may first need to be employed, to hasten resorption of the calcium deposits. However, isometric exercises are usually very effective under these conditions. Progress to concentric progressive resistance exercises as the pain-free arc expands.

In the early stages of rotator cuff injury rehabilitation, full-range exercises are inappropriate (2, p. 464). Some of the other muscles of the shoulder girdle are too powerful to perform them in that manner, even if full passive range of motion is allowable. In the treatment of rotator cuff injuries of the shoulder, it is imperative exactly to differentiate the impaired muscle(s) (50). This is because the spatial configuration of the exercises must be altered to fit the line of action of the specific muscle(s) involved.

Racquet sports can often cause injury to wrist extensors and retaining ligaments ("racquet wrist") due to rapid acceleration forces, similar to those in a whiplash injury (51). They are common injuries and need a variety of treatments, including strengthening the musculotendinous tissues as soon as the patient is relatively pain free. Exercises usually begin isometrically, to protect the injured area. Then one proceeds to dynamic exercising, preferably of an isokinetic nature, so the patient will be able to handle the high acceleration energies generated during the swing.

Patellar tendinitis ("jumper's knee") can cause pain anywhere from the musculotendinous junction through the infrapatellar region. This kind of injury is most commonly found in athletes who are required to jump high and repeatedly, generating a large amount of sudden force through the quadriceps muscle of the takeoff leg. Jumper's knee may also occur in athletes like basketball players, who land on their feet onto hard boards after jumping high and often. The eccentric contraction thus generated causes an even greater load than usual across the knees. Considering this etiology, it is recommended that, during the early stages of muscle and tendon injuries, negative work be avoided (28, p. 794). The more severe the injury, the longer negative work should be avoided.

Involvement of the rectus abdominus, gluteus maximus and hamstring muscles is also quite common (51). For hamstring injuries, rest may be an important early treatment. Relaxation of hypertonicities and strengthening of weaknesses are essential as soon as possible. Strength training begins with isometric contractions and eventually progresses to isokinetic exercises, as the leg is brought further into normal functioning.

Dislocations and Fractures

In the acute stage, there may not be plastic deformation of the ligamentous structures. In that case, these injuries may be virtually fully rehabilitated. The first phase of rehabilitation in all luxations aims at relaxation of the protective spasming and reduction of fear about moving the joint. The less the ligamentous damage and inflammatory response, the sooner strengthening begins in order to stabilize the joint. After correction, by surgical or nonsurgical means, rehabilitation will consist mainly of improving the muscle tone and articular range of motion, followed by muscle strengthening exercises

Generally, stress fractures are small, well-aligned, and capable of full healing, provided further trauma to the site is avoided. This usually means avoiding protracted and strenuous weight bearing, but not avoiding all activity in the joint. Even in a non-weight-bearing joint, continuous passive and active movements are instituted very early as the first phase of rehabilitation to prevent disuse atrophy. When the bones have knit sufficiently, subsequent rehabilitation includes strength and endurance modes, as appropriate, which are usually weight bearing or, certainly, load bearing.

Rarely is there an osseous fracture without subsequent (or concomitant) soft tissue damage. Even stress fractures have irritated soft tissues around them, and functionally connected with them, because of their etiology. Rehabilitation is necessary not only to restore soft tissue integrity, but to reestablish strength and for muscle reeducation. It is also necessary to place rehabilitative emphasis on surrounding muscular tissue that, as a result of the fracture treatment, suffers from disuse atrophy. As with stress fractures, disuse atrophy is of particular importance. It must be considered when evaluating the rehabilitative program to reestablish normal function (see Chapter 6). The difference here is that immobilization is required for an extended period of time, making atrophy a more probable consequence.

One can contract any voluntary muscle (except those of the face) at will, in an isometric manner (2, p. 918). The initial portion of the contraction is the "muscle setting." It is a most useful procedure when exercise is necessary but motion is undesirable. These situations usually occur in dislocations, casted or uncasted fractures, and early postoperative healing circumstances. An example of this process would be to begin to perform a sit-up and to cease motion just before the back loses contact with the table. The process is useful in toning muscles and facilitating responses. From a physical standpoint, this procedure supplies just about enough energy to overcome the inertia of rest but not enough to generate any momentum. This is one of the safest procedures available, and it is useful to prevent atrophy in situations requiring long-term immobilization. This can be applied in the vast majority of exercises, especially in the early phases of rehabilitation. It should also be an advantage in both warm-up procedures and in the early stage of developing skilled motions.

If properly done, range of motion exercises can be useful even for recent fractures and tendon repairs (12, p. 365). They must be performed at a slow velocity, with very even motion. Bouncing can produce a tendon reflex, and one also wishes to avoid contraction of the antagonist muscle.

Many fractures demand special considerations. For example, patellar fractures can be extremely difficult, especially if the fragments are comminuted and alignment is not maintained. Isometric exercises are begun as soon as possible, on the casted leg, combined with kinetic exercises for the proximal and distal joints. A recommended program includes the following exercises, performed on an hourly basis, as soon as possible after a 24-hr waiting period postinjury or postsurgery (52). Isometrically contract the quadriceps, perform a straight leg raise to about 45° and hold for several seconds, isometrically contract the hip extensors, exercise the hip through the other motions available, and exercise the ankle through its allowable motions. Note that the quadriceps contraction is actually a setting exercise and, as such, is performed at moderate intensity. Exercises are all performed to tolerance.

Cartilage Injuries

Although spinal discs are mainly cartilaginous in nature, their problems are discussed under "Low Back Pain" (see below). However, the temporomandibular joint (TMJ) also contains a cartilaginous disc. The TMJ is also a postural joint, but weight bearing is generally minimal. Therefore, active or passive exercises, other than isometrics, do not impose significant loads, if the patient is not chewing. This joint is more delicately arranged than spinal joints, and exercises should be performed at a slower rate and at less than the full allowable motion. Knee cartilages, especially the medial ones, like the TMJ discs, are much more likely to become physically displaced. Therefore, one needs to be appropriately cautious in exercises not to move forcefully in the direction that causes such displacement. In all knee exercises, be careful not to compress the patella into the groove of the femoral condyles (4, p. 204). Such compressive action, especially during weight bearing, may hasten cartilaginous degeneration.

There is a simple physical means of diagnosing a torn knee cartilage, which has an accuracy of 95% or better (53). The maneuvers listed below are performed in such a manner as to produce a submaximal load on the menisci. The inability to perform any of these exercises is a positive finding. The ability to perform all of these exercises is a negative finding.

The maneuvers are as follows: (a) jumping from one leg to the other, with weights attached to the legs, while holding a 3- to 5-lb medicine ball; (b) squatting while holding the medicine ball; (c) squatting, then pointing the lower extremities to the left and to the right; (d) jumping over a medicine ball and jumping over a gymnasium bench, rebounding with both legs; (e) high jumping or jumping while reaching up; (f) exercises involving resistance of the quadriceps; and (g) running up and down stairs.

Chondromalacia patellae has several characteristics that are important to know for rehabilitative purposes. This condition is more common in females and is the most common running injury. It is most usually related to biomechanical imbalances in one or more joint areas, from the feet through the spine (54). Furthermore, imbalances in the long muscles of the thigh and hip, such as the tensor fascia lata (iliotibial band), the psoas, the adductors, the quadriceps, and the hamstring group, can cause the patella to "track" improperly, thus irritating the underlying cartilage. Sometimes, manipulation is the first treatment of choice. However, at some point, there are usually soft tissues that need stretching and/or strengthening.

Progressive resistance exercises for the quadriceps and hamstrings are proposed for such degenerative conditions as chondromalacia patellae. Hamstring exercises are performed in the usual isotonic manner, and quadriceps exercises are performed isometrically (55). Quadriceps atrophy is not an uncommon finding in chondromalacia, due to disuse secondary to pain (56). Whenever there is knee instability or abnormal motion, there should be a general check of all related musculature and a program applied to strengthen any muscles that are weak.

Neck Pain

Whiplash Injury

Hyperflexion and hyperextension injuries are typically produced by accidents involving collisions. They are frequently found together clinically in "whiplash" injuries. Such injuries often include damage to all related soft tissues, including nerves. Small fractures, such as of oncovertebral processes, or avulsions of tendinous insertions may be associated with them. Depending upon the head position at the time of impact, most acceleration/deceleration injuries involve the majority of cervical musculature and even the temporomandibular joints. The greater the amount of tissue damage and inflammatory response, the less the load allowed in early rehabilitative stages. One may not be able to begin significant rehabilitation until the cervical collar is removed. Relaxation procedures can begin almost immediately and will make the patient more amenable to other treatments, including manipulation.

It should be pointed out that the amount of vehicular damage in an auto accident is a highly inaccurate measure of the magnitude of spinal (especially cervical) damage. Spinal injuries are due to the rapid acceleration forces that suddenly drive the body's joints through the resistance of the softer tissues. (57). Therefore, when determining the proper and necessary treatment plan, give significant weight to the patient's symptoms and to examination findings and little weight to the circumstances of the accident. Too much motion, too early, can be deleterious to the final patient outcome.

Before hyperflexion or hyperextension injuries can rupture ligaments, either body compression fracture or neural arch fracture must take place (58, p. 24). However, rotational and horizontal shearing forces can cause considerable soft tissue and discal damage without osseous disruptions. This is another reason for eliciting a detailed history, including head position at the time of impact. Depending upon the tissues involved and the nature of their pathology, one may treat this injury in a manner similar to a sprain/strain, a fracture, a dislocation, or a disc injury.

Treatment for whiplash type syndromes always depends upon the extent and severity of soft tissue injury. Assuming that one has reached the stage of allowable motion, relaxation and improvement of motion are the initial goals. Subsequently, isometric exercises are used for strength development. They may be modified, in the beginning, by reducing the intensity and the frequency or duration, according to the patient's pain response. If tolerated, these exercises may be begun simultaneously with the weaning of the patient from the immobilizing collar (59).

Torticollis

The rule of thumb in torticollis (in most of its varieties) is that the resultant fixed cervical motion is rotated opposite and laterally flexed toward the contracted muscle. Therefore, one aims at reducing tendency toward contraction in the homolateral muscle and increasing tone and strength in the contralateral muscle. This can be tested manually or mechanically or confirmed with electromyographic studies, but it is usually evident on palpation. The types of exercises employed can be quite varied and depend somewhat on the causes of the problem. There are congenital types that may be due to a whole or partial lack of muscle tissue. In congenital cases due to trauma at birth, there is often a considerable deposition of fibrous tissue in and about the muscle. Some congenital situations may require surgery, whereas long-term exercise therapy may suffice for others. In hemiplegia, exercise will work if there is innervation to the involved muscle (4, p. 472).

Cervical Arthritides

Because a hypolordotic cervical curve predisposes one to degenerative spurs (57), exercises that aim to produce a normal lordosis are in order when treating (and attempting to prevent) most spinal arthritides. A whiplash injury may result in a hypolordotic cervical curve, and it should be treated with this potential long-range consequence in mind. When performing exercises in the supine position, it may be desirable to have the patient lie upon a cervical pillow and/or a lumbar pillow to help maintain normal lordoses.

Cervical Subluxation Complexes

When attempting to isolate atlanto-occipital motion, for rehabilitative purposes, remember that these joints are essentially only capable of flexion-extension (sagittal plane motion) (60). The specific motion accomplished here is often referred to as "nodding," and it contributes to the total sagittal (θ_x) motion. Therefore, one can reasonably assume that rotatory (θ_y) and lateral flexion (θ_z) maneuvers will affect these joints very little, if at all. The same is true for motion anywhere in the body. First, one must understand exactly what motions are allowed by a specific joint, then direct the exercise into those motions.

The need to provide exercises to promote normal spinal curvature is accentuated by the discovery of an anterior cervical subluxation complex. There are a number of hallmarks to this clinical impression, including increased posterior disc height, decreased anterior disc height, anterior body translation (as little as 1 to 2 mm), nonparallel facet surfaces, spinous process altered spacing, and a kyphotic angulation of at least 11° (61). Although this complex is usually of traumatic origin, it is sometimes not apparent for months or years. This position is unstable and is prone to degenerative change. The inherent combination of precarious ligamentous support and foraminal or canal stenosis tends to lead to the expression of neurological dysfunction. These latter factors are also a relative contraindication to certain exercises, especially those with high force and high velocity. Therefore, we favor modifying the normal isometric protocols to moderate or mild intensity, especially in the early stages. This will have little or no strengthening effect but will help to tone the muscles and promote normal neuromuscular responses.

Spinal Curvature

Spinal biomechanical stability, particularly in the dynamic mode, requires an optimum lordotic structure. These curves affect the spine's ability to resist axial pressures. This relates to the spine as a model spring and, thus, to the aforementioned Hooke's law. However, the resistance to axial pressure is described in the following equation (66, p. 6):

$$r = c^2 + 1$$

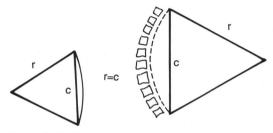

Figure 5.12 Formula for optimal spinal curvature. r = resistance to axial pressure. c = number of curvatures.

where r = resistance to axial pressure and c = number of curvatures. Normally, $r = 3^2 + 1 = 10$. If even one of these curves is lost, then $r = 2^2 + 1 = 5$, a reduction of 50%. This equation is somewhat different from the linear model proposed by Hooke for spring action. The biomechanical reality often is different from the predicted physical model.

In engineering, the strongest and most functional curvature or arc is one in which the radius of curvature equals the cord across the arc of curvature (66, p. 7) (Fig. 5.12). For the cervical spine, one measures from the posterior inferior part of the anterior arch of C1 to the anterior superior aspect of the body of T2. For the thoracic spine, one measures from the line parallel to the T1 endplate, projecting anteriorly to another parallel to the T12 inferior endplate. If perpendiculars are drawn to these two lines, they normally intersect at an angle of approximately 55°. For the lumbar spine, mark the inferior anterior aspect of the body of T12 and another at the same aspect of L5. One can use a compass to measure the distance between any of the points mentioned. The point of all this is that it is important to maintain optimum spinal curvatures and to restore them when they have been altered. Spinal curvatures are easier to evaluate and monitor using the guidelines suggested here.

Low Back Pain

Inasmuch as back pain is the scourge of society, it is reasonable and necessary to question the medical model of analgesics, muscle relaxers, rest, and surgery as the standard treatment protocol. Not only is planned active rehabilitation not contraindicated, it is the treatment of choice (67).

It is suggested that restoration of function, rather than reduction of pain, be the chief clinical objective.

From a large Scandinavian study, weak trunk extensors were associated with a history of sciatica and weak trunk flexors with back injuries and with current backache at work/exercise. Also, weak leg extensors were associated with a history of low back insufficiency, with use of sick leave due to the back, and with current hip pain (68). This gives one a perspective on cause and a direction for therapeutic application.

In a large Finnish study, about 5% of the adult population were deemed to suffer from lumbar disc syndrome and about 6% of the population's work disability was found to stem from it (69). There is always the question of proper diagnosis with such studies, but modern diagnostic tools—particularly magnetic resonance imaging (MRI), discography, thermography, and electronic neuromuscular functional studies—are now much more effective in producing accurate diagnoses. They also found that one-third of the patients with the disc syndrome had been previously hospitalized for it, and one-fifth of them already had surgery for it. We believe that this indicates the necessity of a basic rehabilitation program for all such conditions. *The authors believe that any condition in which there is a high recidivism rate points strongly toward the lack of proper rehabilitative procedures.*

Pain researchers at the University of California, Berkeley, indicated that subjects who participated in athletics had higher pain thresholds (70). This was either because of their increased tolerance, due to learned behavior (or biochemical factors, such as endorphin release) or because high pain threshold people tended more to participate in sports. Increased frequency of activity, in decreasing order of effect, for weight lifting, running, and stretching tended to decrease low back pain.

Changes in the vertebrae and discs are apparent on MRI after 5 weeks of bed rest. Specifically, there is a decrease in the nucleus that is theorized to be caused by water loss (71). Therefore, some form of motion, even passive or assistive, in the gravity field is suggested whenever possible.

Evidence shows that low back pain may accompany 85% of acceleration/deceleration injuries within the first year. In fact, greater than 70% showed a delayed onset of more than 4 months, the "delayed low back syndrome" (72). The significance here is that it is all too common to ignore the lower back when complaints are minimal or absent in traumatic cervical injuries. Our suggestion is to examine the so-called "asymptomatic" low back even more thoroughly and include it in the rehabilitation program with the least excuse to do so.

The following weaknesses and imbalances are to be addressed in most low back injuries: hamstrings, lower back muscle groups, hip flexors, and abdominals (3, p. 295). In low back rehabilitation programs, the rather seldom used abdominals and the gluteal muscles usually need to be strengthened to perform such important activities as climbing stairs and ladders and getting up from sitting or lying down. Together, these muscle groups act as a force couple, causing the pelvis to flex (posteriorly), reducing the lumbar lordosis, and relaxing the tension on the low back (73).

Intervertebral Disc Syndromes

Intradiscal pressures change dramatically with body postural changes. Therefore, when rehabilitating someone with moderate to severe discopathies, with or without radiculalgias, we strongly recommend that exercises be initiated in positions that stress those joints least. Intradiscal pressure is least while lying supine, increases by nearly 50% when sitting with the knees and hips flexed, and almost doubles if one leans forward while sitting (4, p. 459). Additionally, due to gravitational and imbibitional effects, the disc swells during prolonged recumbent periods or while in traction (74, p. 335). Therefore, as soon as one resumes weight bearing, the intradiscal pressure is far greater until one can ambulate and normalize it again. This is why intermittent traction is favored over static traction and why sustained bed rest should whenever possible be interspersed with periods of activity. Rather than forceful motions, we recommend beginning the program with gentle, non-weight-bearing isotonic type motions, with gravity providing the main resistance. This is much of the basis for the success of the Cox-McManus type treatments on tables of those names

(75). Tractioning and mild loosening type maneuvers are usually effective and safe in the early stages as well. Some decisions are based upon the nature of the injury, such as the absence or presence of a disc fragment somewhere within the canal or foraminal confines. The usual moderate to severe muscle guarding can also increase intradiscal pressure and can even inhibit the venous drainage which might otherwise relieve it. Therefore, gentle stretching and massage procedures are indicated at this stage.

As the situation becomes subacute and then chronic, gradually increase range of motion by extending the thoracolumbar exercises into the allowable ranges. Whichever motion is most limited or produces most symptoms is begun last and needs the most work. Paying strict attention to the antalgic positions indicates what the patient will allow now and what will be necessary to accomplish later. As more motion is allowed, proceed to strengthening exercises. Many of the same principles apply for other types of injuries or injuries to other parts of the spine, although they may not all lead to the same possible neurological considerations.

Lumbar Vertebral Subluxation Complexes

Similar considerations apply to the lumbar spine, with three notable differences. (a) Anterior lumbar subluxations are usually of the spondylolisthesis variety, often accompanied by spondylolysis or congenitally anomalous structures. These are unlikely to be corrected, but they may be compensated. (b) Even though there is far greater incumbent load upon the lumbar segments normally there is an even greater amount of anatomical support for such a load. (c) The allowable normal motion is less in the lumbar spine; therefore, less dynamic stress exists. However, whenever there is a real or potential stenosis, all motion (and thereby exercise) must be considered with caution and clinical judgment.

Radiographic evidence of deficiencies in the rotational and lateral flexion mechanics of the lumbar spine is one of the earliest signs of degenerative disease (62). The authors use radiographic and goniometric evidence to demonstrate the progress of exercise programs, particularly in arthritides.

The main components of some degree of pathomechanics in the lumbar spine are inadequate contralateral spinous rotation (i.e., away from concavity) and disc wedging, which improperly reflects the side and degree of lateral flexion. Of course, the normal mechanical relationships are reversed in the lumbar spine. In other words, underrotation, over-rotation, or lack of rotation, concomitant with lateral flexion is aberrant (63). This may be demonstrable by thermographic techniques as well as radiographically (64, 65). Besides specific adjustive procedures, the authors highly recommend an equally specific exercise program to correct the dysfunction(s). As always, diagnostic and analytic procedures must precede treatment and corrective procedures.

Facet Syndromes

Approximately 75% of all static (postural) low back pain is directly related to hyperlordosis (76). Often, a hyperlordotic posture causes excess weight bearing and loading stresses upon the facets. In facet joint problems, extension can be a major problem and should generally be avoided, especially during weight bearing and heavy resistance type exercises. Eventually, with slow stretching and gentle small oscillations, this situation can be improved considerably. In other words, modifying frequency and spatial configuration can make an otherwise undesirable exercise successful. A strong determinant in rehabilitation of facetal irritations is whether there is associated hypomobility. The more chronic the hypomobility is, the more likely there will be adjacent hypermobility. Such excess motion must be handled carefully, because exercise could tend to exacerbate the fault produced secondarily by the fixated area(s). This is a typical problem in which postural improvement is a must, so that muscles are not strengthened in aberrant posture. Strengthening exercises themselves are not likely to improve posture on a long-term basis (77, p. 154). Other modifications are necessary when there is a concomitant arthritic disorder. This is particularly significant when osteophytic processes are likely to impinge upon nerves within the neuroforaminal confines. X-rays help to determine the motions and positions most likely to cause such interference and, therefore,

the exercises that are indicated or contraindicated.

Other Common Causes of Low Back Pain

The piriformis syndrome, which seems to have a much higher incidence in females (6:1), is a cause of low back pain which seems to defy the usual etiologies (78). It responds well to typical manual therapies, followed by exercise routines.

Some causes of the "failed back surgery syndrome" are reflex sympathetic dystrophy, soft tissue dysfunction, facet syndrome, internal disc disruption, pseudarthrosis, and metallic implants (79). Of these, probably only metallic implants and facet syndrome with severe arthrosis receive little help from therapeutic exercises. In most cases, severity of condition, complicating factors, patient tolerance to pain, and general physical health largely determine what success will be achieved in rehabilitation.

Neurologic Lesions

In upper motor neuron conditions, there is a loss of motor units, resulting in a loss of muscle tension feedback, which diminishes the capacity of the system to regulate force. As a result, rehabilitative exercises should be designed to allow for slow (tonic) muscle control, which is associated with low-threshold motor units (12, p. 176). In patients suffering from cerebral vascular accidents, there may be a reduction in the sensory threshold and an increased response to stimulus, resulting in an increase in tendon reflex reactions. The musculature of these patients is hyperreflexive, and this must be taken into consideration when designing an exercise program. Because a relatively small force can result in reflex spasm, over-reactions, or even myoclonus, very low intensities and relatively slow frequencies and short durations are best tolerated.

A few situations that demand variations in the exercise program. If the premotor cortex is injured, postural exercises may need to be initiated early to improve muscle tone for later exercises. The cerebellum is best benefited by exercises aimed at improving coordination. This is an oversimplification, but it serves as a starting point in developing a regimen.

In conditions involving nerve damage, rehabilitative exercises for the muscles are necessary after the nerve has healed. Sometimes exercise is initiated as soon as hypesthesia turns into pain, so long as it is not exacerbated by the procedures. There are many causes of chronic pain, including symptoms of a burning sensation, which courses a nerve pathway. The etiology may be a hyperactive sympathetic nervous system. Causalgia is the result of a partial injury to a major nerve, with subsequent symptoms of an overactive sympathetic nervous system. Reflex sympathetic dystrophy is often the result of a minor injury, or in some cases no apparent injury, with symptoms of an overactive sympathetic nervous system. Sudek's atrophy is also in this category. A common feature of all these type of disorders is a certain amount of osteopenia, along with muscle and inflammatory changes. Actually a more accurate name for all of them might be reflex autonomic dystonia, which describes all such problems at any stage of development. Symptoms may not correspond to normal dermatomal patterns or neural pathways. Pain may be caused by ischemia and/or any of the normal pathways. It may be the result of neural compression, which can cause lower motor neuron lesions, in this case, due to nerve root impingement. Vertebral subluxation complexes, spinal canal stenosis, and entities causing encroachment in the vertebral foraminal confines are common etiologies for neural compression syndromes.

Traction stretch injuries to nerves may be produced by excessive joint motion. This motion must produce a centrifugal force vector parallel to the anatomical line of the neural axon. An example may be the overstretching of the peroneal nerve after the lateral ligaments of the knee are sprained by an excessive varus force applied to the knee joint. Again, it is imperative that the rehabilitation is not only directed at the damaged nerve and ligaments, but at the associated musculature that may have been affected. Regular evaluation of the strength of the muscles served by the hypertractioned nerve indicates which muscles are affected and to what degree, and what

progress has been made. Care must be taken not to generate a significant force vector parallel to that causing the injury. The early phases of rehabilitation concentrate on reestablishing the neuromuscular connection. Strength and endurance training come during a later phase since a (partially) denervated muscle cannot be strengthened, in any case. It may take 6 weeks or more for phase one to be completed, following the pattern of Wallerian degeneration and regeneration.

In patients with lower motor neuron lesions, perform strengthening exercises cautiously, because there is increased injury risk from loading a joint controlled by an inactive or weakened muscle (12, p. 357).

It is recommended that muscle reeducation programs for such illnesses as poliomyelitis begin as soon as possible after the diagnosis is made (2, p. 558). Depending upon how much degeneration has already taken place, one may need to begin on a reflex level, initiating proprioceptive pathways by moving joints passively. Numerous exercise procedures are applicable to such rehabilitation, including sensory stimulation of the overlying skin, loosening, shaking, coordination maneuvers, and variations of these. Continuous and constant stimulation, as done in the creations of engrams, is very important, so long as intact pathways can be established. When incoordination occurs with an active motion, it is necessary to backtrack to assistive or even passive modes to correct the motion before returning to the current level of functioning. Inasmuch as coordination (or muscle balancing) is essentially a supraspinal function, strength and endurance training obviously occur later (2, p. 560). In muscle reeducation, avoid substitutions whenever possible by singular attention to form and by carefully palpating and observing the entire action.

The main function of muscle reeducation in the lower extremities is the production of a satisfactory gait for locomotion. The most important muscles relative to gait are those of the trunk, those of the upper extremities (needed for crutches, if the lower extremities are braced), and, in the lower extremities, the hip extensors, other thigh muscles (except quadriceps), ankle muscles, and quadriceps (2, p. 577–8). It is usually important to pay great attention to rehabilitating the gluteal muscles, which are often weak in such disorders, as attested by a positive Trendelenburg test (43, p. 7). Relationships of the entire kinetic chain that produces locomotion must be considered and attended to, or gait is highly altered.

Cardiovascular Rehabilitation

This section presents recommendations from several sources, which tend to reflect the general opinion, within narrow tolerances, of the academic community. Whether you chose one, amalgamate from all, or find your own sources is not important. A viable and safe cardiovascular rehabilitation program can be developed based on these principles. In this area the risk:benefit ratio may be challenged and specific emergency medical procedures may be required, so the clinic must be prepared to handle such exigencies, either internally or externally. It is a good idea to have a backup system for such situations.

The following recommendations from the National Athletic Health Institute in conjunction with a hospital staff. They reflect the concepts espoused from many diverse sources (80, pp. 19–21).

1. Regular exercise is imperative, because sporadic exercise appears to increase the body's clotting mechanism and the chance for overexertion.
2. Alcohol consumption tends to decrease the blood flow through the coronary arteries and is to be avoided for at least 4 hr before exercising.
3. Smoking decreases the amount of oxygen available and its transport across alveolar/capillary membranes. Total abstention is recommended.
4. Long duration and low intensity exercise is preferable over the inverse of this.
5. Do not end the workout with a sprint or other high demand activity; this can be catastrophic.
6. Avoid isometric exercises, because they increase blood pressure and cardiac work, while simultaneously increasing intrathoracic pressure, the latter decreasing venous return. Even exercises with isometric components — i.e., push-ups, pull-ups, water

skiing, and weight lifting—must be properly supervised.
7. Large meals are prohibited prior to exercising because they cause blood flow to be greatly increased to the gut and reduced proportionately elsewhere.
8. Be more cautious at high altitudes, because there is a reduced partial pressure of oxygen in the atmosphere.
9. Avoid temperature extremes that further increase cardiac output. This includes the use of a sauna or a hot or cold shower immediately following exercise.
10. Rubberized suits are contraindicated, due to increased water loss and increased heat retention. Use sweat clothes for warm-up and in cold weather only.
11. Do not chew gum while exercising, since this interferes with breathing and can be swallowed and lodge in an airway.
12. Allow at least 1 month of training for each year of inactivity.
13. Wear cool and unrestrictive clothing.

Program Parameters

In 1979 Froelicher made recommendations for cardiovascular fitness, that hold true today, with the possible exception of the duration (81). The frequency suggested was 3 to 5 days/week, evenly spaced. The intensity suggested was about 75% of the maximum heart rate (and/or maximum oxygen uptake). The duration suggested was from 15 to 60 min, either continuously or at intervals with short rest periods. There is some question as to whether there is significant cardiovascular benefit after 15 to 20 min of continuous activity. The modes of activity suggested were running, jogging, walking, bicycling, swimming, rowing, arm cranking, or endurance sports activities. Both activity and intensity may be modified according to any physical restrictions or abnormalities that coexist.

Intensity and duration are often dependent variables. The increase of one may signal the decrease of the other, in order to maintain the level of work. In addition, when the level of activity is elevated, one or both can be altered to affect the result. For beginners or those who are more severely injured, lower intensity and longer duration exercise is probably desirable. For beginners to enjoy, profit, and accomplish sufficient continuous training, the intensity level should be from 60 to 75% of the heart rate (HR) max reserve when walking briskly and from 75 to 85% of the HR max reserve when jogging (3, p. 250). A reasonable program for beginners alternates levels of intensity, i.e., as ability increases, the jogging periods increase proportionately. Periodic reevaluations and careful monitoring aid in determining when to make changes in the program.

The necessary frequency of cardiovascular exercise is three to four times a week, and the duration is 30 to 40 min/session. (80). Increased benefits can accrue beyond this, but not in proportion to the effort and not without significant risk. The intensity should be at such a level as to produce a target heart rate of between 70 and 85% of maximum. Below this is of little benefit and above this is of considerable risk (80, p. 8). Take the pulse rate every 5 min during the session 10 sec after exercise stops. Exercises are increased at regular intervals to the next level of each parameter, but not if the patient is markedly fatigued 1 to 2 hr after a workout (80, p. 16).

Cardiovascular respiratory fitness prescriptions have been developed by studying oxygen-carrying and utilization capacities. Improvement in maximum oxygen uptake is proportional to the frequency of training, although improvements with exercising more than 5 days/week are minimal and probably not worth pursuing (3, p. 55–6).

Exercise increases arterial blood pressure and can be useful for patients with peripheral vascular insufficiencies. Increased arterial pressure is a disadvantage for those with hypertension, and this must be considered.

Many disorders of structures of the neck, upper-mid back, and thoracic cage (i.e., chest wall syndrome) can mimic cardiac pain. Before exercises are decided upon, one must differentiate those causes from cardiovascular etiologies (82). For noncardiac conditions, appropriate exercise programs should be instituted immediately. However, in patients with cardiovascular disorders, stress testing and appropriate examinations and laboratory procedures should first be performed to discover the extent of damage and the relative ability to exercise.

Respiratory Function

Rehabilitation of respiratory function has two distinct components, which merge at the neurological level. The biomechanical functioning of the physical parts and the functional element within the cardiovascular and pulmonary systems can be involved together or separately. Eventually, when the situation is sufficiently chronic, they are both involved.

Proper upright posture and maintenance of respiratory function depend upon strong vertebral, scalenus, and thoracic cage muscle groups (83). There is generally noted an increased sense of strength and vitality when a person throws back his shoulders and straightens his spine, while taking a deep breath, from an initially mildly flexed, slouching posture. Nilsson postulated that such a result is too rapid for the coursing circulation (8 to 18 seconds) to be a factor, thereby suggesting that this effect is due to the relief of some amount of nerve root pressure (83). This emphasizes the necessity of creating and reinforcing good static posture, as well as postural mechanics, in the course of most exercise programs.

Dynamic exercises should be performed rhythmically and in a manner that does not impede normal forced breathing (3, p. 269). When performed rhythmically, the parameters are easier to follow and the chances of injury are reduced. Also remember that the heavier the load, the more the impedance of respiration and circulation becomes a consideration. This is a self-limiting factor in any exercise program. There is no specific cadence to recommend for any particular condition or type of person. However, it is usually easy to match exercises with some phase of or ratio to one's respiratory actions. There is much said about in which phase of respiration to perform exercises or manipulations, but this will not be discussed here. The authors do recommend that exertive exercises, like those to build strength, be performed in the expiratory phase. This maximizes and focuses strength and protects the lower abdomen from overstress.

One can reduce the asthmogenicity of exercises by attending to two factors (84), diaphragmatic breathing and exhalation against pressure, which reduce trapped air and prevent asthma.

Prone exercises should be modified or eliminated for patients with chronic respiratory distress syndromes. Sometimes, soft pillows can make the position comfortable enough. Even supine exercises can be arduous, unless the arms are elevated above the head, thus expanding the capacity of the thoracic cage. Such patients may be assisted by partially propping them up at the cephalad end. This is a virtual necessity when the patient is orthopneic. Also, such patients are easily "winded," have low endurance, and are easily placed in oxygen debt, thus fatiguing more quickly. Therefore, exercise intensity, frequency and duration may start at lower levels and progress more slowly than in patients whose problems are more mechanical. Most of these concepts apply equally well to patients with cardiovascular problems.

Mechanical Respiratory Considerations

The thoracocostal facet syndrome is one in which a rib or ribs are subluxated, with respect to their relationships with the thoracic vertebrae. The following muscles are involved in this syndrome: pectoralis minor, pectoralis major (particularly the sternal division), serratus anterior, intercostales externi, intercostales interni, transversus thoracis, rectus abdominis, and diaphragm (85). In an acute situation, usually precipitated by trauma, keep the joint(s) mobilized and the muscles toned, provided bone pathology is ruled out. In a chronic situation, strengthening of these muscles is a must. The obvious connection with respiration increases the importance of these lesions.

Properly conducted breathing exercises help to correct the problem. Maintaining efficient posture has a direct bearing on the correction of a chronic misalignment of this nature, and poor posture can worsen the condition. The lesion is more typically in the posterior elements of articulation than in the anterior elements (85). Therefore, exercise should emphasize utilizing the stronger, more stable, anterior joints as fulcrums of motion for the more labile posterior ones. This type of lesion may need to be rehabilitated after surgery for cardiopulmonary disorders. These situations are often produced or exacerbated by a sudden motion (such as a sneeze or cough) while in a yawn or stretch type position. This position is best described as sitting or standing with both arms abducted about 90°, both elbows flexed about 135°, and the arms extended and scapulae adducted simultaneously, in a slow stretching motion. Because of the potential to disturb the breathing apparatus, relaxation exercises are usually recommended as well. The thoracocostal facet syndrome is most commonly found at the sixth thoracic level (85), if for no other reason than this is near the apex of the normal thoracic kyphosis.

Miscellaneous Considerations

One must provide adequate recovery time after every resistive exercise session in the program. Normal recovery times vary from about 1 hr to remove lactic acid to several days to replenish glycogen stores (4, p. 73). It has been shown that fatigue recovery occurs faster when light exercise is performed during the recovery period than it does with total rest (4, p. 74). This relates to the warm-down period.

Trick Actions

Vicarious motions are those motions which either deceive the therapist (examiner) into believing a muscle or group is working, when it is paralyzed, or successfully replace the function lost by obvious paralysis (2, pp. 117–27). Because of their nature, they are also referred to as "trick movements" or "trick actions." An example of the first type is the simulation of finger abduction by the long extensors when there is an ulnar nerve paralysis (2, p. 117). The second type is shown in the abduction and elevation of the shoulder, despite total paralysis of the deltoid.

There are several modes by which these trick actions take place (2, pp. 117–8). (a) There can be direct substitution of one muscle for another. For example, the biceps, pectoralis, and rotator cuff muscles can effectively abduct an arm in the absence of a functioning deltoid. Such substitution will usually be accompanied by an alteration in the normal motion, which can then appear "jerky" and limited. (b) Sometimes, an accessory insertion, from another muscle, like the abductor pollicis brevis has into the extensor aponeurosis of the thumb, can produce the desired action, in this case, thumb extension by an abductor despite a loss of extensor tone due to a radial nerve palsy (2, p. 118). Just as in substitution, the alternate contractor cannot function as efficiently as the paralyzed prime mover did normally. Therefore, the resultant contraction is diminished, at best. (c) Another mode is via the tendon action secondary to an antagonist's contraction. An example of this is the way wrist extension can cause a slight passive flexion of the fingers, even though finger flexors are otherwise paralyzed by a discontinuity in their typical nerve supply. (d) A rebound phenomenon occurs when a strong contraction of the antagonist is followed by a sudden relaxation, giving the appearance and feel of a contraction in the prime mover. The neurological basis for such events is discussed in Chapter 2. (e) Trick actions may also be due to the effects of gravity. According to the muscle testing system, the weakest strength of a muscle refers to its inability to move against gravity. (86). An example of this is the inability to extend the elbow or knee while the shoulder is abducted and the hip is flexed, due to a gross weakness in the triceps or quadriceps, respectively.

Rehabilitating Neuronal Injuries

It must be remembered that no trick movement truly fills in for the physiological motor unit (PMU) that is injured; it can only approximate the appropriate response. However, it has been said that movements, not muscles, are represented in the brain (2, p. 121). Therefore, during the long recuperative period, while awaiting nerve regeneration, if the proper movement patterns are produced, the reeducation process is facilitated and the deficit in activities of daily living is lessened. Often, an appropriate, movable splinting device is used both to guide the motion and to support the anatomical motor units involved. The splint also helps to prevent the deformity that would normally be caused by the relatively (or absolutely) hypertonic antagonist. Early therapeutic aims in such palsies are to strengthen the synergists, maintain range of motion, and keep the normal motion path active, for facilitation purposes. For permanent injuries, this is all one can expect. When the injury is deemed recoverable, one gradually integrates the weakened muscle into the program, lessening support

(both mechanical and human) as soon as possible. Then one works on coordination and endurance as the injured PMU becomes capable of such action. During the course of rehabilitation, especially in the early stages, stretching the hypertonic antagonist is necessary to prevent debilitating contractures and injuries to other structures. In some permanent injuries, surgical transplantation of an active tendon can be a useful and functional solution when all else fails. It is a most helpful rule that the earliest sign of recovery in a lower motor neuron lesion is the elimination of trick movements, even though little or no actual movement may be seen (2, p. 127).

Visualization Techniques

There has been a great deal of research on visualization procedures, and the results of such mental imaging are well documented by noted Stanford brain researcher Karl Pribram (87). We believe this mechanism is as great an aid in exercising for rehabilitation as in rehearsing for a performance. People of all ages and types, from pianists to high jumpers, have utilized this process to enhance performance (87).

First, a proper knowledge and visual image in one's head of the nature and location of the structures in the body that are being trained allows one to perform with superior accuracy. Second, the patient gets the sense, and the reality, of control over his or her performance, even in the earliest stages. Last, and most importantly, the brain does not know the difference between an activity in physical space and the same activity conducted within the confines of its neural tissues alone (87).

Thinking in terms of engram formation, this is a very powerful concept. Once a physical process is known by a patient, in intimate detail, it can be reproduced within one's brain while sitting still. This means one can, to a certain extent, perform one's exercises or practice one's skills virtually anywhere and nearly all day. This kind of focus will definitely speed up a healing or learning process, but it must be done precisely to be effective. The difficulty is in knowing that one has performed the activity according to specifications, without the three-dimensional feedback normally received from the physical body. That is the present limitation, apparently; and, more research needs to be done in this area to see exactly what proportion of training can be accomplished by visualization techniques.

Nutrition

Nutritional factors are numerous, with respect to exercise. An example of a biochemical substance that naturally enhances performance is the incremental effect of potassium-magnesium aspartate on endurance (88). There should also be sufficient protein in the diet to supply the demands of the resultant muscle hypertrophy. Certainly, obesity or general malnutrition interferes with any rehabilitation program and needs to be considered and, hopefully, corrected. The authors recommend regular and continuous monitoring of progress during the exercise program. This protects the patient and the doctor and informs all concerned, including third party payers. Mechanical, computerized muscle strength testing is a favored mode of neuromuscular evaluation. One of the important findings of this testing is that when purified chondroitin sulfates are added to the patient's diet during rehabilitation, healing time is shortened and strength gain is improved (89). Nutritional requirements for an individual vary with age, gender, special considerations (like pregnancy), and overall condition.

Exercise during Pregnancy

Exercises for pregnant women have a few distinct purposes. In the prenatal period, exercises can be designed to relieve back pain and to improve conditioning and muscle tone in order to facilitate delivery. Some traditional obstetricians believe that continuous, daily, prenatal exercising can help to maintain a woman's figure (90, pp. 112–3). Because of the effort required during the actual delivery, the authors recommend endurance type exercises for about 6 to 8 weeks prior to the birth. Virtually all pregnant women suffer from a certain degree of back pain during gestation (90, p. 97). The combination of increased load (i.e., weight bearing), altered postural demeanor (both static and dynamic), and hormonally induced ligamentous laxity produces the majority of problems. The ligamentous laxity makes it unlikely (and even contraindi-

cated) that stretching exercises would be of benefit. However, strengthening and endurance conditioning are definitely in order, as are postural exercises. Furthermore, because most natural delivery methods involve regulated breathing, respiratory exercises are equally important. In this situation, breathing exercises often do not involve the abdominal breathing because it might interfere with uterine contractions. Strengthening of the pelvic floor and perineal musculature is also recommended, usually by bearing-down exercises, which are a form of isometric contractions.

In the postnatal period, exercises are mainly to retone the muscles and to help the tissues and body recover normal form and function. These may be termed restorative exercises. Postnatal exercises are to be performed at four bouts and two sessions daily, for at least 1 month postpartum (90, p. 211).

Observe certain precautions in exercises for pregnant women. The maternal heart rate should not exceed 140 beats/min, and strenuous activities should not exceed 15 min in duration. The woman should drink liberal amounts of liquids before and after exercising. Deep flexion or extension of joints or vigorous stretching of muscles and tendons is to be avoided due to hormonally induced joint laxity. Prone exercises are contraindicated after the fourth month of gestation. Avoid exercises employing the Valsalva maneuver, and stop if maternal temperature exceeds 38°C. If the patient is very athletic and has been highly active prior to pregnancy, most of these proscriptions can be modified to a certain extent.

In the gravid female, due to the necessary alteration in weight-bearing mechanics and probable shift of center of mass, some automatic changes take place in muscle dynamics. For instance, the accentuated calcaneal weight bearing stresses the hip flexor and knee extensor groups, in their attempt to sustain an erect posture (91). This causes a muscle imbalance to ensue, as these muscles dominate their antagonists, and causes the sacral base angle to increase. The result of this is that facets and spinous processes become compressed increasingly, in direct proportion to the lumbar lordosis. Such a situation may be counteracted by the use of isometric and/or isotonic exercises of hip extensors and knee flexors. This would support the adjustive and therapeutic aspects of a treatment program and may even be used preventively. It is also a good idea to use range of motion exercises to keep the spinal segments mobilized.

Relaxation Exercises

There is evidence that performing relaxation exercises prior to surgery reduces post-surgical pain (92). Furthermore, progressive relaxation techniques can be utilized in controlling pain ratings. They seem to be able to block chronic pain even better than biofeedback, acting as a behavioral modification process (93).

Several aspects of relaxation that are related to this or any exercise program. First, some exercises are specifically aimed at relaxing the person, as a whole. This refers essentially to psychosomatic features. For example, the effects of anxiety are well known. The central nervous system is hyperstimulated, causing prolonged myospasms, among other results. Second, there is often a relaxation period between actual contractions, or between sets or cycles in a given session. Third, each given exercise is generally intended for a specific anatomical location, thus requiring relaxation of the rest of the body. Last, some patients are either overtense or asthenic, and they may benefit from short, intermittent rest periods at selected times.

The first step in a progressive relaxation program is to recognize the amount of tension that exists in a given area. The muscle is gradually relaxed on a voluntary basis, then tension is gradually increased voluntarily again (2, p. 919). This is most useful when there is muscle spasm in a normal joint.

Elderly Patients

Exercise programs for the elderly can be as variable as they are for any other group, with the same relative precautions. Those who have remained quite active with a relatively high level of fitness will, of course, have little difficulty with most rehabilitative procedures. The main consideration is in the relative length of the healing process. Compared to others who have been relatively inactive for some time, it may take older people longer than average to perform most tasks and they will probably be more susceptible to secondary injury. In general, the longer someone has been inactive, the more difficult it will be to motivate them to perform regular exercise maneuvers.

Adolescent Patients

The main concern with adolescents is that strength training not be performed at too high an intensity level. The emphasis should be placed on higher repetition and lower load endeavors. Loads should not be increased until at least 15 repetitions can be performed in perfect form, and increments should be smaller than for adults.

Neural Regeneration

The newest evidence indicates that nerve cell regeneration is probably possible. It has been shown in the lamprey (94), and in axonal regeneration via neuronal grafts (95) that such results may be possible. Borgens' et al regenerated dorsal nerve axons and cell bodies in a guinea pig, with the application of weak electrical fields (96). These electrical fields were postulated to approximate the kind of fields present during embryonic development. Whether they apply to humans is uncertain, but they are moving gradually up the evolutionary scale. It is also questionable whether function can be restored, even though structure has been regenerated. This is "where there's life, there's hope" issue, because structure and function are each believed to give birth to the other under proper circumstances. Among these proper circumstances is the application of therapeutic movements (i.e., exercising) for the purpose of stimulating appropriate neuroanatomical substrate formation and neurophysiological responses. Where there is no function, one would obviously initiate this process with passive actions and work through the spectrum of activities.

Cross–Crawl Exercises

The addition of cross-crawl type exercises to the exercise program tends to improve overall performance. Also, changing exercises which tend toward homolateral extremity activity into ones with a cross-crawl nature tends to prevent recidivism and shorten the time needed for correction of a problem (97).

Thoracic Outlet Syndrome

In thoracic outlet syndrome (TOS), one of the following muscles is usually tight and requires stretching: scalenus group, levator scapulae, or pectoralis minor. (4 p. 474). Additionally, such muscles as the subclavius, biceps (short head), and the coracobrachialis may play a minor role in altering the space available in the thoracic outlet. The sternoclavicular and glenohumeral joints need to be mobilized, and the scapulocostal area needs to be freely movable. Postural training, free movement, and development of proper curvatures in both the cervical and thoracic spines are usual procedures for this condition. Teaching proper abdominal-diaphragmatic breathing and relaxation of the thoracic cage is also necessary to produce lasting results.

Hundreds of different conditions could be considered here. However, the information presented is the basis for developing an exercise program appropriate for any patient's needs. Think in terms of a proper differential diagnosis, including the specific tissues that have been injured and the nature of the pathophysiology produced. Once those entities are determined, use the information and concepts provided in this chapter to design an appropriate program. Specific exercises are presented in the following chapters.

References

1. Applied Kinesiology: The Advanced Approach in Chiropractic. Pueblo, CO; D. Walther Systems, Pueblo, CO, 1976.
2. Basmajian JV, Wolf SL: Therapeutic Exercise. 5th ed. Baltimore:Williams & Wilkins, 1990.
3. Pollock ML, Wilmore JH, Fox SM III: Exercise in Health and Disease. Philadelphia:WB Saunders, 1984.
4. Kisner C, Colby LA: Therapeutic Exercise. Philadelphia:FA Davis, 1985.
5. Waters B, Goodheart G: Applied Kinesiology. Workshop Manual. Detroit, 1972.
6. Workbook, Seminar on Chiropodiatrics. Long Beach, CA: American Orthotic Laboratories, 1985.
7. Bates BT, Osternig LR, Mason B, James LS: Foot orthotic devices to modify selected aspects of lower extremity mechanics. Am J Sports Med. 1979;7(6):338–42.
8. Goodheart GJ: Posture: 30 years of observation and some logical chiropractic conclusions. Part III. Dig Chiropract Econ Nov/Dec 1987:62–7, 128–9.
9. Williams M, Worthingham C: Therapeutic Exercise for Body Alignment and Function. Philadelphia, WB Saunders, 1960:33–6.
10. Martin JP: A short essay on posture and movement. J Neurol Neurosurg Psychiatry 1977; 40:25–9.
11. Brennan MJ: Adaptations to bipedalism. ACA J Chiropract November 1980;14:24–33.
12. Delisa JA: Rehabilitation Medicine. Philadelphia:JB Lippincott, 1988.
13. Perry L: Spring into action: make your exercise workouts safe. ICA J 1986;2(1):1.
14. Feagin J, Hlavac H, Miller HS, Walsh W: Helpful hints for joggers' doctors. Patient Care, April 30, 1979: 130–167.
15. Kottke FJ, Stillwell KG, Lehman JF: Krusen's Handbook of Physical Medicine and Rehabilitation. 3rd ed. Philadelphia:WB Saunders, 1982.
16. Harvey JS: Rehabilitation of the Injured Athlete. Clinics in Sports Medicine. Philadelphia, WB Saunders, July 1985, vol 4, no 3.
17. Daniels L, Worthingham C: Therapeutic Exercise for Body Alignment and Function. 2nd ed. Philadelphia:WB Saunders, 1977.
18. Perrine JJ: Isokinetic exercise and the mechanical energy potentials of muscle. J Health Phys Ed Rec 1968;39:40–4.
19. Marras WS, Wongsam PE: Flexibility and velocity of the normal and impaired lumbar spine. Arch Phys Med Rehabil 1986;67:213–7.
20. Vahl RJ, Bettermann-Vahl DE: Some biomechanical basis of therapeutic exercise. Dig Chiropract Econ, March/April 1987; 14–18, 116–117.
21. Pollock ML: How much exercise is enough? Physician Sports Med, June 1978; 50–64.
22. Payne FE Jr: A practical approach to effective exercise. Am Fam Prac 1979;19(6):76–81.
23. Gemmell HA: Myofascial pain syndrome. Am Chiropract Aug 1988; vol. 3, 64–6.
24. Cavanagh PR, Komi PV: Electromechanical delay in human skeletal muscle under concentric and eccentric contractions. Eur J Appl Physiol 1979;42(3):159–63.
25. Bosco C, Komi PV, Ito A: Prestretch potentiation of human skeletal muscle during ballistic movement. Acta Physiol Scand 1981;111(2):135–40.
26. Bosco C, Komi PV: Potentiation of the mechanical behavior of the human skeletal muscle through prestretching. Acta Physiol Scand 1979; 106(4):467–72.
27. Komi PV, Viitasalo JT: Changes in motor unit activity and metabolism in human skeletal muscle during and after repeated eccentric and concentric contractions. Acta Physiol Scand 1977; 100(2):246–54.
28. O'Donoghue DH: Treatment of Injuries to Athletes. 3rd ed. Philadelphia:WB Saunders, 1976.
29. Hakkinen K, Komi PV, Alen M: Effect of explosive type strength training on isometric force- and relaxation-time, electromyographic and muscle fibre characteristics of leg extensor muscles. Acta Physiol Scand 1985;125(4):587–600.
30. Hakkinen K, Komi PV: Training-induced changes in neuromuscular performance under voluntary and reflex conditions. Eur J Appl Physiol 1988; 55(2):147–55.
31. Bosco C, Tihanyi J, Komi PV, et al: Store and recoil of elastic energy in slow and fast types of human skeletal muscles. Acta Physiol Scand 1982; 116(4):343–9.
32. Michaud T: Pedal biomechanics as related to or-

thotic therapies: an overview. Part I. Dig Chiropract Econ, Nov/Dec 1986;20–25.

33. Loeser JD: Almost any therapy relieving acute pain worsens chronic pain. Fam Practice News, December 1–14, 1985.

34. Kuprian W, ed: Physical Therapy for Sports. Philadelphia:WB Saunders, 1982.

35. Manniche C, Hesselsoe G, Bentzen L, et al: Clinical trial of intensive training for chronic low back pain. Lancet. 1988;2:1473–6.

36. Harvey JS: Rehabilitation of the Injured Athlete. Clinics in Sports Medicine. Philadelphia:WB Saunders, July 1985 vol 4, no 3.

37. Douglas JE, Wilkes T, David I: Reconditioning cardiac patients. Am Fam Prac, Jan 1975;123–9.

38. Simonelli C, Eaton RP: Cardiovascular and metabolic effects of exercise. Postgrad Med 1978; 63(2):71–7.

39. Wilbur A: Woes of the weekend jock. Sci Dig, Mar 1986; 18.

40. Olson DW: Iliotibial band friction syndrome. Athletic Train 1986;21:32–5.

41. Christensen K: Shin splints. Dig Chiropract Econ, Jan/Feb 1988;68.

42. Bonamo JJ: More than just a sprained ankle. Emerg Med, 1977;97–9, 105–6, 111–12.

43. Janse J, Kissinger RN: The relationship of the mechanical integrity of the feet, lower extremities, pelvis, and spine to the proper function of the various structural and visceral systems of the body. Chicago, National College of Chiropractic, 1975.

44. Murphy DJ: Whiplash and Spinal Trauma Notes. 2nd ed. Privately published, 1985.

45. Cyriax J: Textbook of Orthopaedic Medicine. volume 1. Diagnosis of Soft Tissue Lesions. 6th ed, Baltimore:Williams & Wilkins, 1975.

46. Keim HA: Low Back Pain. Clinical Symposia. Ciba Pharmaceutical Company, 1973, vol 25, no 3.

47. Hanus SW: The anterior cruciate ligament dilemma. Dig Chiropract Econ, March/April, 1987;126–31.

48. Schoenholtz F: Conservative management of selected shoulder problems. ACA J Chiropract. 1979;13:91–8.

49. Lawrence DJ: The frozen shoulder: conservative management. ACA J Chiropract 1981;15:49–51.

50. Hammer WI: Specificity in soft-tissue diagnosis and treatment. ACA J Chiropract, 1986;20:38–9.

51. Mladenoff E: Sports injuries: diagnosis and treatment of racquet wrist and jumper's knee. Am Chiropract, May 1986;52–6, 61.

52. Dickerson CR: Postfracture treatment of the patella. Dig Chiropract Econ, March/April 1987; 64–9.

53. Wejsflog A, Dubowski A: Stern cartilage test. Med Tribune, September 25, 1985.

54. Jeffers K: The "running doctor" reports on "overuse injuries." Dynamic Chiropractor, July 15, 1989;28.

55. Dehaven KE, Dolan WA, Mayer PJ: Chondromalacia patellae in athletes. Am J Sports Med 1979;7(1):5–11.

56. Christensen K: Chondromalacia patellae—the runner's knee. Success Express, April/June 1981; 12–9.

57. Harrison DD: Mechanisms of injury during whiplash accidents. Am Chiropract, May 1987;16–29.

58. Cailliet R: Soft Tissue Pain and Disability. Philadelphia:FA Davis, 1977.

59. Janecki CJ, Lipke JM: Whiplash syndrome. Am Fam Prac 1978;17(4):144–151.

60. Phillips RB: Upper cervical biomechanics. ACA J Chiropract 1976;X:127–35.

61. Croft AC, Foreman SM: The anterior subluxation: a subtle manifestation of soft tissue damage. Am Chiropract, Oct 1987;10–4.

62. Cassidy DJ: Roentgenological examination of the functional mechanics of the lumbar spine in lateral flexion. J CCA, July 1976;13–16.

63. Aragona RJ: Lateral bending lumbar x-rays. ASBE course notes, lumbar section, 1987;70.

64. Kneebone WJ, Grand LS: A correlation of lateral flexion lumbar spinal radiographs and thermograms on chiropractic patients: a pilot study. Second Opinion: J Int Acad Clin Thermol; 1989; 1(2):12–5.

65. Aragona RJ: Normal lumbar biomechanics. ASBE course notes, lumbar section, 1987;50–78.

66. Christensen KD: Clinical Chiropractic Biomechanics. 2nd ed. Va:Foot Levelers, 1984.

67. Waddell G: A new clinical model for the treatment of low-back pain. Spine 1987;12:632–44.

68. Karvonen MJ, Viitasalo JT, Komi PV, et al: Back and leg complaints in relation to muscle strength in young men. Scand J Rehabil Med 1980; 12(2):53–9.

69. Heliovaara M, Impivaara O, Sievers K, Melkas T, et al: Lumbar disc syndrome in Finland. J Epidemiol Commun Health 1987;41:251–8.

70. Kirk RO: Pain thresholds in athletes. Today's Chiropractic, Dec/Jan 1987; 71.

71. LeBlanc AD, Schonfeld E, Schneider VS, Evans HJ, Taber KH: The spine: changes in T2 relaxation times from disuse. Radiology 1988;169:105–7.

72. Neel SS, Mercer B, Young G: The relationship between whiplash injury and subsequent lower back complications. Chiropractic 1988; 1:86–8.

73. Christensen K: Therapeutic exercise and evaluation of muscle strength. Success Express, Jan/Mar 1981;46–51.

74. White AA, Panjabi MM: Clinical Biomechanics of the Spine. Philadelphia:JB Lippincott, 1978.

75. Cox JM: Low back pain diagnosis and treatment. Today's Chiropractic, Nov/Dec 1987;67–70, 111.

76. Shamos DE: Hyperlordosis and low back pain. Dig Chiropract Econ, Jan/Feb 1989;48.

77. Torg JS, Vegso JJ, Torg E: Rehabilitation of Athletic Injuries. Chicago:Year Book Medical Publishers, 1987.

78. Neel SS, Jheeta GS: Pyriformis Syndrome. ACA J Chiropract, 1987;20(12): 32–5.

79. Pate D: The failed back surgery syndrome. Part II. Dynamic Chiropractic, Sept 1, 1989;26.

80. National Athletic Health Institute staff: Exercise for a Healthy Heart, Presented as part of a community health education program in coordination with the Daniel Freeman Hospital Department of Education, 1984.

81. Froelicher VF: Benefits and risks of exercise programs for cardiac patients. Med Times, May 1979;79–84.

82. Epstein SE, Gerber LH, Borer JS: Chest wall syndrome: a common cause of unexplained cardiac pain. JAMA 1979;241(26): 2793–7.

83. Nilsson AV: The price man pays for being ortho-

static. The ACA Journal of Chiropractic, August 1975;IX:98–101.

84. Sheehan GA Letters JAMA 1977;237(2):120.
85. Maurer EL: The thoraco-costal facet syndrome with introduction of the marginal line and the rib sign. ACA J Chiropract, 1976;X:151–64.
86. Kendall HO, Kendall FP, Wadsworth GE: Muscle Testing and Function. 2nd ed. Baltimore:Williams & Wilkins, 1971;10–1
87. DeVore S.: The Neuropsychology of Self-Discipline. New York:SyberVision Systems, 1985.
88. Gupta JS, Srivastava KK: Effect of K-Mg aspartates on endurance work in man. Presented at the Defense Institute of Physiology and Allied Sciences, Delhi, India, April 1973.
89. Christensen KD: Quantification of lumbar function via mechanical muscle testing. Dig Chiropract Econ, March/April 1987;74–8.
90. Benson RC: Handbook of Obstetrics and Gynecology. Fifth Edition. Lange Medical Publications, California, 1974.
91. Blankenship T, Blankenship VG: Biomechanics of back pain in the gravid female. ACA J Chiropract, 1980;14:113–5.
92. Lawlis GF, Selby D, Hinnant D, McCoy CE: Reduction of postoperative pain parameters by pre-surgical relaxation instructions for spinal pain patients. Spine 1985;10:649–51.
93. Linton SJ: Behavioral remediation of chronic pain: a status report. Pain 1986;24:125–41.
94. Borgens R, et al: Nerve regeneration using electronic fields in the lamprey. Proc Natl Acad Sci, USA 1980;77:1209–13.
95. Medical Tribune, March 6, 1985; 16.
96. Borgens R, et al: J Compar Neurol, 1986; 247–8.
97. Stevenson RW: Cross crawl pattern: an adjunct to other exercise programs. Dig Chiropract Econ, January/February 1977; 9, 114.

6

Specific Conditions by Body Area

The following conditions are discussed according to body areas. The muscles involved with each condition and, in some cases, the mechanics of the injury are discussed. There is a description of the rehabilitative exercises recommended for each area (Table 6.1). Rehabilitative exercises listed are potential recommendations only. A complete analysis of the patient's condition is necessary to determine the proper series and sequence of exercises and the parameters utilized. Furthermore, not all muscles associated with an area may be in need of rehabilitation. The clinician must assess the extent of muscle involvement in the injury. However, lack of direct involvement in the injury may not rule out the need to rehabilitate a muscle as a functional component in the supportive mechanism for the injured unit.

Cervical Spine

Acute Cervical Sprain Syndrome

An acute cervical sprain is a common traumatic neuromuscular type condition. It may be the result of an automobile accident, a work-related injury, or a sports injury. The patient may complain of having his neck "jammed," pain in the cervical spine, inability to move his neck, and radiating pain into the shoulders and/or upper extremities. Sometimes, cephalgia is a primary feature of this injury. The specific rehabilitative exercise program prescribed

will depend on whether the injury involved flexion, extension, rotation, or lateral bending. It is also necessary to determine the status of the musculature at the time of the injury, i.e., whether they were loaded in anticipation of the impending trauma, or were in a relaxed state.

Hyperflexion Injury

The sternocleidomastoid, scalenus, splenius, levator scapulae, and cervical paravertebral muscles are involved. Exercises for flexion rehabilitation are 7.1.1, 7.1.2, 7.3, 7.3.1, 7.6, 7.10, and 7.13 (see Chapter 7).

Hyperextension Injury

The sternocleidomastoid, scalenus, splenius, semispinalis capitis, trapezius, levator scapulae, and intrinsic muscles are involved. Exercises for extension rehabilitation are 7.1.1, 7.1.2, 7.1.3, 7.1.4, 7.3, 7.4, 7.5, 7.5.1, 7.6, 7.7, 7.8, 7.9, 7.10, 7.11, and 7.12 (see Chapter 7).

Rotation injuries

Muscles involved are the sternocleidomastoids and the small intrinsic muscles. Exercises for rotation rehabilitation are 7.1.2, 7.3, 7.3.1, 7.4, 7.6, 7.8, 7.9, and 7.12 (see Chapter 7).

Lateral Flexion Injuries

Muscles involved are the scalenus anticus, scalenus medius, scalenus posticus,

Table 6.1. Specific Conditions

Condition	Muscles Involves	Exercises
Cervical spine		
Flexion injury	Sternocleidomastoid, scalenus, paravertebral	7.1.1, 7.1.2, 7.3, 7.3.1, 7.6, 7.10, 7.13
Extension injury	Levator scapulae, splenius, semispinalis, capitis, trapezius, intrinsic	7.1.1, 7.1.2, 7.1.3, 7.1.4, 7.3, 7.4, 7.5, 7.5.1, 7.6, 7.7, 7.8, 7.9, 7.10, 7.11, 7.12
Rotation injury	Trapezius, sternocleidomastoid, small intrinsic	7.1.2, 7.3, 7.3.1, 7.4, 7.6, 7.8, 7.9, 7.12
Lateral flexion injuries	Trapezius, levator scapulae, scalenus anticus, scalenus medius, scalenus posticus, small intrinsic	7.2, 7.2.1, 7.3, 7.3.1, 7.4, 7.6, 7.8, 7.9, 7.10, 7.12, 7.14
Brachial plexus, axonotmesis/neuropraxis	Muscles of upper extremity, including shoulder girdle	8.1, 8.2, 8.3, 8.4, 8.5, 8.6, 8.8, 8.9, 8.10, 8.11, 8.12, 8.13, 8.15, 8.16, 8.17, 8.18, 8.19, 8.22
Torticollis	Intrinsic cervical muscles, sternocleidomastoid	7.1, 7.2, 7.3, 78.4, 7.6, 7.8, 7.9, 7.12
Scalenus syndrome	Anterior, middle, posterior scalene	7.1, 7.1.2, 7.2, 7.2.1, 7.3, 7.3.1, 7.6, 7.10, 7.13, 7.13.1, 7.13.2, 7.14
Shoulder		
Rotator cuff tear	Biceps, supraspinatus, infraspinatus, teres minor, subscapularis	8.1, 8.2, 8.3, 8.4, 8.5, 8.6, 8.7, 8.8, 8.9, 8.10, 8.11, 8.12, 8.13, 8.14, 8.15, 8.16, 8.17, 8.18, 8.19, 8.21, 8.22
Acromioclavicular sprain	Shoulder girdle	8.1, 8.2, 8.3, 8.4, 8.5, 8.6, 8.7, 8.8, 8.9, 8.10, 8.11, 8.12, 8.13, 8.14
Adhesive capsulitis	Infraspinatus, supraspinatus, deltoid, coracobrachialis, pectoralis major, biceps, latissimus dorsi, teres major, teres minor, triceps, subscapularis, shoulder girdle	8.1, 8.2, 8.3, 8.4, 8.5, 8.6, 8.7, 8.8, 8.9, 8.10, 8.11, 8.12, 8.13, 8.14
Bursitis	Deltoid, coracobrachialis, pectoralis major, subscapularis, latissimus dorsi	8.1, 8.2, 8.3, 8.4, 8.5, 8.6, 8.7, 8.8, 8.9, 8.10, 8.11, 8.12, 8.13, 8.14
Swimmer's shoulder	Shoulder flexors and internal rotators, teres major	8.1, 8.2, 8.5, 8.6, 8.7, 8.8, 8.11, 8.14
Elbow		
Medial and lateral epicondylitis	Wrist flexors and extensors, extensor carpi radialis brevis, elbow pronation and supination, shoulder abduction/adduction, internal/external rotators	8.3, 8.4, 8.6, 8.9, 8.10, 8.12, 8.13, 8.15, 8.16, 8.17, 8.18, 8.19, 8.22, 8.23, 8.26
Sprain or strain	Medial collateral ligament, flexor and pronator muscles	8.15, 8.16, 8.17, 8.18, 8.19, 8.20, 8.21, 8.22, 8.23, 8.26

Table 6.1. Specific Conditions (*continued*)

Condition	Muscles Involves	Exercises
Wrist		
Carpal tunnel syndrome	Medial nerve entrapment	8.23, 8.24, 8.25, 8.26, 8.29, 8.30
Tenosynovitis	Extensor tendons	8.23, 8.24, 8.25, 8.26
Fractures		While casted: 8.16, 8.27, 8.29. After cast removal: 8.15, 8.16, 8.17, 8.18, 8.19, 8.20, 8.20.1, 8.21, 8.22, 8.22.1, 8.23, 8.24, 8.24.1, 8.25, 8.26, 8.27, 8.28, 8.29, 8.30
Intersection syndrome	Extensor tendons	8.23, 8.26, 8.30, 8.31, 8.31.1
Rotatory subluxation of scaphoid		8.23, 8.26, 8.28, 8.29, 8.30, 8.31
Finger		
Mallet finger	Extensor tendon	8.29, 8.30
Gamekeeper's thumb	Radial collateral ligament	8.28, 8.29, 8.30
Chest		
Asthma	Muscles of respiration	7.1.1, 7.1.2, 7.2, 7.3, 8.2, 8.5, 9.7, 9.8, 9.9, 9.12, 9.13, 9.14, 9.15, 9.16, 9.17, 9.19
Emphysema	Shoulder muscles, muscles of respiration	7.1.1, 7.1.2, 7.2, 7.3, 8.2, 8.5, 9.7, 9.8, 9.9, 9.12, 9.13, 9.14, 9.15, 9.16, 9.17, 9.18, 9.19
Thoracic spine		
Hyperkyphosis	Posterior longitudinal ligament, thoracic erector spinae, scapular retractors	9.1, 9.2, 9.3, 9.4, 9.5, 9.7, 9.8, 9.9, 9.11
Hypokyphosis	Erector spinae anterior thorax	9.1, 9.2, 9.3, 9.7, 9.8, 9.9, 9.10, 9.12
Lower back and pelvis		
Spondylosis, idiopathic low back pain	Rectus abdominis, external oblique, internal oblique, erector spinae, intrinsic muscles	10.1, 10.2, 10.3, 10.4, 10.5, 10.6, 10.7, 10.8, 10.9, 10.11, 10.12, 10.13, 10.14, 10.15, 10.16, 10.17, 10.18, 10.19, 10.21, 10.22, 10.23, 10.24, 10.25, 10.26, 10.27, 10.28, 10.29, 10.30, 10.31, 10.32, 10.33, 10.34, 10.35
Scoliosis	Postural muscles	10.2, 10.6, 10.12, 10.14
Lumbar facet syndrome		10.1, 10.2, 10.6, 10.6.1, 10.7, 10.9, 10.11, 10.11.1, 10.13, 10.15, 10.27, 10.27.1, 10.34
Hip		
Hip pointer	External oblique, tensor fascia lata, gluteus medius, gluteus maximus	10.4, 10.6, 10.6.1, 10.7, 10.8, 10.10, 10.11, 10.12, 10.18, 10.18.1, 10.19, 10.20, 10.21, 10.26.1, 10.27, 10.27.1, 10.32.1

(*continued*)

Table 6.1. Specific Conditions (*continued*)

Condition	Muscles Involves	Exercises
Hip strain	Abdominal muscles, gluteal muscles, tensor fascia lata	10.4, 10.7, 10.8, 10.10, 10.10.1, 10.10.2, 10.10.3, 10.18, 10.18.1, 10.19, 10.20, 10.21, 10.27, 10.27.1, 10.32.1
Groin strain	Sartorius, adductor magnus, adductor brevis, adductor longus, gracilis, iliopsoas, rectur femoris	10.2, 10.7, 10.8, 10.11.1, 10.12, 10.18, 10.21, 10.27, 10.32.1
Knee		
Chondromalacia patellae	Articular cartilage	10.18, 10.19, 10.19.1, 11.1, 11.3, 11.4, 11.6, 11.8
Patellar tendinitis	Infrapatellar tendon	10.19, 10.19.2, 11.1, 11.3, 11.4, 11.4.1, 11.4.2, 11.5, 11.6, 11.7, 11.8
Strain or sprain	Knee joint ligaments	10.5, 10.8, 10.19, 10.19.2, 10.32.1, 11.2, 11.3, 11.4, 11.4.1, 11.4.2, 11.5, 11.6, 11.7, 11.8, 11.9
Hamstring strain	Semimembranosus, semitendinosus, biceps femoris	10.11, 10.11.1, 10.18.1, 10.19, 10.19.2, 10.32.3, 11.2, 11.3, 11.6, 11.7.1
Quadriceps contusion	Quadriceps	10.4, 10.5, 10.18, 10.19, 10.19.2, 11.2, 11.3, 11.4, 11.4.1, 11.4.2, 11.5, 11.6, 11.8
Leg		
Anterior "shin splint" compartment syndrome	Tibialis anterior, extensor hallucis longus, extensor digitorum longus	11.5, 11.6, 11.7.1, 11.10, 11.13, 11.14, 11.19
Posterior "shin splint" compartment syndrome	Posterior tibialis longus, flexor digitorum longus, flexor hallucis longus	11.5, 11.6, 11.7.1, 11.11, 11.13, 11.14, 11.16, 11.17, 11.18, 11.19
Ankle and foot		
Ankle strain or sprain		11.10, 11.11, 11.13, 11.14, 11.16, 11.17, 11.18, 11.19
Turf toe	Metatarsophalangeal joint sprain	11.12, 11.13, 11.15, 11.19
Metatarsal stress fractures		11.12, 11.13, 11.14, 11.15, 11.19
Plantar fasciitis		11.12, 11.13, 11.14, 11.16, 11.17, 11.18

and the small intrinsic muscles. Exercises for lateral flexion injuries are 7.2, 7.2.1, 7.3, 7.3.1, 7.4, 7.4.1, 7.6, 7.8, 7.9, 7.10, 7.12, and 7.14 (see Chapter 7).

Brachial Plexus Injuries

Cervical disc herniations or severe stretching injuries of the brachial plexus may cause degeneration of the peripheral nerve roots with subsequent loss of function to the associated musculature. Treatment is aimed at the reduction of causative factors, and rehabilitation is aimed at reducing the effects. Additionally, the subserved muscles need strength and endurance training, proportionate to the duration of injury and the amount of atrophy that has occurred. Exercises for the muscles of the upper extremity, including the shoulder girdle, are 8.1, 8.2, 8.3, 8.4, 8.5, 8.6, 8.8, 8.9, 8.10, 8.11, 8.12, 8.13, 8.15, 8.16, 8.17, 8.18, 8.19, and 8.22 (see Chapter 8).

Torticollis (Wry Neck)

There are many varieties of this condition, including a congenital type that usually requires surgical alteration and is due to a developmental abnormality. Otherwise, stress reduction programs are useful in keeping normal muscle tone and preventing a preloading situation that predisposes to this condition. Muscles involved are primarily the sternocleidomastoids. Intrinsic cervical and suboccipital musculature and even the levator scapulae can be secondarily involved. Exercises for torticollis are 7.1, 7.2, 7.3, 7.4, 7.6, 7.8, 7.9, and 7.12 (see Chapter 7).

Scalenus Anticus Syndrome

Neurovascular compression syndromes, such as this one, usually have associated vertebral subluxation complexes that precipitate tonic hypertonicity. They generally do not reach the contracture state, but it is not always easy to break the feedback loop. Relaxation exercises and strengthening of weakened distal muscles served by the neurovascular bundles are necessary components of rehabilitation. Muscles involved are the anterior, medial, and posterior scalene muscles. Exercises for the scalene musculature are 7.1, 7.1.2, 7.2, 7.2.1, 7.3, 7.3.1, 7.6, 7.10, 7.13, 7.13.1, 7.13.2, and 7.14 (see Chapter 7).

Shoulder

Rotator Cuff Tear

The muscles of the rotator cuff are the supraspinatus, infraspinatus, teres minor, and subscapularis. An actual tear involves a long-term healing process. Active and resistive exercises are limited for 2 to 8 weeks, depending on the severity of the injury. More often, the muscle or tendon is severely strained with some torn fibers, or the myotendinous junction is somewhat elongated. This can be complicated by calcific deposits and/or periosteal reactions, causing the rehabilitation to be modified accordingly. Exercises for a rotator cuff tear are 8.1, 8.2, 8.3, 8.4, 8.5, 8.6, 8.7, 8.8, 8.9, 8.10, 8.11, 8.12, 8.13, 8.14, 8.15, 8.16, 8.17, 8.18, 8.19, 8.21, and 8.22 (see Chapter 8).

Acromioclavicular Sprain

Acromioclavicular joint sprains involve the rehabilitation of all of the muscles of the shoulder girdle. To avoid restrictive shoulder sequelae, one may attempt to exercise the shoulder joints isometrically while firmly bracing the joint. This is true for most serious shoulder injuries, since even medium-term immobilization can result in a very long-term recovery of the full range of motion. Exercises for the shoulder girdle are 8.1, 8.2, 8.3, 8.4, 8.5, 8.6, 8.7, 8.8, 8.9, 8.10, 8.11, 8.12, 8.13, and 8.14 (see Chapter 8).

Frozen Shoulder/Adhesive Capsulitis

This is the most serious consequence of shoulder immobilization subsequent to a moderate to severe injury. In fact, most of the other rehabilitation programs are aimed initially at avoiding this consequence. The muscles that can be involved in adhesive capsulitis are the anterior, middle, and posterior fibers of the deltoid, coracobrachialis, pectoralis major (clavicular and sternal portions), biceps, latissimus dorsi, supraspinatus, infraspinatus, serratus anterior, teres major, teres minor, triceps, subscapularis, and pectoralis minor. Exercises for shoulder flexion, extension, abduction, adduction, and external and internal rotation are 8.1, 8.2, 8.3, 8.4, 8.5, 8.6, 8.7, 8.8, 8.9, 8.10, 8.11, 8.12, 8.13, and 8.14 (see Chapter 8).

Bursitis

There are three types of bursitis in the shoulder region: acute and chronic subacromial, subdeltoid, and subscapularis bursitis. Exercises are for the entire shoulder girdle as described under "Acromioclavicular Sprain." However, according to which bursa is inflamed, exercises are varied to avoid irritation of that bursa. Exercises can be modified by decreasing the load, reducing the frequency, and reducing the rate of contraction relative to the surrounding muscles.

Swimmer's Shoulder

Internal rotation and forward flexion restrict the swimmer's shoulder. Increased tenderness is found along the coracoacromial ligament and under the acromion. Exercises for internal rotation and forward flexion are 8.1, 8.2, 8.5, 8.6, 8.7, 8.8, 8.11, and 8.14 (see Chapter 8).

Elbow

Tennis Elbow (Medial and Lateral Epicondylitis)

In a classic tennis elbow, pain is elicited at the musculotendinous junction of the extensor carpi radialis brevis muscle and/or at the tendinous insertion. There are partial tears of the tendons at their origin. A medial epicondylitis is more likely to occur in a sport such as golf, where flexion is the paramount activity. Exercises for tennis elbow, which involve the wrist, forearm, elbow, and shoulder, are 8.3, 8.4, 8.6, 8.9, 8.10, 8.12, 8.13, 8.15, 8.16, 8.17, 8.18, 8.19, 8.22, 8.23, and 8.26 (see Chapter 8).

Elbow Strain of Sprain

Elbow strains and sprains include such conditions as medial collateral ligament strain and flexor-pronator strains. Elbow sprains are best exercised by not loading the joint in early phases and by utilizing maximal isometric contractions. Elbow strains require minimizing contraction and mobilizing joints through full ranges of motion. Exercises for elbow strains and sprains are 8.15, 8.16, 8.17, 8.18, 8.19, 8.20, 8.21, 8.22, 8.23, and 8.26 (see Chapter 8).

Wrist

Carpal Tunnel Syndrome

This syndrome is the result of entrapment of the median nerve in the carpal tunnel. Pain and tingling sensations are elicited along the median nerve distribution, usually distal, but occasionally proximal, to the lesion site. Activity requiring prolonged wrist dorsiflexion, particularly while weight bearing, tends to produce and exacerbate this condition. Unfortunately, wrist ranges of motion need to be improved, and strength in the appropriate distal muscles needs to be regained. Exercises for carpal tunnel syndrome are 8.23, 8.24, 8.25, 8.26, 8.29, and 8.30 (see Chapter 8).

Tenosynovitis

Wrist tenosynovitis is a chronic inflammatory condition affecting the extensor tendons of the wrist. One of the more common forms of this condition, associated with racquet sports, is De Quervain's tenosynovitis. There is an inflammation of the abductor pollicis longus and extensor pollicis brevis tendons where they pass through a fibro-osseous tunnel at the radial styloid. Exercises should initially be performed at slower rates and not through the full ranges of motion, until inflammation has subsided. Exercises for tenosynovitis are 8.23, 8.24, 8.25, and 8.26 (see Chapter 8).

Wrist Fractures

Carpal navicular, hamate, hamate hook, radius, and ulna (Colles' fracture) are a few of the common types of fractures found within the wrist joints. When casting has been performed, we recommend exercising synergists homolaterally and contralaterally, while the cast is in place. Exercises for wrist fractures while in a cast are 8.16, 8.27, 8.28, and 8.29. Following removal of the cast, exercises for wrist rehabilitation are 8.15, 8.16, 8.17, 8.18, 8.19, 8.20, 8.20.1, 8.21, 8.22, 8.22.1, 8.23, 8.24, 8.24.1, 8.25, 8.26, 8.27, 8.28, 8.29, and 8.30 (see Chapter 8).

Intersection Syndrome (Squeaker's Wrist)

This is the result of a peritendinous bursitis, occurring at the junction where the first extensor compartment tendons cross over the radial wrist extensor tendons. Symptoms are crepitation and pain with movement and a weak grasp. Edema can be severe. This condition primarily occurs in rowers and power lifters and has also been found in squash players. Exercises are designed to avoid palmar flexion and to minimize ulnar and radial deviation, such as 8.23, 8.26, 8.30, 8.31, and 8.31.1 (see Chapter 8).

Rotatory Subluxation of the Scaphoid

This condition is usually the result of avoiding a collision with a wall during racquetball type games, where the athlete will block the collision with his arms and hands. The patient will develop pain and weakness of the wrist, along with a "clicking" of the wrist with movement. This is due to a continual subluxation of the scaphoid bone, which is the primary bridge between the proximal and distal carpal rows. As with all chronic subluxations and dislocations, exercises are aimed at strengthening the entire area to support the hypermobile joint. Exercises are designed to avoid wrist dorsiflexion and radial deviation, such as 8.23, 8.26, 8.28, 8.29, 8.30, and 8.31 (see Chapter 8).

Hand

Mallet Finger

Hyperflexion injury against resistance results in damage to the extensor tendon. This can be difficult to rehabilitate, because either the tendon is split or it tends to slip off its mooring or gliding place on the bone. Since surgical intervention is generally necessary, exercises may have to be performed postsurgically. (see Chapter 5). Exercises for mallet finger are 8.29 and 8.30 (see Chapter 8).

Gamekeeper's Thumb

Injury to the radial collateral ligament results in an avulsion from its attachment to the proximal phalanx. Exercises for gamekeeper's thumb are 8.28, 8.29, and 8.30 (see Chapter 8).

Chest

In all chronic respiratory disorders, endurance (especially cardiovascular) is a pri-mary objective. Also, since breathing is labored and secondary respiratory muscles are engaged, sometimes for long periods of time, relaxation exercises are of paramount importance.

Asthma

Asthma is an obstructive lung disease resulting in acute bronchospasms and increased mucus production. It is most difficult to exhale, thereby creating a greater than normal dead air space. Exercises for asthma are 7.1.1, 7.1.2, 7.2, 7.3, 8.2, 8.5, 9.7, 9.8, 9.9, 9.12, 9.13, 9.14, 9.15, 9.16, 9.17, and 9.19 (in Chapters 7 to 9).

Emphysema

Emphysema is a chronic inflammation and thickening causing destruction of the respiratory bronchiolus and alveoli. It is usually more debilitating than asthma, with permanent scarring and hyperinflation of lungs, making inspiration and oxygenation very difficult. It is also necessary to rehabilitate shoulder musculature to aid the rehabilitation of inspiration. Breathing exercises are 7.1.1, 7.1.2, 7.2, 7.3, 8.2, 8.5, 9.7, 9.8, 9.9, 9.12, 9.13, 9.14, 9.15, 9.16, 9.17, 9.18, and 9.19 (in Chapters 7 to 9).

Thoracic Spine

Hyperkyphosis

Hyperkyphosis is an increase in the thoracic kyphotic curve, with concomitant protraction of the scapulae. Symptoms include pain elicited along the posterior longitudinal ligament, fatigue of the thoracic erector spinae and rhomboid musculature, and thoracic outlet syndrome. It may be due, in part, to osteoporosis and, therefore, tends to afflict postmenopausal women more than any other group. Strengthening of supportive musculature, particularly postural exercises, is very important in at least maintaining the status quo. Exercises for hyperkyphosis are 9.1, 9.2, 9.3, 9.4, 9.5, 9.7, 9.8, 9.9, and 9.11 (see Chapter 9).

Hypokyphosis

Hypokyphosis is a decrease in the thoracic kyphotic curve, with concomitant depressed scapulae and clavicle. Symptoms include fatigue of the postural musculature with depression of the thoracic outlet neurovascular bundle between the clavicle and the ribs. This is normally accompanied by significant muscle spasm, relief of which is an early rehabilitative objective. Exercises for thoracic hypokyphosis are 9.1, 9.2, 9.3, 9.7, 9.8, 9.9, 9.10, and 9.12 (see Chapter 9).

Lower Back and Pelvis

Spondylolysis

Stress fracture involving the pars interarticularis are most often seen in pole vaulter's, gymnasts, interior football linemen, swimmers, and divers. Spondylolysis may be asymptomatic. However, when symptomatic, pain may be localized to the area of the posterior superior iliac spine, resulting in hamstring spasm, loss of the normal lumbar lordosis, and limited dorsilumbar extension. When this condition is traumatically induced it can heal 100%. When it is due to a congenital lack of ossification in or elongation of the pars it will not heal. In any case, strengthening of adjacent supporting structures is the primary objective. Exercises for spondylolysis are 10.1, 10.2, 10.3, 10.4, 10.5, 10.6, 10.7, 10.8, 10.9, 10.11, 10.12, 10.13, 10.14, 10.15, 10.16, 10.17, 10.18, 10.19, 10.21, 10.22, 10.23, 10.24, 10.25, 10.26, 10.27, 10.28, 10.29, 10.30, 10.31, 10.32, 10.33, 10.34, and 10.35 (see Chapter 10).

Scoliosis

Most scoliotic conditions are idiopathic. Their key feature, other than the intersegmental curve, is intrinsic and extrinsic muscle imbalance, from left to right. The sequence of rehabilitation is as follows: tone the flaccid side, relax the hypertonic side, and mobilize fixated areas. Postural exercises are in order, especially when the scoliosis is functional, i.e., it changes with posture. Often there is no pain, but a new engram needs to be formed and muscular components need to be strengthened. Exercises for scoliosis are 10.2, 10.6, 10.12, and 10.14 (see Chapter 10 and Appendix).

Lumbar Facet Syndrome

Low back pain is most frequently due to hyperflexion injuries to the lumbar spine. Studies have shown that 82% of the population suffers from this condition. Exercises for low back pain are 10.1, 10.2, 10.6, 10.6.1, 10.7, 10.9, 10.11, 10.11.1, 10.13, 10.15, 10.27, 10.27.1, and 10.34 (see Chapter 10).

Hip

Hip Pointer

Hip pointers are due to contusions caused by direct blows to the rim of the iliac crest. Severe pain results from contraction of the external oblique muscle. There may also be injury to the tensor fascia lata or gluteus medius/maximus. Exercises for hip pointers are 10.4, 10.6, 10.6.1, 10.7, 10.8, 10.10, 10.11, 10.12, 10.18, 10.18.1, 10.19, 10.20, 10.21, 10.26.1, 10.27, 10.27.1, and 10.32.1 (see Chapter 10).

Hip Strain

Strain of the muscles inserted into the iliac crest is characterized by pain with contraction of the abdominal muscles. Strain of the gluteal, tensor fascia lata, or lateral abdominal muscles will cause pain with abduction or extension of the leg. Exercises for hip strain are 10.4, 10.7, 10.8, 10.10, 10.10.1, 10.10.2, 10.10.3, 10.18, 10.18.1, 10.19, 10.20, 10.21, 10.27, 10.27.1, and 10.32.1 (see Chapter 10).

Groin Strain

Groin strain involves the adductor muscles (sartorius, adductor magnus/brevis/longus), gracilis, iliopsoas, and rectus femoris. The injury is due to overuse or overexertion without sufficient warm-up. Exercises for groin strain are 10.2, 10.7, 10.8, 10.11.1, 10.12, 10.18, 10.21, 10.27, and 10.32.1 (see Chapter 10).

Knee

Chondromalacia Patellae

Chondromalacia is a deterioration of the articular cartilage of the posterior surface of the patella. Exercises for chondromalacia in the initial phase are 10.18, 11.1, and 11.3. Care is taken to avoid motions, especially while weight bearing, that permit grinding upon the cartilage, as evidenced by crepitus and pain. After the initial phase, the following exercises are added: 10.19, 10.19.2, 11.4, 11.6, and 11.8 (see Chapters 10 and 11).

Patellar Tendinitis (Jumper's Knee)

Patellar tendinitis is an overuse injury causing microtears at the attachment of the infrapatellar tendon. This can be related to Osgood-Schlatter's disease, which is more of an avulsion of the tibial tuberosity. The rehabilitation programs for overuse injuries and Osgood-Schlatter's disease are similar. However, the latter affects mainly teenage boys, in fast growth phases, and one must be extra careful not to accelerate the program too rapidly. Exercises for patellar tendinitis are 10.19, 10.19.2, 11.1, 11.3, 11.4, 11.4.1, 11.4.2, 11.5, 11.6, 11.7, and 11.8 (see Chapters 10 and 11).

Knee Strain or Sprain

Knee sprain results in a loss of the integrity of the joint capsule, due to a loss of stability of the various ligaments of the knee joint. Exercises for knee sprain are 10.5, 10.8, 10.19, 10.19.2, 10.32.1, 11.2, 11.3, 11.4, 11.4.1, 11.4.2, 11.5, 11.6, 11.7, 11.8, and 11.9 (see Chapters 10 and 11).

Hamstring Strain

Hamstring strains are traction type injuries to the hamstring muscle group, which includes the semimembranosus, semitendinosus, and biceps femoris. These injuries often occur as an athlete decelerates. When contracting eccentrically (negatively) as a braking mechanism, the hamstrings have greater tension on them than when they contract concentrically. This is why eccentric exercises can be more dangerous to perform. Exercises for the hamstrings are 10.11, 10.11.1, 10.18.1, 10.19, 10.19.2, 10.32.3, 11.2, 11.3, 11.6, and 11.7.1 (see Chapters 10 and 11).

Quadriceps Contusion

Quadriceps contusion are caused by a direct trauma from an external force to the thigh. Exercises for the quadriceps are 10.4, 10.5, 10.18, 10.19, 10.19.2, 11.2, 11.3, 11.4, 11.4.1, 11.4.2, 11.5, 11.6, and 11.8 (see Chapters 10 and 11).

Leg

Anterior "Shin Splint" Compartment Syndrome

Anterior shin splints result from irritation and inflammation due to overuse of the tibialis anterior, extensor hallucis longus, and extensor digitorum longus. Exercises for anterior shin splints are 11.5, 11.6, 11.7.1, 11.10, 11.13, 11.14, and 11.19 (see Chapter 11).

Posterior "Shin Splint" Compartment Syndrome

Posterior shin splints result from irritation and inflammation due to prolonged or abnormal pronation affecting the posterior tibialis longus, flexor digitorum longus, and flexor hallucis longus. Exercises for posterior shin splints are 11.5, 11.6, 11.7.1, 11.11, 11.13, 11.14, 11.16, 11.17, 11.18, and 11.19 (see Chapter 11).

Ankle and Foot

Ankle Strain or Sprain

Ankle strains and sprains are classified as inversion or eversion types, and exercises depend upon which ligaments and tendons have been injured. Inversion types are far more common, because full eversion requires a complete tearing of the medial ligament. Opinions as to the best treatment method vary from complete immobilization for extended periods to weight-bearing exercises as soon as possible. Immobilization is used only if the sprain is third degree and the patient needs to be weight bearing. Exercises for ankle strains and sprains are 11.10, 11.11, 11.13, 11.14, 11.16, 11.17, 11.18, and 11.19 (see Chapter 11).

Turf Toe

Turf toe is a sprain of the metatarsophalangeal joint of the great toe. It is especially common in athletes who exercise on the newer artificial surfaces that have little give. It is a result of direct impact with that surface. Exercises for turf toe are 11.12, 11.13, 11.15, and 11.19 (see Chapter 11).

Metatarsal Stress Fractures

Metatarsal stress fractures are due to significant pressure to the area from various athletic activities. Exercises for the metatarsals after the fracture has healed are 11.12, 11.13, 11.14, 11.15, and 11.19 (see Chapter 11).

Plantar Fasciitis

Plantar fasciitis has an insidious onset with low-grade pain along the medial plantar fascia, distal to the calcaneus. It is found in those who perform activities requiring frequent maximal ankle plantar flexion, with metatarsophalangeal dorsiflexion occurring at the same time. Exercises for plantar fasciitis are 11.12, 11.13, 11.14, 11.16, 11.17, and 11.18 (see Chapter 11).

7

Cervical Spine

Action	Muscle	Exercise
Flexion	Sternocleidomastoid, scalenus anterior, prevertebral muscles	7.1.1, 7.1.4, 7.8, 7.8.1, 7.10, 7.12, 7.13, 7.13.1
Extension	Splenius, semispinalis, rectus capitis posterior, upper trapezius, intrinsic, erector spinae	7.1.2, 7.1.3, 7.1.4, 7.4, 7.4.1, 7.5, 7.5.1, 7.6, 7.7, 7.11, 7.12
Rotation	Sternocleidomastoid, small intrinsic	7.3, 7.3.1, 7.5.1, 7.9
Lateral flexion	Scalenus anticus, scalenus medius, scalenus posticus, small intrinsic, sternocleidomastoid	7.2, 7.2.1, 7.13.1, 7.14

The treatment of various neck injuries, specifically those causing a strain or sprain of the cervical spine and surrounding capsular supportive tissue, is directed toward the restoration of full function. Therefore, rehabilitative exercises must be included.

The fundamental purposes of these exercises are to strengthen the paravertebral musculature, to elongate the soft tissues to their proper or functional lengths, to minimize the periarticular fibrous contracture or adhesions within the zygapophyseal joints, and, by muscle action, to increase circulation to the deep neck tissues. Another objective, and perhaps the most important, is to increase the flexibility and/or mobility of the neck, thereby maximizing cervical function.

The entire cervical spine is involved with motion of the head and neck. However, up to 50% of flexion/extension occurs between the occiput and the atlas (C1), with the remainder of the cervical spine contrib-

uting to the remaining 50%, primarily at C5-C6 (1, p. 114). Rotation occurs primarily between the atlas and the axis (C1 and C2), with the remaining cervical vertebrae involved with the balance of rotational movement (1, p. 114).

The cervical spine ranges of motion are flexion, extension, lateral flexion, and rotation. Primary cervical spine flexors are the sternocleidomastoids, assisted by the secondary flexors, the three pairs of scalenus muscles and the cervical paravertebral musculature (Fig. 7.1) (1, p. 116).

The primary extensors are the paravertebral extensor mass, composed of the splenius capitis and cervicis, semispinalis, rectus capitis group, and upper trapezius. The secondary extensors are the intrinsic muscles (Fig. 7.1) (1, p. 117).

Primary rotators of the cervical spine are the sternocleidomastoids; secondary rotators are the small intrinsic muscles (Fig. 7.1) (1, p. 117).

142

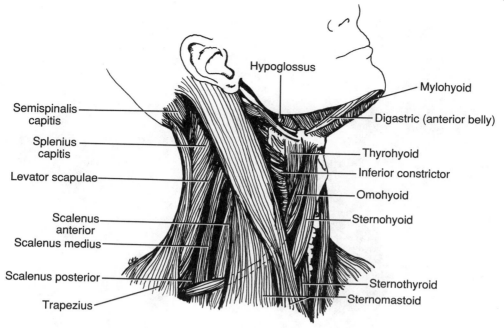

Figure 7.1 Cervical spine musculature.

Primary lateral flexors are the scalenus anticus, medius, and posticus. The secondary lateral flexors are the small intrinsic muscles (Fig. 7.1) (1, p. 117).

In order for the paravertebral musculature to stabilize the cranium and cervical spinal column, assistance is necessary from the synergistic and antagonistic muscles. The longus capitis, the suboccipital muscles, and the suprahyoid and infrahyoid muscles, act as synergistic and antagonistic muscles by initially flattening the cervical lordotic curve (2, p. 244). A synergistic-antagonistic action is seen between the sternocleidomastoid muscles and the paravertebral muscles when the cervical spine is kept rigid, cervical lordosis is reduced, and

extension of the cranium is prevented by the anterior suboccipital muscles, and the suprahyoid and infrahyoid muscles. At that point, flexion of the cervical spine on the thoracic spine is maintained by the two sternocleidomastoid muscles (2, p. 244)

Table 7.1 describes the cervical ranges of motion.

The cervical plexus is formed by the anterior rami of C1, C2, C3, and C4. The motor branches of the cervical plexus innervate the infrahyoid (strap) muscles of the neck, levator scapulae, and scalene muscles, with contributory branches to the trapezius and sternocleidomastoid muscles (3, p. 338).

The brachial plexus is formed by the ventral rami of C5, C6, C7, C8, and T1. Collat-

Table 7.1. Cervical Spine Ranges of Motion (ROM)[a]

Motion	ROM	Anatomical	Cartesian
Flexion	65°	Sagittal	Positive θ_x
Extension	50°	Sagittal	Negative θ_x
Right lateral flexion	40°	Frontal	Negative θ_z
Left lateral flexion	40°	Frontal	Positive θ_z
Right rotation	55°	Transverse	Positive θ_y
Left rotation	55°	Transverse	Negative θ_y

[a] Reprinted with permission from Licht S, ed: Therapeutic Exercise, 2nd ed. Baltimore: Williams & Wilkins, 1976; 138.

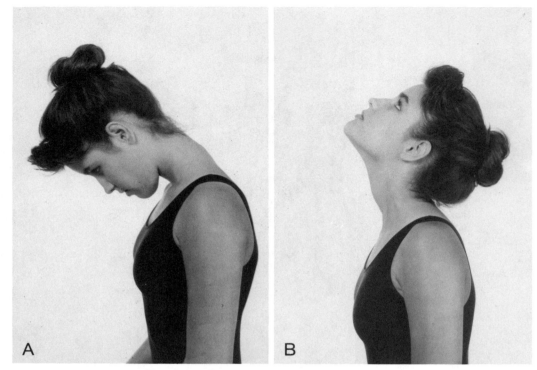

Figure 7.2 Cervical flexion (**A**) and extension (**B**).

eral branches of the brachial plexus supply the scalenus medius and scalenus anterior muscles (3, pp. 338–9).

CERVICAL SPINE EXERCISES

For each cervical exercise, an isokinetic variant is established for each of the three cervical planes of motion. It is produced by performing the exercise in a rhythmic cadence at approximately 1 sec for each half of the axis of motion, with a brief pause at the neutral position. (See chapter 5 for design modifications.)

7.1. Cervical Flexion and Extension (Fig. 7.2)

7.1.1 Description

Stand or sit, with head in neutral position, with therapist restricting extraneous movement caudally from T2 by placing hands at the T2 level posteriorly and midsternally anteriorly. Initially inhale, then slowly exhale while gradually allowing the cervical spine to flex toward chest to its maximum. Return to neutral position.

Exercise format. Standard function 1.

7.1.2 Variant

Maintain same starting position as in 7.1.1. During inspiration, extend the cervical spine to the maximum range and maintain this position for 5 to 10 sec.

Exercise format. Standard function 1.

Area affected. Cervical spine, cervical musculature, flexors and extensors.

Action mode. Active stretching, isotonic.

Intent. Flexibility, mobility, strength, relaxation.

7.1.3 Variant—Occipital Rock

Initially tuck chin toward chest, then repeat 7.1.1 and 7.1.2.

Exercise format. Standard function 4.

Area affected. Suboccipital muscles and atlanto-occipital joints.

Action mode. Active stretching, isotonic.

Intent. Mobility, flexibility, strength.

7.1.4 Variant

Perform flexion and/or extension against the resistance of the therapist.

Exercise Format. Standard function 6.

Action Mode. Isometric.

Intent. Strengthening.

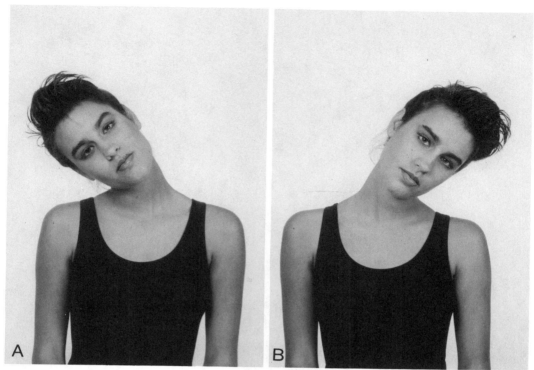

Figure 7.3 Cervical lateral flexion.

7.2. Cervical Lateral Flexion (Fig. 7.3)

Description

Stand or sit, with head in neutral position, with therapist restricting motion at shoulders. Laterally flex the head to the left as far as possible and maintaining this position for 5 to 10 sec. Return to neutral position then laterally flex to the right, maintaining the position 5 to 10 sec.
Exercise format. Standard function 1.
Area affected. Cervical spine, cervical lateral flexors.
Action mode. Active stretching, isotonic.
Intent. Flexibility, mobility, strength, relaxation.

7.2.1 Variant

Perform lateral flexion against resistance by the therapist.
Exercise format. Standard function 6.
Action mode. Isometric.
Intent. Strengthening.

7.3. Cervical Spine Rotation (Fig. 7.4)

Description

Circumduct the cervical spine, first in a clockwise direction and then counterclockwise.

Exercise format. Standard function 2.
Area affected. Cervical spine, all cervical musculature.
Action mode. Active stretching, isotonic.
Intent. Flexibility, mobility, relaxation, strength.

7.3.1 Variant

Against resistance applied by a therapist, rotate cervical spine clockwise and then counterclockwise.
Exercise format. Standard function 6.
Action mode. Isometric.
Intent. Strengthening.

7.4. Cervico-occipital Glide (Fig. 7.5)

Description

Hold head and cervical spine erect, with therapist restricting anterior and posterior movement at shoulders. Move the occiput anteriorly while attempting to keep the cervical spine in place. Repeat posterior glide accomplished with reverse motion.
Exercise format. Standard function 2, with the variation that one performs anterior and posterior glide each for half of the duration of the exercise.
Area affected. Suboccipital musculature, atlanto-occipital joints.

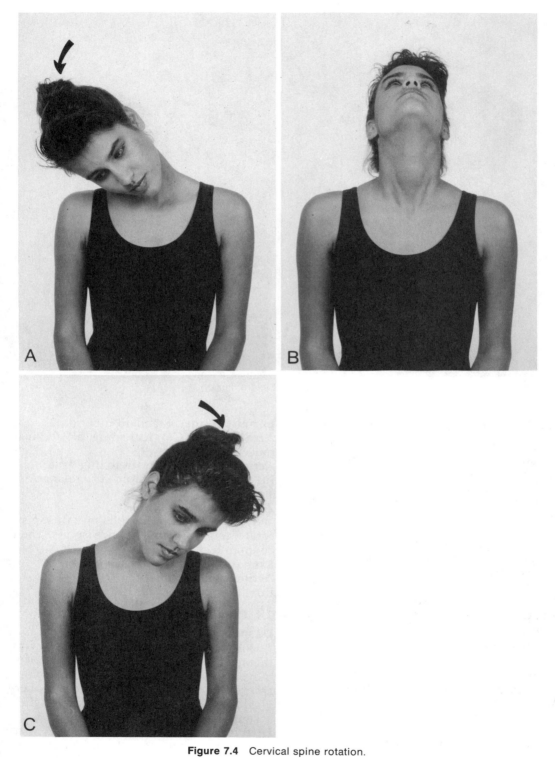

Figure 7.4 Cervical spine rotation.

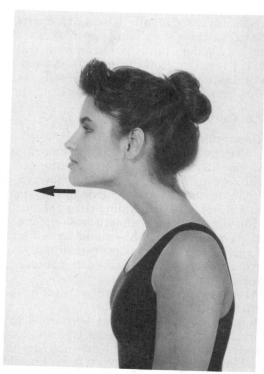

Figure 7.5 Cervico-occipital glide.

Action mode. Active stretching.
Intent. Flexibility, mobility.

7.4.1 Variant

Applying resistance by the therapist changes the action mode to isometric and the intent to strength.
Exercise Format. Standard function 6.

7.5. Cervical Hand Resistance (Fig. 7.6)

Description

Hold head and cervical spine erect. Clasp both hands together on the posterior occipital area. Extend the occiput, while at the same time applying anterior pressure with the hands.
Exercise format. Standard function 4.
Area affected. Cervical spine extensors.
Action mode. Isometric resistance.
Intent. Strength.

7.5.1 Variant

Initially rotate head approximately 20° to either side, which will change the area affected to cervical spine rotators and unilateral extensors.
Exercise format. Standard function 6.
Precaution. Moderate to severe cervical spine injuries will preclude performing ex-

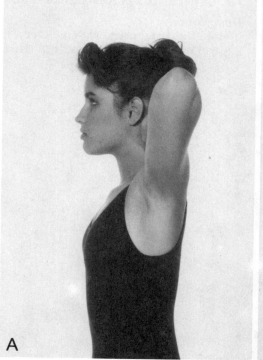

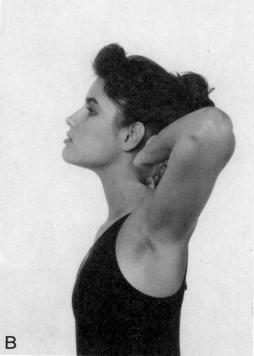

A   B

Figure 7.6 Cervical hand resistance.

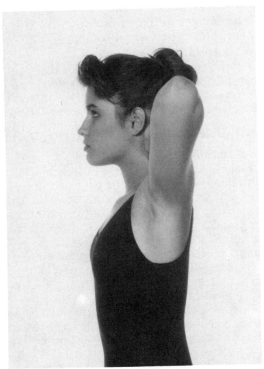

Figure 7.7 Cervical mobilizer.

ercise in this manner. Initially exercise with therapist stabilizing upper thorax, anteriorly and posteriorly. Therapist will also apply resistance on the anterior occiput to eliminate rocking motion. This will make this exercise a cervical mobilizer.

7.6. Cervical Mobilizer (Fig. 7.7)

Description

Patient is seated with head in neutral position. Place both hands on posterior cervical area, using index finger contact. Apply light pressure anteriorly upon one segment at a time, while extending the neck posteriorly and making contact across the posterior portion of each functional motor unit.
Exercise format. Standard function 1.
Area affected. Cervical spine functional motor units.
Action mode. Assistive/active stretch.
Intent. Mobilization.
Note. This is often better performed passively with one of the therapist's hands posteriorly on the neck and the other on the patient's forehead. This way, other muscles are not recruited, the surrounding structures are properly stabilized, and the parameters of technique are better produced.

7.7. Cervical Towel Resistance (Fig. 7.8)

Description

Hold head and cervical spine erect. Hold a towel on the posterior aspect of the occi-

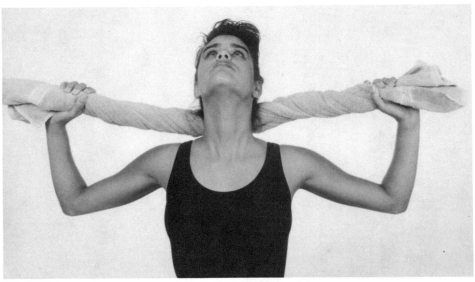

Figure 7.8 Cervical towel resistance.

DYNAMICS OF CLINICAL REHABILITATIVE EXERCISE

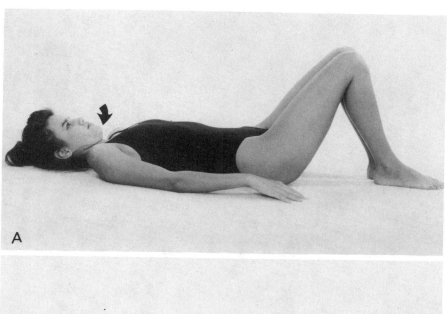

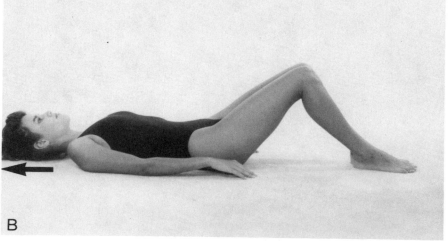

Figure 7.9 Supine, occipital stretch.

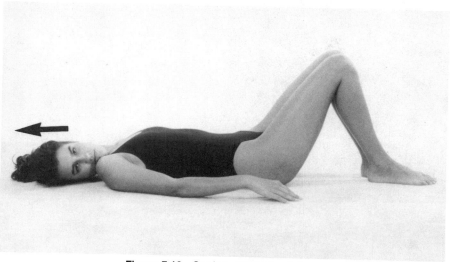

Figure 7.10 Supine, cervical rotation.

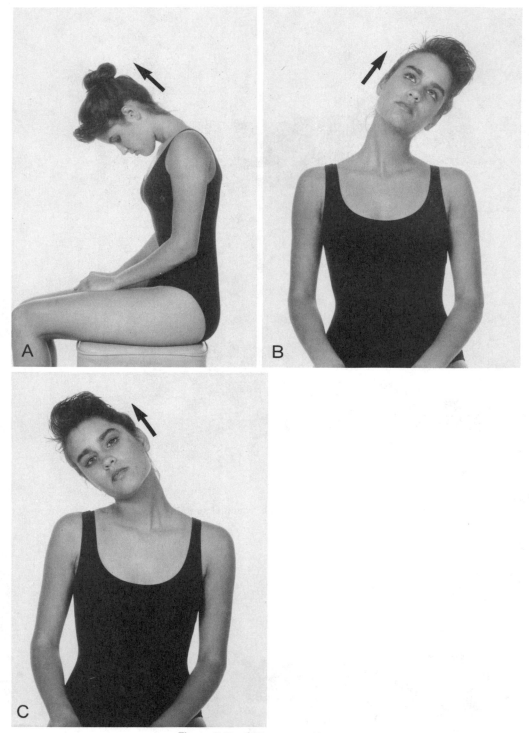

Figure 7.11 Sitting cross-legged.

put, grasping each end with the hands at shoulder width. Resistance can be increased by bringing the hands closer together on the towel and decreased by spreading the hands apart. While in this position, extend the occiput against the resistance of the towel.

Exercise format. Standard function 6.
Area affected. Cervical spine extensors.
Action mode. Isometric resistance.
Intent. Strength.
Note. Variations of this exercise can be performed for cervical spine flexors and lateral flexors, but they should only be performed in the assisted mode.

7.8. Supine, Occipital Stretch (Fig. 7.9)

Description

In the supine position, with arms at sides, feet on the floor, and knees in flexion, flex occiput with chin on chest and the shoulders in contact with the floor. Stretch the posterior occiput cephalward.

Exercise format. Standard function 4.
Area affected. Cervical and suboccipital paravertebral musculature.
Action mode. Active stretch, isometric.
Intent. Flexibility, strength.

7.8.1 Variant

Action mode can be made isotonic by making the exercise weight bearing and employing standard function 2.

7.9. Supine, Cervical Rotation (Fig. 7.10)

Description

In the supine position, with arms at sides, feet on the floor, and knees in flexion, rotate the head toward the right shoulder while stretching the posterior occiput cephalward. Return to the neutral position and repeat this exercise to the left.

Exercise format. Standard function 4.
Area affected. Bilateral cervical and suboccipital paravertebral musculature.
Action mode. Active stretching, isometric.
Intent. Flexibility, mobility, strength.

7.9.1 Variant

Action mode can be made isotonic by making the exercise weight bearing and employing standard function 2.

7.10. Sitting Cross-Legged (Fig. 7.11)

Description

Assume sitting position in chair or with legs crossed upon the floor, keeping the en-

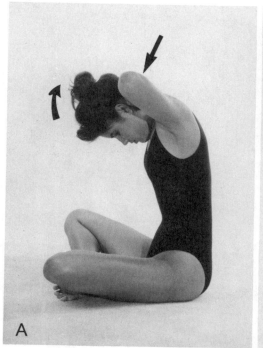
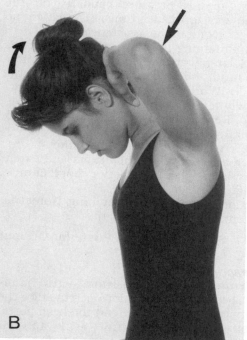

Figure 7.12 Sitting, hands on posterior occiput.

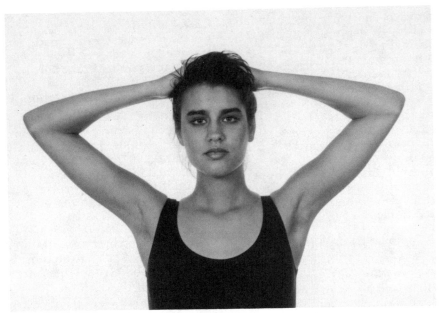

Figure 7.13 Standing, hands on head.

tire spine and head erect. While fully flexing the cervical spine, attempt to lengthen the neck cephalward. Do not further flex or extend the neck or occiput during this maneuver. Maintain this tension for 6 to 10 sec, then slowly relax the neck, and return it to the neutral position. Initially the therapist applies pressure caudally on the shoulders, until such time as the patient no longer requires the assistance.

Maintaining the same position, flex the neck laterally to the right side (do not rotate the head) and then attempt to lengthen the neck. While maintaining this tension, slowly return the neck to the neutral position. Repeat the exercise, flexing the neck laterally to the left side.

Exercise format. Standard function 4.
Area affected. Cervical flexors and extensors, lateral flexors, superior shoulder musculature.
Action mode. Active stretching, isometric.
Intent. Flexibility, strength.

7.11. Sitting, Hands on Posterior Occiput (Fig. 7.12)

Description

From a sitting position, with hands clasped on the posterior occiput, flex the cervical spine then extend the head posteriorly. At the same time, apply anterior pressure with the hands against this movement.

Exercise format. Standard function 6.
Area affected. Cervical spine extensors.
Action mode. Isometric resistance.
Intent. Strength.

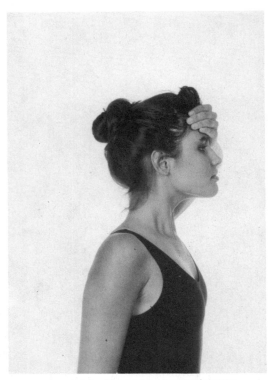

Figure 7.14 Cervical flexion resistance.

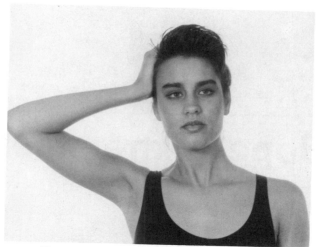

Figure 7.15 Cervical lateral flexion resistance.

7.12. Standing, Hands on Head (Fig. 7.13)

Description
Standing with head and spine erect, clasp hands over the head, elongating the neck cephalward, with pressure applied caudally by the hands.
Exercise format. Standard function 6.
Area affected. Cervical paravertebral musculature.
Action mode. Isometric resistance.
Intent. Strength.
Precaution. This exercise may be contraindicated with cervical spine disc protrusions, healing fractures (even lower in the spine), and lateral canal stenosis.

7.13. Cervical Flexion Resistance (Fig. 7.14)

Description
From a sitting position with hands clasped on the frontal bone, flex head anteriorly. At the same time, apply posterior pressure with the hands against this movement.
Exercise format. Standard function 6.
Area affected. Cervical spine flexors.
Action mode. Isometric resistance.
Intent. Strength.

7.13.1 Variant
Rotate head approximately 30° to one side then apply pressure as above. Repeat to opposite side.
Area affected. Scalenus muscles.
Exercise format. Standard function 6.

7.13.2 Variant
Rotate head approximately 90° to one side, and apply pressure perpendicular to contralateral side of head. Repeat to opposite side.
Area affected. Sternocleidomastoid muscles.
Exercise format. Standard function 6.

7.14. Cervical Lateral Flexion Resistance (Fig. 7.15)

Description
From a sitting position with one hand placed on the right temporal area, the patient attempts to flex the head laterally to the right. At the same time the therapist applies resistance with the hand. Repeat, flexing the head contralaterally and resisting left lateral flexion.
Exercise format. Standard function 6.
Area affected. Cervical spine lateral flexors.
Action mode. Isometric resistance.
Intent. Strength.
Note. The patient can do this himself, but it will cause contraction of homolateral upper shoulder musculature and may be counterproductive to the contralateral contraction desired.

References
1. Hoppenfeld S: Physical Examination of the Spine and Extremities. New York:Appleton-Century-Crofts, 1976.
2. Kapandji IA: The Physiology of the Joints. 2nd ed. New York:Churchill Livingstone, 1982, vol 3.
3. Basmajian JV: Primary Anatomy. 8th ed. Baltimore:Williams & Wilkins, 1982.

8

Upper Extremities

Action	Muscle[a]	Exercise
Flexion	Biceps brachii, coracobrachialis, pectoralis major, deltoid anterior	8.1, 8.1.1, 8.1.2, 8.2, 8.2.1, 8.5, 8.5.1, 8.7, 8.8, 8.11, 8.11.1
Extension	Latissimus dorsi, teres major, deltoid posterior, triceps	8.2, 8.5, 8.5.1, 8.7, 8.14
Abduction	Deltoid, supraspinatus, long head of biceps	8.2, 8.3, 8.4, 8.5, 8.9, 8.12, 8.12.1
Adduction	Short head of biceps, coracobrachialis, pectoralis major, latissimus dorsi, teres major, long head of triceps	8.2, 8.4, 8.5, 8.5.1, 8.6, 8.14
External rotation	Infraspinatus, teres minor, deltoid posterior	8.2, 8.2.1, 8.5, 8.5.1, 8.10, 8.13, 8.14
Internal rotation	Subscapularis, pectoralis major, latissimus dorsi, teres major, deltoid anterior	8.2, 8.5, 8.5.1, 8.6, 8.10.1

[a] See table at beginning of Chapter 9 for scapular involvement.

Shoulder Girdle

The glenohumeral joint is a spheroid joint supported by the articular capsule, coracohumeral ligament, glenohumeral ligament, glenoidal labrum, and transverse ligament (1, p. 501).

The entire shoulder girdle is composed of the glenohumeral joint along with two other joints, and the scapulothoracic articulation (2, pp. 85–9): (a) sternoclavicular joint, and (b) acromioclavicular joint. The coexistence of these enables the uninhibited rhythm of the shoulder, allowing all of its ranges of motion.

The ranges of motion for the shoulder are flexion, extension, abduction, adduction, and internal and external rotation. Table 8.1 describes the shoulder ranges of motion.

The primary flexors are the anterior portion of the deltoid muscle and the coracobrachialis. They are innervated by the axillary nerve (C5) and musculocutaneous nerve (C5/C6), respectively. The muscles of the shoulder girdle are innervated by branches of the brachial plexus. The secondary flexors are the pectoralis major, the biceps, and the anterior portion of the deltoid muscle (Fig. 8.1) (3, p. 25).

Table 8.1. Shoulder Ranges of Motion (ROM)

Motion	ROM	Anatomical	Cartesian[a]
Flexion	90°	Sagittal	$-\theta_x$
Extension	45°	Sagittal	$+\theta_x$
Abduction	180°	Frontal	$\pm\theta_z$
Adduction	45°	Frontal	$\pm\theta_z$
Internal rotation	55°	Transverse	$\pm\theta_y$
External rotation	40–45°	Transverse	$\pm\theta_y$

[a] ± depends upon side of body.

The primary extensors are the latissimus dorsi, teres major, and the posterior portion of the deltoid muscle. They are innervated by the thoracodorsal nerve (C6,C7,C8), the lower subscapular nerve (C5,C6), and the axillary nerve (C5,C6), respectively. The secondary extensors are the teres minor and the long head of the triceps (Fig. 8.2) (3, p. 26).

The primary abductors are the midportion of the deltoid muscle and the supraspinatus. They are innervated by the axillary nerve and the suprascapular nerve (C5,C6), respectively. The secondary abductors are the anterior and posterior portion of the deltoid muscle and the serratus anterior (Fig. 8.2) (3, p. 27).

The primary adductors are the pectoralis major and the latissimus dorsi. They are innervated by the medial and lateral anterior thoracic nerve (C5,C6,C7,C8,T1) and the thoracodorsal nerve, respectively. The secondary adductors are the teres major and the anterior portion of the deltoid muscle (Fig. 8.2) (3, p. 27).

Primary external rotators of the shoulder are the infraspinatus and the teres minor, the secondary external rotator being the posterior portion of the deltoid muscle. The primary external rotators are innervated by the suprascapular nerve and a branch of the

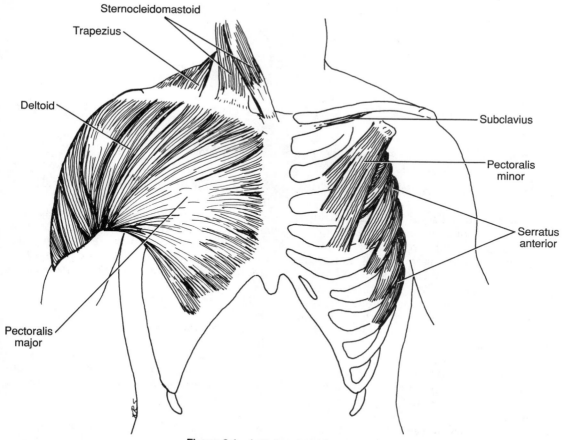

Figure 8.1 Anterior shoulder girdle.

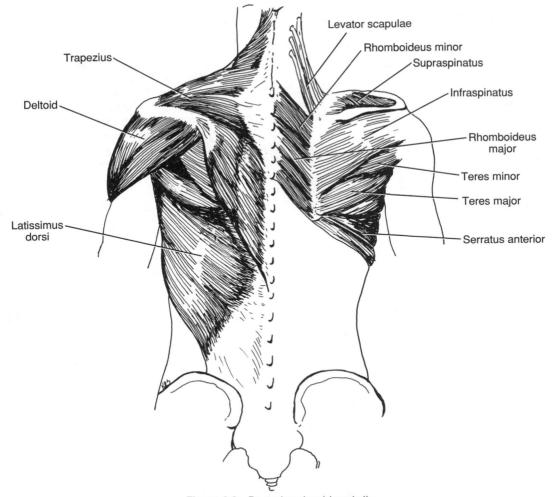

Figure 8.2 Posterior shoulder girdle.

axillary nerve (C5), respectively (Fig. 8.2) (3, p. 28).

Primary internal rotators of the shoulder are the subscapularis, pectoralis major, latissimus dorsi, and teres major. They are innervated by the upper and lower subscapular nerves (C5,C6), the medial and lateral anterior thoracic nerves, the thoracodorsal nerve, and the lower subscapular nerve, respectively. The secondary internal rotator is the anterior portion of the deltoid muscle (Figs. 8.1 and 8.2) (3, p. 28).

The primary elevators, trapezius and levator scapulae, and the secondary elevators, rhomboids major and minor, provide scapular elevation (shoulder shrug) (Fig. 8.2). The primary elevators are innervated by the spinal accessory nerve (cranial nerve XI) and C3, C4 branches of the cervical plexus,

with possible branches from the dorsal scapular nerve (C5), respectively (3, p. 29).

The primary retractors, rhomboids major and minor, and the secondary retractor, the trapezius, provide scapular retraction (position of attention) (Fig. 8.2). The primary retractors are innervated by the dorsal scapular nerve (3, p. 30).

The serratus anterior provides scapular protraction (reaching) and is innervated by the long thoracic nerve (C5,C6,C7) (Fig. 8.2) (3, p. 11).

Flexion of the shoulder is assisted by upward rotation and protraction of the scapulae. Extension of the shoulder is assisted by downward rotation and retraction of the scapulae. Abduction of the shoulder is assisted by upward rotation of the scapulae, while adduction of the shoulder is assisted by downward rotation of the scapulae. Medial rotation of the shoulder is assisted by protraction of the scapulae, and external rotation of the shoulder is assisted by retraction of the scapulae. According to *Gray's Anatomy*, "independent movements of the scapulae are elevation by the Levator scapulae and upper part of the Trapezius; depression by the Pectoralis minor, lower Trapezius and lower Serratus anterior; drawing it forward (abduction of scapulae) by the Serratus anterior, as in pushing; drawing it backward (adduction of scapulae) by the Rhomboidei and Trapezius." As an added note, the subclavius muscle assists in the ventral and caudal motion of the shoulder. For further explanation of the contribution of the motion of the clavicle relative to the scapulohumeral rhythm, one may refer to any authoritive kinesiological text (1, pp. 500–5).

Of primary concern with the shoulder girdle is the necessity to isolate the exact soft tissue requiring rehabilitation to avoid further injury, and to ensure a proper return to a pretraumatic state.

SHOULDER EXERCISES

8.1. Shoulder Flexor (Fig. 8.3)

Description

Bilaterally fully flex shoulders, keeping the elbows in extension.

Exercise Format. Standard function 2.
Area Affected. Shoulder flexors.
Action Mode. Isotonic.
Intent. Strength, mobility, flexibility.

8.1.1 Variant

Therapist adds weights, then repeats exercise as above.

8.1.2 Variant

Proprioceptive neuromuscular facilitation, standard function 9.

8.2. Shoulder Mover (Fig. 8.4)

Description

Standing, suspend arm perpendicular to the floor. Begin to allow arm and shoulder to move freely through a pattern of flexion, extension, internal and external rotation (i.e., circumduction), while keeping elbow extended.

8.2.1 Variant

Repeat above exercise, with suspended hand grasping a 1- to 3-lb weight.
Exercise Format. Standard function 2.
Area Affected. Shoulder girdle.
Action Mode. Isotonic, active stretch.
Intent. Mobility, flexibility, strength.

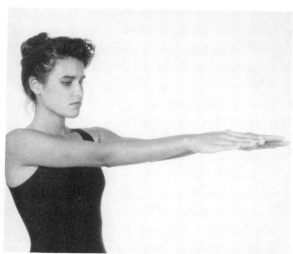

Figure 8.3 Shoulder flexor.

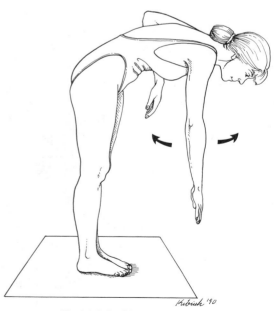

Figure 8.4 Shoulder mover.

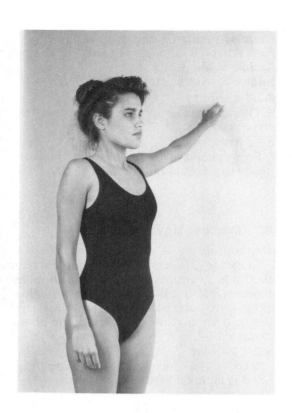

8.3. Shoulder Climber (Fig. 8.5)

Description

Standing laterally to a wall, abduct arm, elbow in extension, with fingers on wall. Finger-walk arm up wall cephalward, abducting arm and shoulder into maximum range. Hold position for 5 to 10 sec, then gradually relax arm.

Exercise Format. Standard function 1.
Area Affected. Shoulder abductors.
Action Mode. Active stretching.
Intent. Flexibility, mobility.

8.4. Shoulder Mobilizer (Fig. 8.6)

Description

Standing with shoulders abducted and elbows flexed 90°, grasping a towel on both ends posteriorly, extend right elbow, pulling the left shoulder into further abduction. Alternate exercise by extending left elbow, pulling the right shoulder into abduction. Hold end position.

Exercise Format. Standard function 4 (modify load mild to moderate).
Area Affected. Shoulder abductors and adductors.
Action Mode. Active stretching, isotonic (with some isometric component).
Intent. Flexibility, mobility, strength.

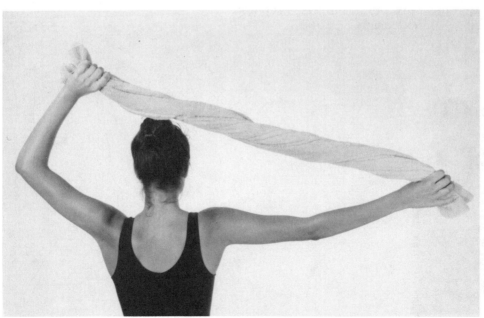

Figure 8.6 Shoulder mobilizer.

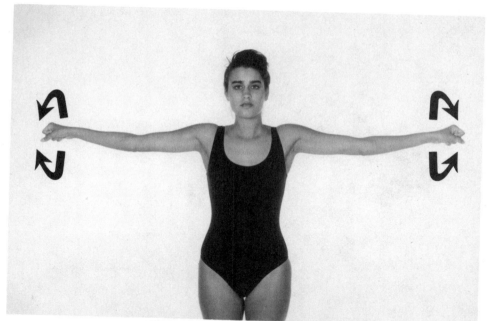

Figure 8.7 Shoulder circumduction.

8.5. Shoulder Circumduction (Fig. 8.7)

Description

Standing, arms bilaterally abducted to 90° with elbows in extension, begin to bilaterally circumduct arms clockwise 5 to 10 times, then counterclockwise 5 to 10 times, in the sagittal plane, beginning with small circles and gradually increasing the radius. What is clockwise for the right side is actually counterclockwise for the left. Therefore, one of each is performed simultaneously.

Exercise Format. Standard function 2.
Area Affected. Shoulder girdle.
Action Mode. Isotonic.
Intent. Flexibility, mobility, strength, endurance.

8.5.1 Variant

Repeat exercise 8.5, with patient holding weights. The greater the weight, the more strength is emphasized over endurance.
Exercise Format. Standard function 5.

8.6. Shoulder Internal Rotator (Fig. 8.8)

Description

Standing, hands clasped posteriorly, adduct scapulae and extend elbows, forcing clasped hands inferiorly.
Exercise Format. Standard function 3.

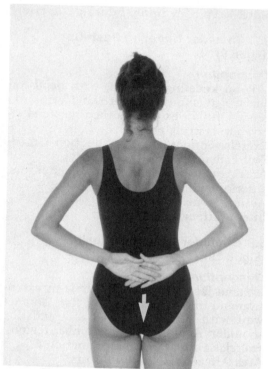

Figure 8.8 Shoulder internal rotator.

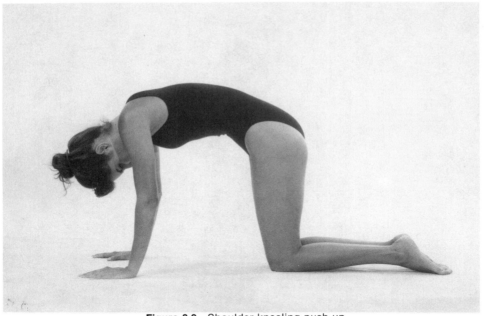

Figure 8.9 Shoulder kneeling push-up.

Area Affected. Shoulder internal and external rotators and adductors.
Action Mode. Active stretching.
Intent. Flexibility, mobility, strength.
Note. Keep body upright during exercise.

8.7. Shoulder Kneeling Push-Up (Fig. 8.9)

Description
From kneeling position, with hands on surface at shoulder width and arms extended, fully flex elbows then reextend elbows to starting position.
Exercise Format. Standard function 5 (modify frequency to patient's ability).
Area Affected. Shoulder flexors, extensors, anterior and posterior upper thorax.
Action Mode. Isotonic.
Intent. Strength, endurance.

8.8. Shoulder Isometric Flexion (Fig. 8.10)

Description
Stand facing wall with elbow in extension and fingers flexed into a fist. Contact wall with thenar area of hand, and flex shoulder. Avoid extending lumbar region.
Exercise Format. Standard function 6.
Area Affected. Shoulder flexors.
Action Mode. Isometric.

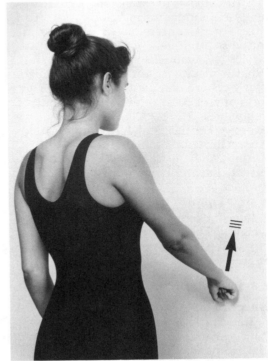

Figure 8.10 Shoulder isometric flexion.

DYNAMICS OF CLINICAL REHABILITATIVE EXERCISE

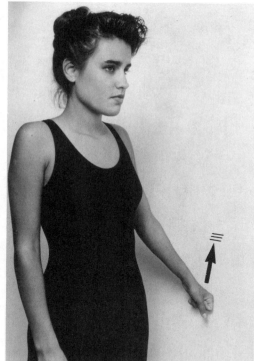

Figure 8.11 Shoulder isometric abductor.

Intent. Strength.
Precaution. This exercise may be contraindicated for patients with elbow problems.

8.9. Shoulder Isometric Abductor (Fig. 8.11)

Description
Standing with wall lateral to body, arm flexed and slightly abducted, contact wall with dorsal aspect of hand, and abduct shoulder.
Exercise Format. Standard function 6.
Area Affected. Shoulder abductors.
Action Mode. Isometric.
Intent. Strength.

8.10. Shoulder Isometric Rotator (Fig. 8.12)

Description
Standing with wall lateral to body, shoulder at 0°, and elbow flexed, contact wall with dorsal aspect of hand, and push hand against wall without moving arm.
Exercise Format. Standard function 6.
Area Affected. Shoulder external rotators.
Action Mode. Isometric.
Intent. Strength.

8.10.1 Variant
Area affected becomes internal rotators by positioning body so that resisting surface is at ventral aspect of arm and hand and pushing against wall in that direction.

Figure 8.12 Shoulder isometric rotator.

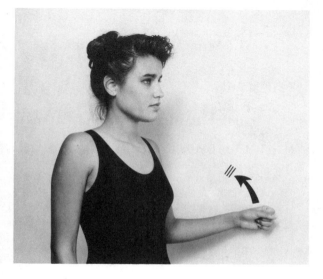

8.11. Shoulder Active Flexor (Fig. 8.13)

Description

Standing with left elbow extended and right hand grasping right arm above elbow, flex right shoulder while gradually increasing resistance. Hold for 5 to 10 sec. Repeat with opposite side.

Exercise Format. Standard function 6.

Area Affected. Shoulder flexors, pectoral muscles.

Action Mode. Isometric.

Intent. Strength.

8.11.1 Variant

Proprioceptive neuromuscular facilitation (PNF), therapist applying resistance in the reverse direction.

Exercise Format. Standard function 9.

8.12. Shoulder Active Abductor (Fig. 8.14)

Description

Standing with right elbow extended and arm at side, with the left hand grasping the right arm laterally above the elbow, abduct the right shoulder while gradually increas-

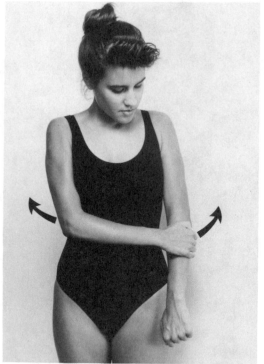

Figure 8.14 Shoulder active abductor.

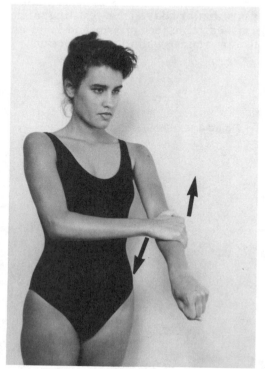

Figure 8.13 Shoulder active flexor.

ing resistance. Hold for 5 to 10 sec, then repeat with left shoulder.

Exercise Format. Standard function 6.

Area Affected. Shoulder abductors, pectoral muscles.

Action Mode. Isometric.

Intent. Strength.

8.12.1. Variant

PNF, therapist applying resistance in the reverse direction.

Exercise Format. Standard function 9.

8.13. Shoulder Active Rotator (Fig. 8.15)

Description

Standing with right shoulder at side, elbow flexed, and right hand grasping the left distal forearm, externally rotate the left shoulder against gradually increasing resistance. Hold for 5 to 10 sec, then repeat with right shoulder.

Exercise Format. Standard function 6.

Area Affected. Shoulder external rotators, pectoral muscles.

Action Mode. Isometric.

Intent. Strength.

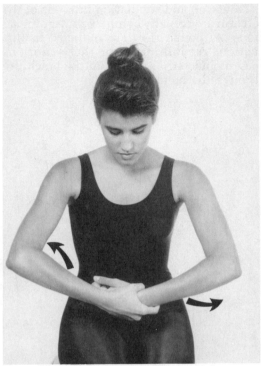

Figure 8.15 Shoulder active rotator.

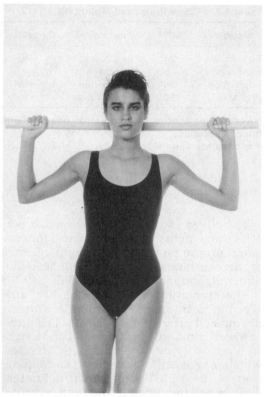

Figure 8.16 Shoulder stretcher.

8.14. Shoulder Stretcher (Fig. 8.16)

Description

Standing with elbows flexed and hands pronated, grasp a pole. Bring the pole posterior to the head and shoulders. Adduct the scapulae, elbows brought caudalward. Have the patient first inhale and then exhale while assuming this position.

Exercise Format. Standard function 4.
Area Affected. Shoulder girdle, anterior chest wall.
Action Mode. Active stretching, isometric.
Intent. Flexibility, mobility, strength, pulmonary enhancer.

Elbow

Action	Muscle	Exercise
Flexion	Brachialis, biceps, brachioradialis, pronator teres, flexor carpi radialis, flexor carpi ulnaris	8.7, 8.17, 8.18, 8.19, 8.20.1, 8.22
Extension	Triceps, anconeus	8.7, 8.17, 8.18, 8.19, 8.20, 8.20.1, 8.21, 8.22
Supination (forearm and wrist)	Biceps, supinator, abductor pollicis longus	8.15, 8.16, 8.22.1, 8.22.2, 8.23, 8.24, 8.24.1, 8.27
Pronation (forearm and wrist)	Pronator teres, pronator quadratus, flexor carpi radialis	8.6, 8.15, 8.16, 8.22.1, 8.22.2, 8.23, 8.24, 8.24.1, 8.27

Table 8.2. Elbow Ranges of Motion (ROM)[a]

Motion	ROM	Anatomical	Cartesian[b]
Flexion	135°	Sagittal	$-\theta_x$
Extension	5°	Sagittal	$+\theta_x$
Supination	90°	Transverse	$\pm\theta_y$
Pronation	90°	Transverse	$\pm\theta_y$

[a] **Assume patient is in anatomical position with thumbs anterior.**
[b] **± depends upon side of body.**

Pronation and supination motions of the forearm are actually complex multijoint actions. Although they are included in this section, rehabilitation of these motions may include structures from the brachium through the hand.

The elbow is a ginglymus joint that permits movements of flexion, extension, supination, and pronation. The joint consists of three articulations: humeroulnar, radiohumeral, and radioulnar (3, p. 36).

The humeroulnar joint is the most susceptible to trauma, consequently limiting flexion and extension. (4, p. 169). The humeroradial joint will limit flexion and extension primarily by way of arthritic changes, which may also limit pronation and supination. (4, p. 169). The proximal radioulnar joint, when involved, limits pronation and supination.

Table 8.2 describes the elbow ranges of motion: flexion, extension, supination, and pronation. The primary flexors are the brachialis and biceps, with the secondary flexors being the brachioradialis and the supinator (Figs. 8.17 to 8.19). The primary flexors are innervated by the musculocutaneous nerve (C5,C6) (3, p. 52).

The primary extensor is the triceps, the secondary the anconeus (Fig. 8.20). The triceps muscle is innervated by the radial nerve (C7) (3, p. 52).

Primary supinators of the elbow are the biceps and supinator, with the secondary supinator being the brachioradialis (Figs. 8.17 and 8.18). The primary supinators are innervated by the musculocutaneous nerve and the radial nerve (C6), respectively (3, p. 53).

Primary pronators are the pronator teres and pronator quadratus. The secondary pronator is the flexor carpi radialis (Figs. 8.17, 8.19 and 8.20). The primary pronators are innervated by the median nerve (C6) and the anterior interosseous branch of the median nerve (C8,T1), respectively (3, p. 53).

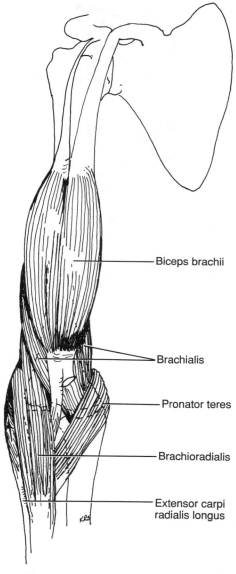

Biceps brachii

Brachialis

Pronator teres

Brachioradialis

Extensor carpi radialis longus

Figure 8.17   Elbow muscles, flexors.

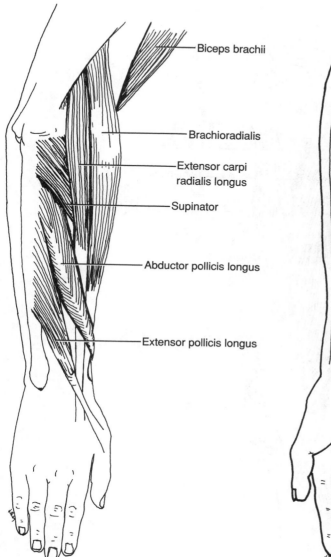

Figure 8.18 Elbow and forearm muscles.

Biceps brachii

Brachioradialis

Extensor carpi
radialis longus

Supinator

Abductor pollicis longus

Extensor pollicis longus

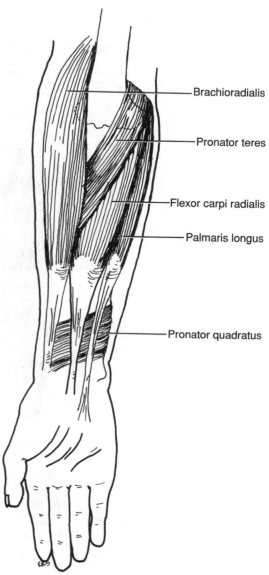

Figure 8.19 Forearm muscles.

Brachioradialis

Pronator teres

Flexor carpi radialis

Palmaris longus

Pronator quadratus

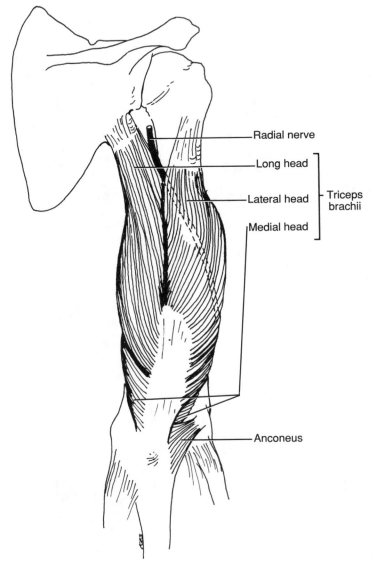

Radial nerve

Long head

Lateral head

Medial head

Triceps brachii

Anconeus

Figure 8.20   Elbow muscles, extensors.

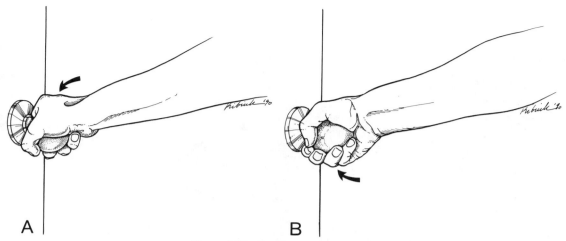

Figure 8.21 Passive elbow rotator.

ELBOW EXERCISES

8.15. Passive Elbow Rotator (Fig. 8.21)

Description
Standing, with elbow extended, grasp a door knob and internally and then externally rotate the arm, limiting shoulder movement.
Exercise Format. Standard function 2.
Area Affected. Elbow and wrist supinators and pronators.
Action Mode. Isotonic.

Intent. Mobility, strength, coordination, endurance.

8.16. Isometric Elbow Rotator (Fig. 8.22)

Description
Standing, with elbow in extension, grasp a stationary object or grasp the hand of the therapist. Against resistance, internally and externally rotate the arm.
Exercise Format. Standard function 6.
Area Affected. Elbow supinators and pronators.
Action Mode. Isometric.
Intent. Strength.

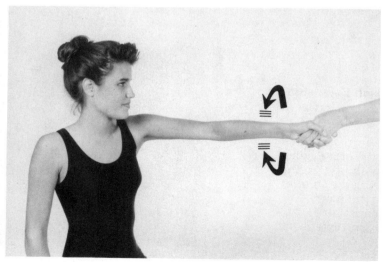

Figure 8.22 Isometric elbow rotator.

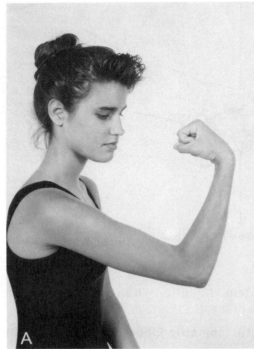

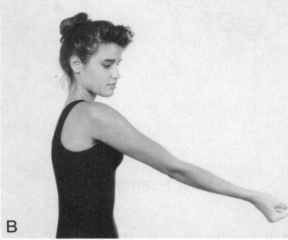

Figure 8.23 Elbow flexion/extension.

8.17. Elbow Flexion/Extension (Fig. 8.23)

Description

Supinate hand, flex fingers into a fist, and alternately flex and extend elbow.
Exercise Format. Standard function 7.
Area Affected. Elbow flexors and extensors.
Action Mode. Isotonic.
Intent. Mobility, endurance, strength.

8.18. Isometric Elbow Flexion/Extension (Fig. 8.24)

Description

Pronate hand, flex fingers into a fist, and grasp proximal to wrist with other hand. Flex and extend the elbow, while at the same time gradually increasing the amount of resistance with the alternate hand.
Exercise Format. Standard function 6.
Area Affected. Elbow flexors and extensors.
Action Mode. Isometric.
Intent. Strength.

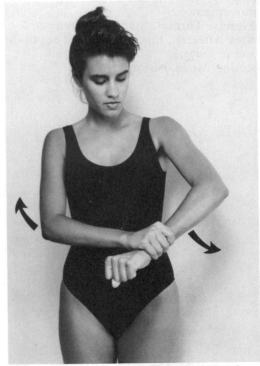

Figure 8.24 Isometric elbow flexion/extension.

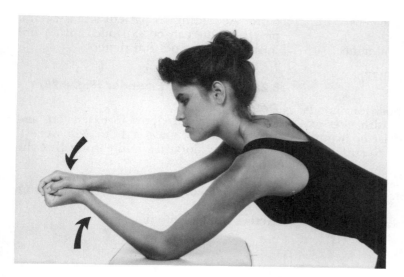

Figure 8.25 Forced elbow extensor/flexor.

8.19. Forced Elbow Extensor/Flexor (Fig. 8.25)

Description

Begin with elbow on table, hand in supination with fingers flexed into a fist, and elbow in flexion. Grasp fist, or proximal to wrist, with other hand, keeping active wrist rigid. While actively flexing elbow, force elbow into extension. Gradually increase the amount of resistance. Repeat, resisting flexion motion.

Exercise Format. Standard function 6.
Area Affected. Elbow extensors and flexors.
Action Mode. Isometric.
Intent. Strength.
Note. A soft pad should be placed under the elbow to avoid further injury and/or discomfort.

8.20. Elbow Extender (Fig. 8.26)

Description

Stand facing wall. Place both hands on the wall at shoulder width, with arms flexed 90° and elbows in extension. Apply pressure against the wall, pushing off with rear foot. Alternate legs, pushing off with rear foot.

Exercise Format. Standard function 6.
Area Affected. Scapular protractors, deltoid, triceps.
Action Mode. Isometric.
Intent. Strength.

8.20.1 Variant: Standing Push-up

From same starting position, push into wall, allowing elbows to flex. Then extend elbows.

Exercise Format. Standard function 5.

Figure 8.26 Elbow extender.

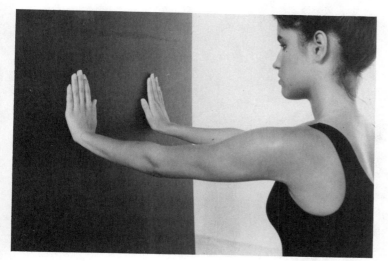

Area Affected. Pectorals and biceps.
Action Mode. Isotonic.
Intent. Strength, mobility, endurance.

8.21. Elbow Push-Ups (Fig. 8.27)

Description
Assume prone push-up position: hands (palms down) at shoulder width, legs extended, contact with toes. Raise up by fully extending arms. Lower body to surface by flexing arms.
Exercise Format. Standard function 5.
Area Affected. Pectorals, biceps, triceps.
Action Mode. Isotonic.
Intent. Strength, mobility, endurance.

Note. According to patient's ability and progress, this can be expanded into a full push-up, or any portion thereof.

8.22. Wrist Elbow Extender (Fig. 8.28)

Description
Standing, with elbow in extension, and arm flexed 90°, grasp a 1- to 3-lb weight. Alternately dorsiflex and palmar flex the wrist.
Exercise Format. Standard function 5.
Area Affected. Wrist and forearm flexors and extenders.
Action Mode. Isotonic.

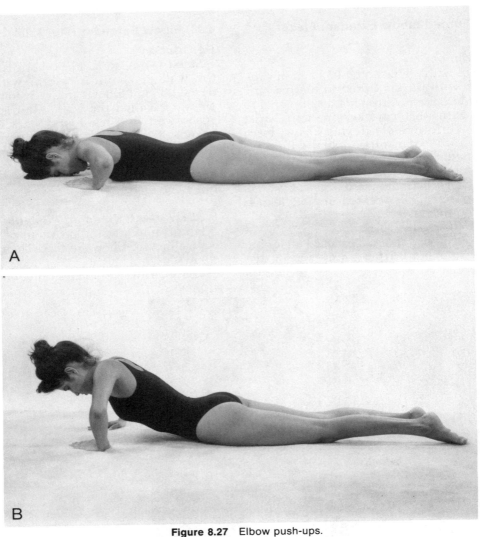

Figure 8.27 Elbow push-ups.

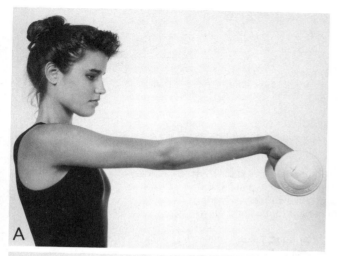

A

Figure 8.28 Wrist elbow extender.

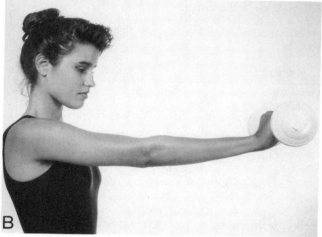

B

Intent. Strength, endurance, mobility, coordination.

8.22.1 Variant

From same position as 8.22, alternately pronate and supinate the elbow.

Exercise Format. Standard function 5.

Area Affected. Elbow and wrist pronators and supinators.

Intent. Strength, mobility, coordination, endurance.

8.22.2 Variant

Assume a starting position halfway between pronation and supination. Therapist grasps the distal forearm, resisting pronation and supination, respectively.

Exercise Format. Standard function 6.

Area Affected. Elbow and wrist pronators and supinators.

Action Mode. Isometric.

Intent. Strength.

Wrist and Hand

Action	Muscle	Exercise
Wrist extension	Extensor carpi radialis longus, extensor carpi radialis brevis, extensor carpi ulnaris, extensor digitorum	8.22, 8.23, 8.24, 8.25, 8.25.1, 8.26, 8.26.1
Wrist flexion	Flexor carpi radialis, flexor carpi ulnaris, palmaris longus, flexor digitorum profundus, flexor digitorum superficialis	8.22, 8.23, 8.24, 8.25, 8.25.1, 8.26, 8.26.1, 8.31
Metacarpophalangeal/ interphalangeal extension	Extensor digitorum communis, extensor indicis, extensor digiti minimi, palmar and dorsal interossei, extensor carpi ulnaris,[a] extensor carpi radialis longus and brevis[a]	8.30
Flexion	Flexor digitorum profundus, flexor digitorum superficialis, lumbricals, flexor digiti minimi brevis, palmar and dorsal interossei	8.29, 8.30, 8.31, 8.31.1
Abduction	Dorsal interossei, abductor digiti minimi, long extensors[b]	8.28, 8.28.1
Adduction	Palmar interossei, long flexors[c]	8.28, 8.28.1, 8.31.1

[a] Act to extend wrist, thereby synergistically allowing maximum flexor contraction.

[b] During metacarpal phalangeal flexion, long extensors are dominant.

[c] During metacarpal phalangeal extension, long flexors are assisting. During flexion, active abduction is not possible.

The radiocarpal articulation is formed by the distal end of the radius and distal articular disc, with the scaphoid, lunate, and triquetrum carpal bones. The stability of the wrist joint is provided by four ligaments (1, pp. 510–1)—palmar radiocarpal, dorsal radiocarpal, ulnar collateral, and radial collateral—and is further enhanced by an encircling synovial capsule and retinaculum.

The wrist and hand are innervated by three major nerves, median, ulnar, and radial, which increase the susceptibility to pain in disease or injury (4, p. 179).

The midcarpal joint, the union of the scaphoid, lunate, triquetrum, and pisiform carpal bones with the trapezium, trapezoid, capitate, and hamate, continues the formation of the wrist into the hand.

The wrist is a condyloid articulation, and therefore enables all movements except rotation (1, pp. 512–13).

The carpal metacarpal joint between the carpals and the second, third, fourth, and fifth metacarpal bones is a gliding joint.

Movements are limited to a minimal gliding motion. The carpal metacarpal articulation of the thumb allows flexion, extension, abduction, adduction, circumduction, and opposition (1, p. 514).

The intermetacarpal articulations are formed where the second, third, fourth, and fifth metacarpal bones articulate with one another, allowing movements of flexion, extension, abduction, adduction, and circumduction (1, pp. 514–15).

The interphalangeal articulations are hinge joints, permitting movements only of flexion and extension (1, p. 516).

The ranges of motion for the wrist are flexion, extension, ulnar deviation, and radial deviation. There are three primary extensors, extensor carpi radialis longus, extensor carpi radialis brevis, and extensor carpi ulnaris (Figs. 8.18 and 8.29). They are innervated by the radial nerve (C6/C7) (3, p. 93).

The primary flexors are the flexor carpi radialis and flexor carpi ulnaris (Figs. 8.19

and 8.20). They are innervated by the median nerve (C7) and the ulnar nerve (C8,T1), respectively (3, p. 94).

The abductor pollicis longus and the extensor pollicis brevis support radial devia-tion (abduction) (Figs. 8.18 and 8.20) (2, p. 156). The adductor pollicis assists ulnar deviation (adduction) (Figs. 8.30 and 8.31) (2, p. 156).

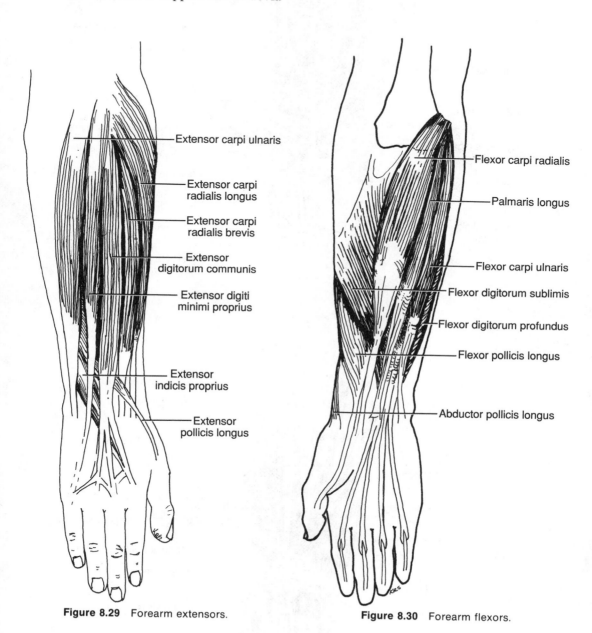

Figure 8.29 Forearm extensors.

Figure 8.30 Forearm flexors.

Extensor carpi ulnaris

Extensor carpi radialis longus

Extensor carpi radialis brevis

Extensor digitorum communis

Extensor digiti minimi proprius

Extensor indicis proprius

Extensor pollicis longus

Flexor carpi radialis

Palmaris longus

Flexor carpi ulnaris

Flexor digitorum sublimis

Flexor digitorum profundus

Flexor pollicis longus

Abductor pollicis longus

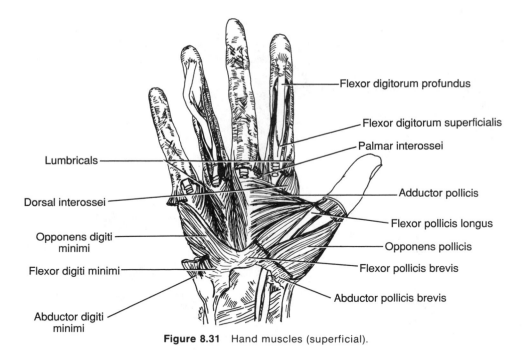

Flexor digitorum profundus

Flexor digitorum superficialis

Palmar interossei

Lumbricals

Adductor pollicis

Dorsal interossei

Flexor pollicis longus

Opponens digiti minimi

Opponens pollicis

Flexor digiti minimi

Flexor pollicis brevis

Abductor digiti minimi

Abductor pollicis brevis

Figure 8.31 Hand muscles (superficial).

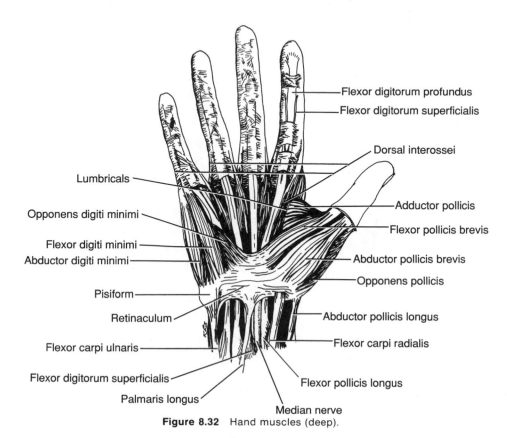

Flexor digitorum profundus

Flexor digitorum superficialis

Dorsal interossei

Lumbricals

Adductor pollicis

Opponens digiti minimi

Flexor pollicis brevis

Flexor digiti minimi

Abductor digiti minimi

Abductor pollicis brevis

Opponens pollicis

Pisiform

Retinaculum

Abductor pollicis longus

Flexor carpi ulnaris

Flexor carpi radialis

Flexor digitorum superficialis

Flexor pollicis longus

Palmaris longus

Median nerve

Figure 8.32 Hand muscles (deep).

Finger

The ranges of motion for the distal and proximal interphalangeal joints are flexion, extension, abduction, and adduction. The primary extensors are the extensor digitorum communis, extensor indicis, and extensor digiti minimi (Fig. 8.29) (3, p. 94).

The primary flexor of the distal interphalangeal joint is the flexor digitorum profundus, and it is innervated by the ulnar nerve (C8,T1) and the anterior interosseous branch of the median nerve. The proximal interphalangeal joint primary flexor is the flexor digitorum superficialis, innervated by the median nerve (C7,C8,T1). Flexors of the metacarpophalangeal joint are the lumbricals. (Fig. 8.32). The lateral lumbricals are innervated by the median nerve (C7), whereas the medial lumbricals are innervated by the ulnar nerve (C8) (3, p. 95).

The primary abductors are the dorsal interossei and the abductor digiti minimi; the primary adductors are the palmar interossei (Figs. 8.30 and 8.31). They are all innervated by the ulnar nerve (C8,T1) (3, p. 95).

Thumb

Action	Muscle	Exercise
Extension	Extensor pollicis brevis, extensor pollicis longus, abductor pollicis longus	8.30
Flexion	Flexor pollicis brevis, flexor pollicis longus, opponens pollicis	8.28, 8.30, 8.31
Abduction	Abductor pollicis longus, abductor pollicis brevis	8.28, 8.28.1, 8.29
Adduction	Adductor pollicis obliquus, adductor pollicis transversus	8.28, 8.28.1
Opposition	Opponens pollicis, flexor pollicis brevis, adductor pollicis,[a] flexor pollicis longus[a]	8.29

[a]Serve to increase oppositional force when grasping.

Ranges of motion for the thumb are extension, flexion, abduction, adduction, and opposition. The extensor pollicis brevis is the primary metacarpophalangeal joint extensor, and the extensor pollicis longus is the primary extensor of the interphalangeal joint (Fig. 8.29). Both are innervated by the radial nerve (C7) (3, p. 97).

The metacarpophalangeal joint primary flexors are the flexor pollicis brevis and longus (Fig. 8.32). The flexor pollicis brevis is innervated by the ulnar nerve (C8) on the medial portion, and by the median nerve (C6,C7) on the lateral side. The flexor pollicis longus is innervated by the median nerve (C8,T1) (3, p. 97).

Primary abductors are the abductor pollicis brevis and longus (Fig. 8.32). They are innervated by the median nerve (C6,C7) and the radial nerve (C7), respectively (3, p. 97).

Primary adductors are the adductor pollicis obliquus and transversus (Figs. 8.30 and 8.31). They are innervated by the ulnar nerve (C8) (3, p. 97).

The opponens pollicis and opponens digiti minimi assist primary thumb opposition (Figs. 8.30 and 8.31) and are innervated by the median nerve (C6,C7) and the ulnar nerve (C8), respectively (3, p. 98).

Table 8.3 describes the ranges of motion of the wrist, fingers, proximal interphalangeal joint, distal interphalangeal joint, thumb metacarpophalangeal joint, thumb interphalangeal joint, and thumb carpometacarpal joint.

WRIST EXERCISES

8.23. Wrist Mover (Fig. 8.33)

Description

Fully flex fingers into a fist and palmar flex wrist to maximum range. Hold position for 5 to 10 sec, and relax.

Fully flex fingers into a fist and dorsiflex wrist to maximum range. Hold position for 5 to 10 sec, and relax.

Fully flex fingers into a fist and abduct (radial deviation) to maximum range. Hold position for 5 to 10 sec, and relax.

Table 8.3. Wrist and Hand Ranges of Motion (ROM)

Motion	ROM	Anatomical	Cartesian[a]
Wrist			
Flexion	80°	Frontal	$\pm\theta_z$
Extension	70°	Frontal	$\pm\theta_z$
Ulnar deviation	30°	Sagittal	$-\theta_x$
Radial deviation	20°	Sagittal	$-\theta_x$
Fingers—Metacarpophalangeal joint			
Flexion	90°	Frontal	$\pm\theta_z$
Extension	30–45°	Frontal	$\pm\theta_z$
Fingers—Proximal interphalangeal joint			
Flexion	100°	Frontal	$\pm\theta_z$
Extension	0°	Frontal	$\pm\theta_z$
Fingers—Distal interphalangeal joint			
Flexion	90°	Frontal	$\pm\theta_z$
Extension	20°	Frontal	$\pm\theta_z$
Fingers			
Abduction	20°	Sagittal	$\pm\theta_x$
Adduction	0°	Sagittal	$\pm\theta_x$
Thumb—Metacarpophalangeal joint			
Flexion	50°	Transverse	$\pm\theta_y$
Extension	0°	Transverse	$\pm\theta_y$
Thumb—Interphalangeal joint			
Flexion	90°	Sagittal	$+\theta_x$
Extension	20°	Sagittal	$-\theta_x$
Thumb			
Palmar Abduction	70°		
Dorsal Adduction	0°		

[a] **Positive/negative depends upon side of body.**

Fully flex fingers into a fist and adduct (ulnar deviation) to maximum range. Hold position for 5 to 10 sec, and relax.
Exercise Format. Standard function 4.
Area Affected. Wrist flexors, extensors, ulnar and radial medial and lateral deviators.
Action Mode. Active stretching, isometric.
Intent. Flexibility, mobility, strength, coordination.

8.24. Wrist Circumductor (Fig. 8.34)

Description
Fully flex fingers into a fist, stabilize arm with opposite hand proximal to wrist, and circumduct clockwise and counterclockwise 5 to 10 times in each direction.
Exercise Format. Standard function 2.
Area Affected. Wrist and forearm.
Action Mode. Active stretch, isotonic.

Intent. Strength, mobility, flexibility, endurance.
8.24.1 Variant
Repeat 8.24 with fingers extended. Area affected includes palm and fingers.

8.25. Wrist Roller (Fig. 8.35)

Description
Grasp a bar with both hands. Keeping both elbows tucked in, rotate bar clockwise 10 to 20 turns, and then counterclockwise 10 to 20 turns, in the sagittal plane.
Exercise Format. Standard function 2.
Area Affected. Wrist and forearm.
Action Mode. Isotonic.
Intent. Flexibility, mobility, endurance, coordination, strength.
8.25.1 Variant
As patient progresses, increase weight of bar.
8.25.2. Variant
Raising elbow of left arm (Fig. 8.35) isolates wrist musculature.

8.26. Forced Wrist Flexor/Extensor (Fig. 8.36)

Description
Therapist grasps dorsum of open hand and passively forces it into maximum palmar flexion. Repeat, forcing hand into dorsiflexion.
Exercise Format. Standard function 10.
Area Affected. Wrist flexors and extensors.
Action Mode. Passive stretch.
Intent. Flexibility, mobility.
8.26.1 Variant
Patient resists therapist with antagonistic motion.
Exercise Format. Standard function 6.
Action Mode. Isometric.
Intent. Strength.

8.27. Hand Slap (Fig. 8.37)

Description
From a sitting position, with arms at sides, elbow flexed 90°, and hands on thighs (palms down), bilaterally alternate slapping thighs with palmar and dorsal sides of hands.
Exercise Format. Standard function 2.
Area Affected. Wrist supinators and pronators.
Action Mode. Isotonic.
Intent. Strength, coordination.

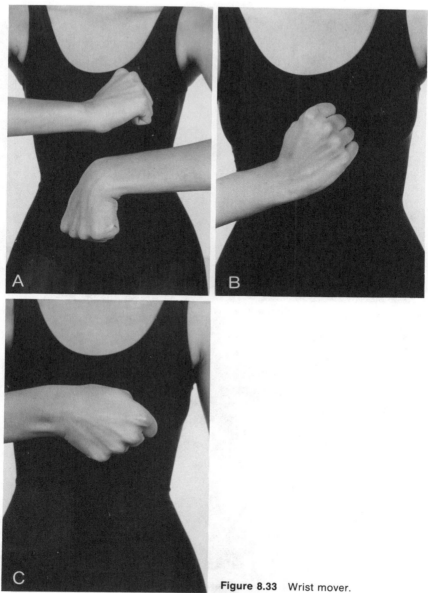

Figure 8.33 Wrist mover.

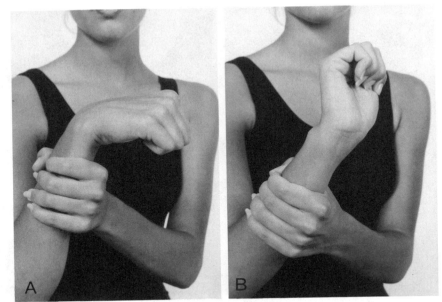

Figure 8.34 Wrist circumductor.

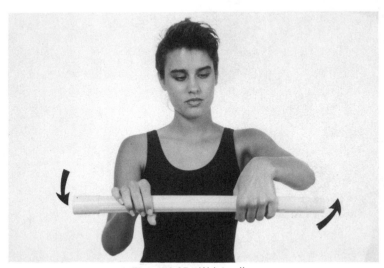

Figure 8.35 Wrist roller.

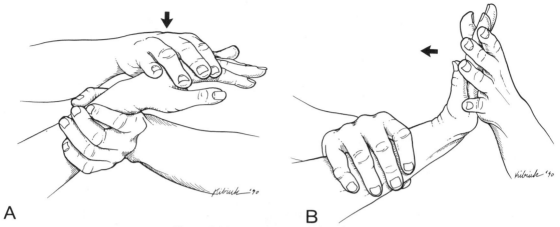

Figure 8.36 Forced wrist flexor/extensor.

A

B

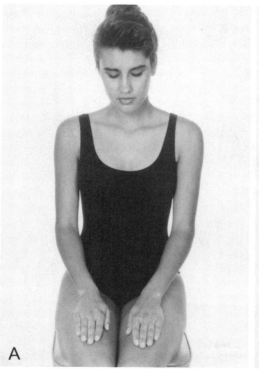

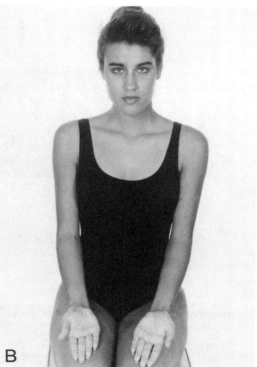

A

B

Finger Exercises

8.28. Finger Abductor (Fig. 8.38)

Description

With carpophalangeal joints in extension, first abduct and then adduct the fingers.

Exercise Format. Standard function 4.
Area Affected. Finger abductors, adductors.
Action Mode. Active stretching, isometric.
Intent. Flexibility, mobility, strength.

8.28.1. Variant

Therapist resists motion.
Exercise Format. Standard function 6.

8.29. Finger/Thumb Opposition (Fig. 8.39)

Description

Contact distal phalanx of the thumb with the distal phalanx of the first digit; apply maximum opposition.

Repeat the above, contacting the distal phalanx of the thumb with the other digits.

Exercise Format. Standard function 6.
Area Affected. Thumb abductors, opposers, and finger flexors.
Action Mode. Isometric.
Intent. Strength, coordination.

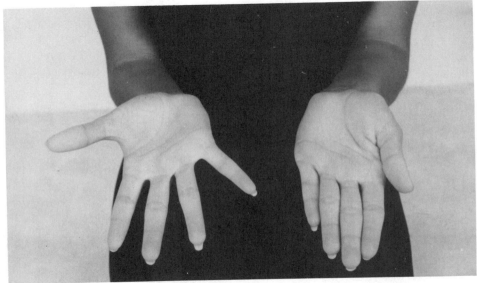

Figure 8.38 Finger abductor.

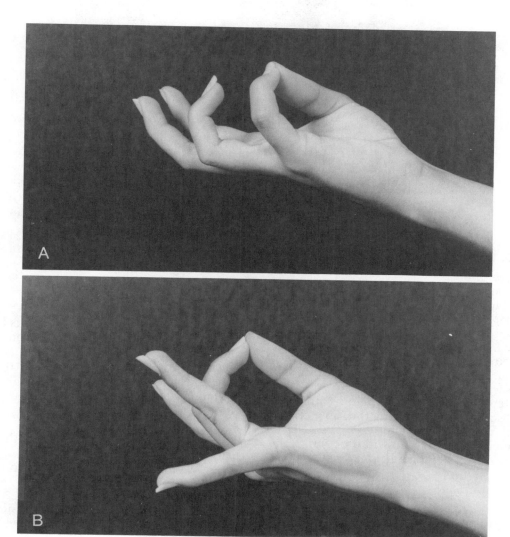

Figure 8.39 Finger/thumb opposition.

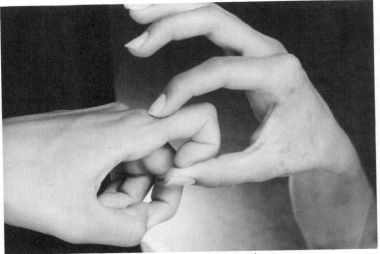

Figure 8.40 Finger isometrics.

8.30. Finger Isometrics (Fig. 8.40)

Description

Contact the carpometacarpal and distal phalanx of the index finger of the active hand, with the distal phalanx of the index finger and thumb, respectively, of the inactive hand.

Extend the index finger of the active hand, at the same time forcing it into flexion with the resistive hand.

Repeat above with remaining fingers of the active hand, utilizing the same contact with the indirect hand.

Exercise Format. Standard function 6.

Area Affected. Finger flexors and extensors.

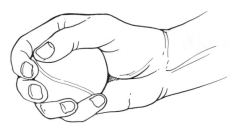

Figure 8.41 Ball squeezer.

Action Mode. Isometric.

Intent. Strength, coordination.

8.31. Ball Squeezer (Fig. 8.41)

Description

Grasp small athletic ball (i.e. tennis ball) in palm of hand, and rhythmically contract and relax fingers.

Area Affected. Forearm flexors, intrinsic hand muscles.

Action Mode. Isotonic.

Intent. Strength and endurance.

8.31.1 Variant

Use soft clay or putty, in place of athletic ball, and knead clay with fingers.

Intent. Coordination and mobilization.

References

1. Williams PL, Warwick R, Dyson M, Bannister LH, eds: Gray's Anatomy. 37th ed. New York: Churchill Livingstone, 1989.
2. Basmajian JV: Primary Anatomy. 8th ed. Baltimore: Williams & Wilkins, 1982.
3. Hoppenfeld S: Physical Examination of the Spine and Extremities. New York: Appleton-Century-Crofts, 1976.
4. Cailliet R: Soft Tissue Pain and Disability. Philadelphia: FA Davis, 1977.

Upper Back and Thorax

Action	Muscle	Exercise
Scapular elevator	Upper trapezius, levator scapulae, upper serratus	9.2, 9.4, 9.6, 9.6.1, 9.11, 9.11.1
Scapular retractor	Rhomboids, latissimus dorsi, trapezius	9.1, 9.2, 9.3, 9.4, 9.5, 9.5.1, 9.5.2, 9.6.1, 9.8, 9.8.1, 9.9
Scapular protractor	Serratus anterior, pectoralis minor, pectoralis major	9.9
Scapular medial rotation (downward)[a]	Levator scapulae, rhomboids, pectoralis minor, pectoralis major, latissimus dorsi	9.2, 9.8, 9.8.1, 9.9
Scapular lateral rotation (upward)[a]	Upper and lower trapezius, serratus anterior	9.4, 9.6, 9.6.1, 9.9, 9.11, 9.11.1
Scapular depression	Lower trapezius, pectoralis minor, pectoralis major, latissimus dorsi, serratus anterior	9.8, 9.8.1

[a] **Glenoid cavity.**

The thoracic spine is that portion of the spine that extends between the cervical and lumbar area. There are 12 thoracic vertebrae. The ribs, 12 sets, connect to the vertebrae anteriorly and posteriorly. This arrangement gives shape to the chest (1, p. 47).

The muscles of the thorax help form a protective cage to house the internal organs, heart, and lungs (2, pp. 335–6). This cage must be capable of alternately expanding during inspiration and expiration. The rib cage is arranged in such a way that with inspiration the chest increases its size in three directions: height, width, and depth (1, p. 48). The muscles of the thorax are also referred to as the muscles of respiration. The muscles of respiration include the internal and external intercostals, levatores costarum, transversus thoracis, serratus posterior superior, serratus posterior inferior, and diaphragm (1, p. 134). These muscles are all innervated by the intercostal nerves (anterior rami of the thoracic spinal nerves) with the exception of the levatores costarum (posterior rami) and the diaphragm (phrenic nerve).

The ranges of motion for the trunk are flexion, extension, lateral flexion, and rotation. These motions can also be described as sagittal (θ_x), frontal (θ_z), and transverse (θ_y).

The flexors are the rectus abdominis, the anterior and lateral fibers of the external obliques, and the lateral fibers of the internal obliques (1, p. 138) (Fig. 9.1). The rectus abdominis is innervated by T5-T12 ventral rami (1, p. 138; 2, pp. 591–2).

The extensors are the erector spinae and the intrinsic spinal muscles (Fig. 8.2).

The lateral fibers of the internal and external obliques, acting unilaterally, provide lateral flexion, as do intrinsic spinal muscles working unilaterally (1, p. 138) (Fig. 9.1). They are innervated by branches from the T8-T12 intercostals, iliohypogastric and ilioinguinal nerves (1, pp. 138–9).

The anterior fibers of the external obliques assist in rotation (Fig. 9.1). Primary rotators of the spine are the external oblique acting contralaterally with the internal oblique (1, p. 138).

The exercises described in this section are for the rehabilitation of the muscles of the upper and middle back (including the shoulder girdle), chest wall, and rib cage. Some of the exercises described may be employed for people with various breathing problems.

For the purposes of anatomical organization we have placed the exercises involving extrinsic scapular muscles in this chapter. This was done because these muscles may be considered to be part of the thoracic structure. However, they are technically interrelated, through the scapulae, with the scapulohumeral mechanism, which we recognize as shoulder motion. Therefore, these exercises will be utilized for the rehabilitation of shoulder problems as well as for thoracic dysfunctions.

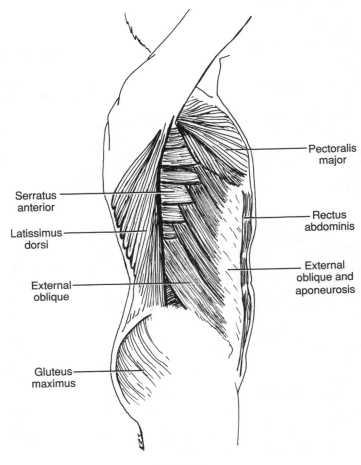

Figure 9.1 Lateral view of thorax.

THORACIC-RIB EXERCISES

9.1. Supine, Arms at Side (Fig. 9.2)

Description

Assume a supine position, with arms by the side and forearms extended and supinated. Flatten both the cervical and upper thoracic spine against the table, externally rotate arms, and then adduct both scapulae. Relax and return to the original position. Make fists, flex both elbows while keeping them at the sides, and again adduct the scapulae.

Exercise Format. Standard function 2.
Area Affected. Scapular retractors, superior anterior thorax, and cervicothoracic junction.
Action Mode. Isotonic, isometric.
Intent. Primary: flexibility, strengthening; secondary: mobility.

9.2. Prone, Arms at Side (Fig. 9.3)

Description

Assume a prone position, with arms at sides. Adduct scapulae, and at the same time pull them inferiorly toward the feet.

Exercise Format. Standard function 1.
Area Affected. Scapular elevators, retractors, glenohumeral joint, anterior thorax.
Action Mode. Active stretching, isometric, isotonic.
Intent. Primary: flexibility, strength; secondary: mobility.

9.3. Prone with Hands Clasped behind Back (Fig. 9.4)

Description

From prone position with hands clasped behind back, adduct scapulae abruptly, and then relax.

Exercise Format. Standard function 2.
Note. Proprioceptive neuromuscular facilitation, standard function 9.
Area Affected. Scapular retractors, shoulder internal and external rotators, anterior thorax.
Action Mode. Active stretching, isokinetic.
Intent. Flexibility, mobility, strength.

9.4. Prone with Arms Elevated (Fig. 9.5)

Description

From prone position with forehead straight down and elbows in flexion, elevate arms and adduct scapulae.

Exercise Format. Standard function 2.
Area Affected. Scapular retractors and elevators.
Action Mode. Active stretching, isokinetic.
Intent. Flexibility, mobility, strength.

9.5. Prone, Arms above the Head (Fig. 9.6)

Description

From prone position with forehead on the table, raise both arms off the floor as high as possible, without lifting chest. Therapist

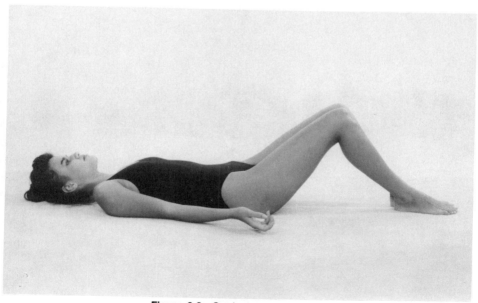

Figure 9.2 Supine, arms at side.

UPPER BACK AND THORAX

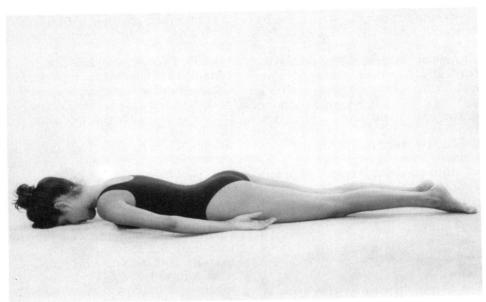

Figure 9.3 Prone, arms at side.

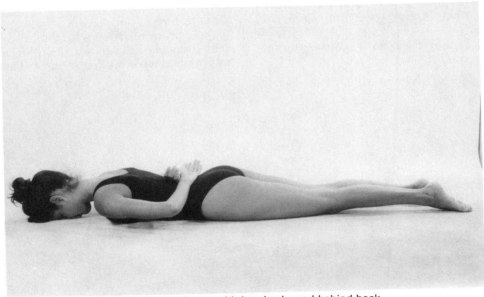

Figure 9.4 Prone with hands clasped behind back.

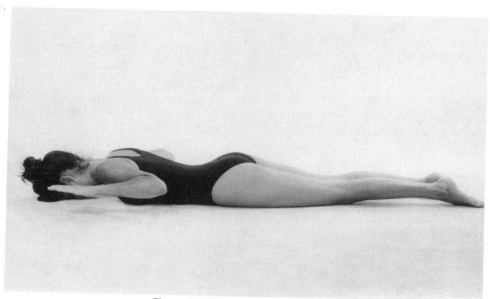

Figure 9.5 Prone with arms elevated.

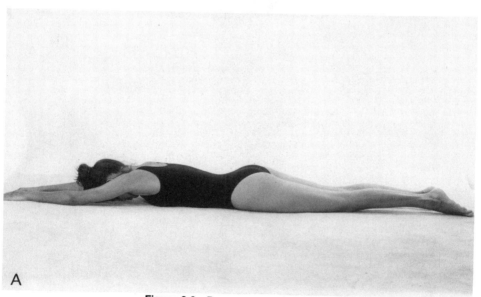

A

Figure 9.6 Prone, arms above the head.

provides stabilization with firm pressure at posterior inferior area of scapulae.

Exercise Format. Standard function 2.

Area Affected. Shoulder external rotators, retractors, thoracic extensors.

Action Mode. Active stretching, isokinetic.

Intent. Flexibility, mobility, strength, posture.

9.5.1 Variant

Adduct arms 30° which moves center of motion in thoracic spine cephalward.

9.5.2 Variant

Raise arms unilaterally, which adds a rotatory component in thoracic spine and also involves intrinsic thoracic musculature, both long and short.

9.6. Prone with Elbows Flexed (Fig. 9.7A)

Description

From prone position with forehead on table, extend elbows, then fully abduct arms cephalward.

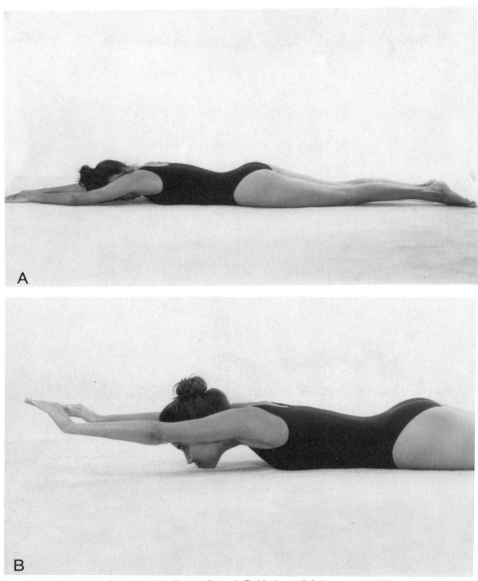

Figure 9.7   A. Prone with elbows flexed. **B.** Variant 9.6.1—prone with arms elevated.

Exercise Format. Standard function 2.

Note. Extension of cervical spine (chin on table) will fix the upper thoracic and cervical regions, thereby isolating the mid and lower thoracic areas for motion. If there is a concomitant cervical injury, this position may be contraindicated.

Area Affected. Shoulder external rotators and elevators.

Action Mode. Isokinetic.

Intent. Flexibility, mobility.

9.6.1. Variant

With arms elevated off the table (Fig. 9.7B), area affected will include thoracic extensors, posterior deltoid, and scapular retractors. Action mode will be isotonic. Intent will be for strength.

9.7. Sitting, Hands around Knees (Fig. 9.8)

Description

Sitting, hands around the knees, relax the spine and allow the head to drop inferiorly toward the knees. Then begin to extend the spine, starting at the lower end of the spine, and advancing toward the occiput.

Exercise Format. Standard function 1.

Area Affected. Primary: thoracic spine; secondary: cervical and lumbar spine.

Action Mode. Isotonic, active stretching.

Intent. Mobility, flexibility.

9.8. Cross-Sitting Position (Fig. 9.9)

Description

From sitting position with legs crossed, raise both arms to shoulder level, flexing the elbows 90°. Extend wrists with volar surface parallel to floor (Fig. 9.9A). Keeping an erect position, extend elbows, adduct arms, and adduct the scapulae (Fig. 9.9B).

Exercise Format. Standard function 2.

Area Affected. Shoulder internal rotators, adductors, depressors, thoracic spine, scapular retractors, anterior thorax.

Action Mode. Active stretching, isotonic.

Intent. Flexibility, mobility, strength, endurance.

9.8.1 Variant: Standard Sitting Position

Note. Lower back should be supported.

9.9. Cross-Sitting, Arms at Sides (Fig. 9.10)

Description

From sitting position with legs crossed, allow the arms to hang free. Circumduct one shoulder into interior rotation, and at the same time circumduct the other shoulder into external rotation.

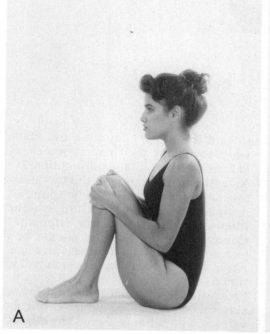
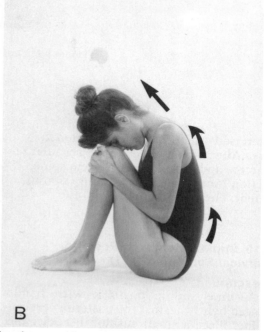

Figure 9.8 Sitting, hands around knees.

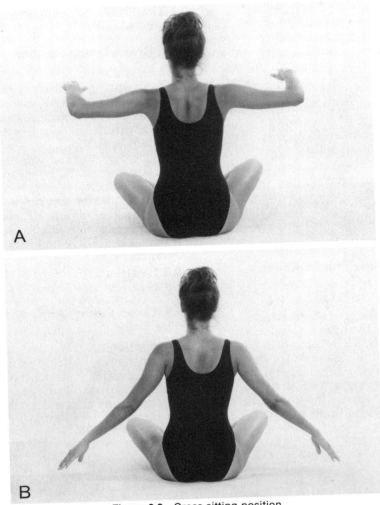

Figure 9.9 Cross-sitting position.

Exercise Format. Standard function 2.
Area Affected. Shoulder girdle, scapular retractors and protractors, thoracic spine.
Action Mode. Active stretching, isotonic.
Intent. Flexibility, mobility.

9.10. Supine, Hands on Posterior Cervical Spine (Fig. 9.11)

Description

Assume supine position with hands placed lightly against the posterior cervical spine. Place a small cushion between the scapulae. Then force the elbows posteriorly toward the table, adducting the scapulae while extending the thoracic spine.

Exercise Format. Standard function 2.
Area Affected. Shoulder adductors and rotators, anterior thorax, thoracic spine.
Action Mode. Active stretching, isokinetic.
Intent. Flexibility, mobility, strength.
Contraindication. Exercise should be performed isometrically if there is an acute anterior thoracic complex. Use standard function 6.
Precaution. Use cervical support for acute cervical conditions, or altered cervical curvatures, adjunctively. Avoid any other than the mildest pressure on the cervical spine.

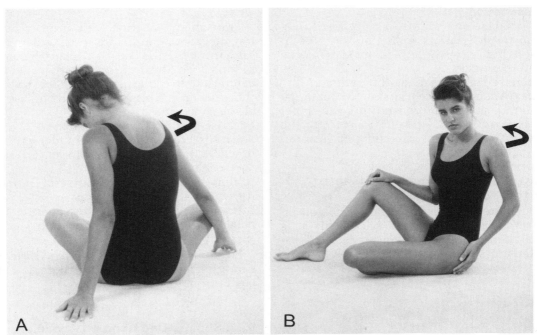

Figure 9.10 Cross-sitting, arms at sides.

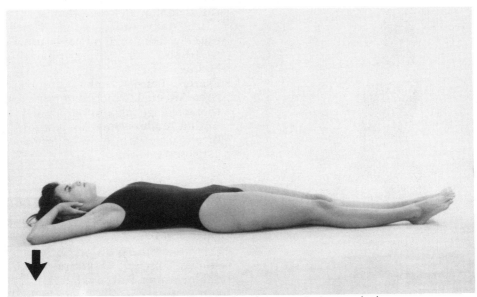

Figure 9.11 Supine, hands on posterior cervical
spine.

9.11. Standing, Arms Extended (Fig. 9.12)

Description

Stand facing a wall with arms raised. Flex arms cephalward, standing on toes, reaching as high as possible. Hold for short a time and then relax.

Exercise Format. Standard function 1.

Area Affected. Primary: shoulder external rotators and elevators, and thoracic spine; secondary: general facilitation of thoracic extensor tonus and stretching of glenohumeral structures.

Action Mode. Active stretching.

Intent. Flexibility, mobility, toning.

9.11.1 Variant: Ladderwalk

Unilaterally flex one arm while contralaterally flexing hip and knee. This adds skill training and neuromuscular reeducation (cross-crawl pattern).

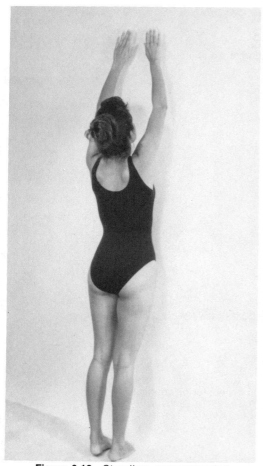

Figure 9.12 Standing, arms extended.

9.12. Supine with Knees Flexed (Fig. 9.13)

Description

From supine position with knees in flexion, elevate one arm anteriorly, and at the same time expand chest with strong inspiration. Then lower the arm, with a gradual expiration at the same time. Repeat with the other arm. Then repeat with both arms at the same time.

Exercise Format. Standard function 2.

Area Affected. Anterior shoulder girdle, brachial flexors, anterior thorax, pulmonary enhancer.

Action Mode. Isotonic, isokinetic, mobility, strength, endurance.

Intent. Flexibility, pulmonary function enhancer, neuromuscular reeducation.

9.12.1. Variant

Flex arms 180°. Increase above with addition of stretching of lateral thoracic and posterior brachium.

9.13. Supine, One Hand on Abdomen (Fig. 9.14)

Description

From supine position with one hand on the abdomen and the other at the side, exhale slowly and completely, while contracting abdominal musculature. Hold for 5 to 10 sec., then allow inhalation by relaxing.

Exercise Format. Standard function 4.

Area Affected. Teach abdominal breathing, thoracic cage, abdominal wall.

Action Mode. Isometric, isotonic.

Intent. Strength, pulmonary function enhancer, relaxation.

9.14. Supine with Two Hands on Abdomen (Fig. 9.15)

Description

From supine position with hands on abdomen, complete inspiration with abdominal breathing. At the same time, apply pressure with the hands inferomedially.

Exercise Format. Standard function 4.

Area Affected. Thoracic cage, abdominal wall.

Action Mode. Active stretching, isotonic.

Intent. Strength, pulmonary function enhancer, relaxation.

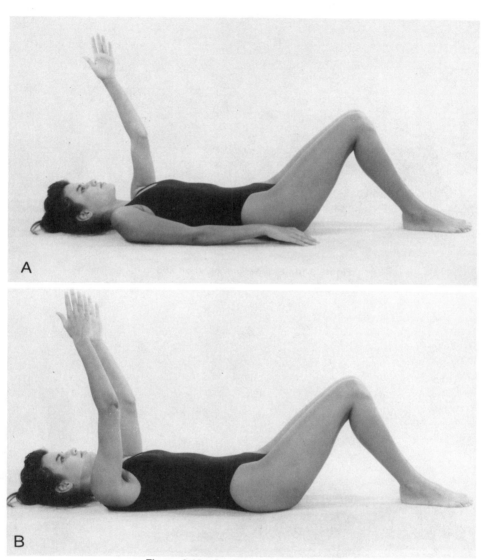

Figure 9.13 Supine with knees flexed.

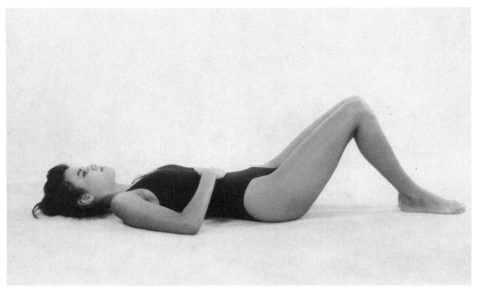

Figure 9.14   Supine, one hand on abdomen.

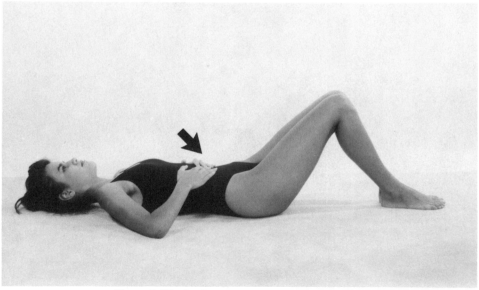

Figure 9.15   Supine with two hands on abdomen.

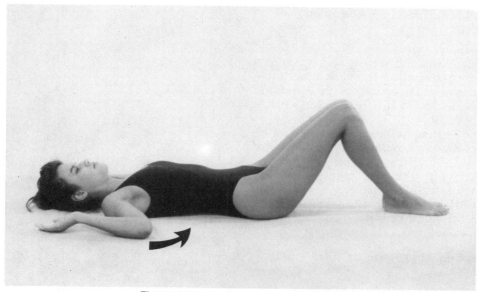

Figure 9.16 Supine with arms elevated.

9.15. Supine with Arms Elevated (Fig. 9.16)

Description

Assume supine position with elbows flexed and arms flexed 180°. Inhale, allowing abdomen to raise and transferring air toward the upper chest. Hold for 5 to 10 sec, then lower arms to side as you fully exhale.
Exercise Format. Standard function 1.
Area Affected. Thoracic cage, abdominal wall, and pulmonary enhancer.
Action Mode. Active stretching, isotonic.
Intent. Strength, pulmonary function enhancer, relaxation.

9.16. Sitting, Hands on Hips (Fig. 9.17)

Description

From sitting position with hands on hips, perform full inspiration, forcing chest superior. At the same time force both hands inferiorly on the hips and allow the abdomen to expand fully.
Exercise Format. Standard function 1.
Area Affected. Thoracic cage, pulmonary enhancer.
Action Mode. Active stretching, isotonic.
Intent. Strength, pulmonary function enhancer, relaxation.
Note. Try to keep the shoulders in a relaxed position during this exercise.

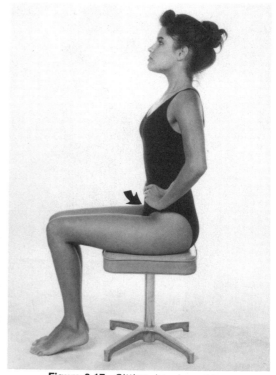

Figure 9.17 Sitting, hands on hips.

9.17. Sitting, Hands on Abdomen (Fig. 9.18)

Description

Sitting with hands across abdomen, fully expire by contracting the abdominal muscles forcefully. Then apply gradual pressure with the hands to slowly exhale as much air as possible.

Exercise Format. Standard function 1 (modify frequency to a maximum of 6 exercises/min).

Area Affected. Thoracic cage, pulmonary system, abdominal muscles.

Action Mode. Isotonic, isometric.

Intent. Strength, pulmonary function enhancer, relaxation.

9.18. Sitting, One Hand on Ribs (Fig. 9.19)

Description

From a sitting position with one hand on ribs, flex laterally toward that same side. Compress ribs with the hand, and exhale deeply, contracting the abdominal muscles

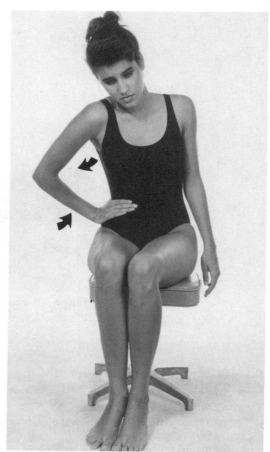

Figure 9.19 Sitting, one hand on ribs.

forcefully. Hold 5 to 10 sec. Repeat on the opposite side.

Exercise Format. Standard function 1.

Area Affected. Thoracic cage, pulmonary system, abdominal muscles.

Action Mode. Isotonic.

Intent. Strength, pulmonary function enhancer, relaxation.

9.19. Sitting, Arms at Sides (Fig. 9.20)

Description

Sitting with arms at side, inhale with abdominal breathing and begin to exhale slowly. Allow the head and upper back to fall forward, flexing the cervical and thoracic spine. At the same time, contract all abdominal muscles forcefully. Return to original position.

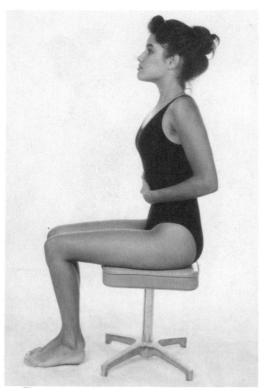

Figure 9.18 Sitting, hands on abdomen.

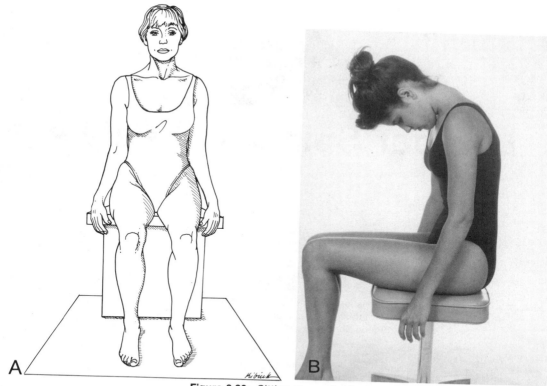

Figure 9.20 Sitting, arms at sides.

Exercise Format. Standard function 1.
Area Affected. Thoracic cage, pulmonary system, abdominal muscles.
Action Mode. Isotonic.
Intent. Strength, pulmonary lung enhancer, relaxation.

References

1. Basmajian JV: Primary Anatomy. 8th ed. Baltimore:Williams & Wilkins, 1982.
2. Williams PL, Warwick R, Dyson M, Bannister LH, Eds.: Gray's Anatomy. 37th ed. New York: Churchill Livingstone, 1989.

10

Lumbar Spine and Pelvis

Action	Muscle	Exercise
Flexion	Rectus abdominis, external obliques (anterior and lateral fibers), internal obliques (lateral fibers), psoas	10.4, 10.9, 10.11, 10.11.1, 10.13, 10.16, 10.23, 10.23.1, 10.26, 10.26.1, 10.26.2, 10.28, 10.34, 10.35
Extension	Erector spinae, intrinsic muscles, quadratus lumborum	10.1, 10.3, 10.13, 10.21.1, 10.23.1, 10.24, 10.28, 10.31, 10.32, 10.32.2
Lateral flexion	External obliques (lateral fibers), internal obliques (lateral fibers), quadratus lumborum, psoas	10.10, 10.10.1, 10.10.2, 10.11.1, 10.12, 10.14, 10.18, 10.21, 10.21.1, 10.22, 10.24, 10.26.1, 10.29
Rotation	External obliques (anterior fibers), erector spinae, intrinsic muscles	10.4, 10.6, 10.6.1, 10.7, 10.8, 10.11.1, 10.22, 10.26.2, 10.31, 10.32.1, 10.33, 10.34

Many conditions related to the lumbosacral area (lumbar spine and pelvis) are due in most part to weakening of the abdominal and erector spinae musculature of the back. Add to this muscle weakness poor posture, caused by improper training and bad habits, along with unusual physical activity, and a predisposition to injury is established.

Of primary importance in the rehabilitation of the low back is to restore the normal rhythm of the lumbar spine and pelvic biomechanics and also to maximize flexibility of the individual vertebral components (1, pp. 23–6, 53–6). This is why we emphasize both static and dynamic exercise circumstances.

The lumbar spine is that portion of the spine that extends between the thoracic spine and the sacrum. The sacrum is surrounded by the pelvis. There is a greater degree of motion between L5/S1 than between L1/L2. Approximately 75% of lumbar flexion occurs at the lumbosacral joint (1, p. 20).

Trunk

The ranges of motion for the trunk are flexion, extension, lateral flexion, and rotation (Table 10.1). The flexors are the rectus abdominis, the anterior and lateral fibers of the external obliques, and the lateral fibers of the internal obliques (Fig. 10.1) (2, pp. 96–101; 3, pp. 201–6).

As there are no ribs to restrict motion in the lumbar spine, flexion and extension are greater than in the thoracic spine, and a greater amount of rotation is possible. Flexion in the lumbar spine is accomplished by the relaxation of the anterior longitudinal ligament and the stretching of the supraspinal and interspinal ligaments, the ligamentum flavum, and the posterior longi-

Table 10.1. Lumbar Spine Ranges of Motion (ROM)[a]

Motion	ROM	Anatomical	Cartesian
Flexion	40°[b]	Sagittal	θ_x
Extension	25°[c]	Sagittal	θ_x
Lateral flexion	20°[d]	Frontal	$\pm\,\theta_y$[f]
Rotation	5°[e]	Transverse	$\pm\,\theta_y$[f]

[a] Reprinted with permission from Delisa JA: Rehabilitation Medicine. Philadelphia: JB Lippincott, 1988; 325.
[b] Combined thoracic and lumbar ROM is 55°.
[c] Combined thoracic and lumbar ROM is 40°.
[d] Combined thoracic and lumbar ROM is 35°.
[e] Combined thoracic and lumbar ROM is 45°.
[f] According to left or right motion.

tudinal ligament. The actual size of the lumbar vertebral bodies affects the amount of flexion possible (4, p. 247). With extension of the lumbar spine, the anterior longitudinal ligament is stretched, while the posterior ligaments are relaxed.

The extensors are the erector spinae and the intrinsic muscles (Fig. 10.2) (5, pp. 135–9; 3, p. 202).

The lateral fibers of the internal and external obliques provide lateral flexion (Fig. 10.1) (3, pp. 202–3).

The anterior fibers of the external obliques assist in rotation (Fig. 10.1) (3, pp. 202–3).

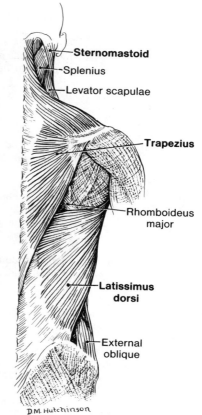

Figure 10.2 Extrinsic muscles of the back.

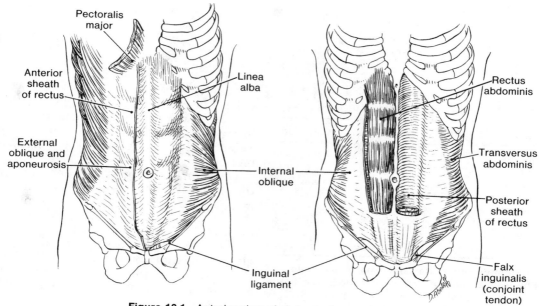

Figure 10.1 Anterior view of abdominal musculature.

Hip

Action	Muscle	Exercise
Flexion	Rectus femoris, psoas major, iliacus, sartorius, pectineus, adductor longus	10.1, 10.4, 10.5, 10.13, 10.14, 10.18, 10.18.1, 10.19, 10.19.2, 10.20, 10.21, 10.21.1, 10.22, 10.26, 10.26.2, 10.27, 10.27.1, 10.32, 10.32.2, 10.32.3, 10.33, 10.34, 10.35
Extension	Gluteus maximus, adductor magnus, semimembranosus, semitendinosus, biceps long head	10.3, 10.5, 10.11, 10.11.1, 10.17, 10.19.2, 10.21, 10.21.1, 10.26.2, 10.32.3, 10.35
Abduction	Gluteus medius, gluteus minimus, gluteus maximus, sartorius, tensor fascia lata, gemelli inferior,[a] piriformis,[a] gemelli superior,[a] obturator internus[a]	10.8, 10.10, 10.10.1, 10.10.2, 10.29, 10.33
Adduction	Adductor longus, adductor brevis, adductor magnus, pectineus, gracilis	10.7, 10.8, 10.10.1, 10.12, 10.26.1, 10.26.2, 10.27, 10.27.1, 10.33, 10.34
Internal rotation	Tensor fascia lata, gluteus minimus, gluteus medius	10.6, 10.6.1, 10.7, 10.8, 10.11.1, 10.26.1, 10.26.2, 10.30.1, 10.30.2, 10.31, 10.32.1, 10.33
External rotation	Psoas major, iliacus, sartorius, obturator externus, gemelli inferior, quadratus femoris, gluteus maximus, piriformis, gemelli superior, obturator internus	10.6, 10.6.1, 10.8, 10.11.1, 10.26.1, 10.26.2, 10.31, 10.33

[a] **All abductors when hip is flexed.**

Table 10.2. Hip Ranges of Motion (ROM)[a]

Motion	ROM	Anatomical	Cartesian
Flexion	120°	Sagittal	$-\theta_x$
Extension	30°	Sagittal	$+\theta_x$
Abduction	45–50°	Frontal	$\pm\theta_z{}^b$
Adduction	20–30°	Frontal	$\pm\theta_z{}^b$
Internal rotation	35°	Transverse	$\pm\theta_y{}^b$
External rotation	45°	Transverse	$\pm\theta_y{}^b$

[a] **Reprinted with permission from Hoppenfeld S: Physical Examination of the Spine and Extremities. New York: Appleton-Century-Crofts, 1976; 155–60.**
[b] **According to side of body.**

The ranges of motion of the hip are flexion, extension, abduction, adduction, and internal and external rotation (4, p. 155). Table 10.2 describes the hip ranges of motion.

The primary flexor is the iliopsoas, and the secondary flexor is the rectus femoris (Figs. 10.3 and 10.4). The iliopsoas muscle is innervated by the femoral nerve (L1,2,3) (4, p. 160).

The primary extensor of the hip is the gluteus maximus, innervated by the inferior gluteal nerve (S1). The secondary extensors are the hamstrings (Figs. 9.1 and 10.1) (4, p. 161).

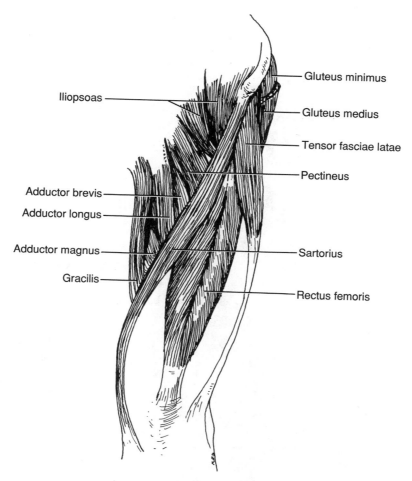

Iliopsoas

Adductor brevis
Adductor longus

Adductor magnus

Gracilis

Gluteus minimus

Gluteus medius

Tensor fasciae latae

Pectineus

Sartorius

Rectus femoris

Figure 10.3 Primary hip flexors.

The gluteus medius and minimis are the primary and secondary abductors respectively (Figs. 10.3 and 10.5). The gluteus medius is innervated by the superior gluteal nerve (L5) (4, p. 162).

The primary adductor is the adductor longus, with the secondary adductors consisting of the adductor brevis and magnus, pectineus, and gracilis (Figs. 10.3 and 10.4). The adductor longus is innervated by the obturator nerve (L2,3,4) (4, p. 163).

Internal rotation is accomplished by the

gluteus minimus, the anterior fibers of the gluteus medius, the tensor fasciae lata, the adductor longus, brevis, and magnus, the pectineus, iliacus, and the psoas major (5, p. 642).

External rotation is performed by the posterior fibers of the gluteus medius, the piriformis, the internal and external obturators, the superior and inferior gemelli, the quadratus femoris, the gluteus maximus, and the sartorius (5, pp. 642–3).

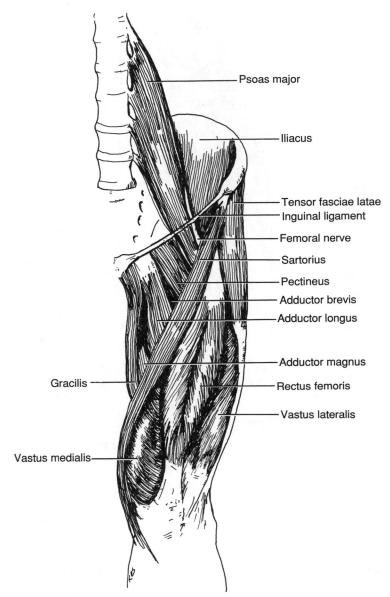

Figure 10.4 Hip muscles.

- Psoas major
- Iliacus
- Tensor fasciae latae
- Inguinal ligament
- Femoral nerve
- Sartorius
- Pectineus
- Adductor brevis
- Adductor longus
- Adductor magnus
- Rectus femoris
- Vastus lateralis
- Gracilis
- Vastus medialis

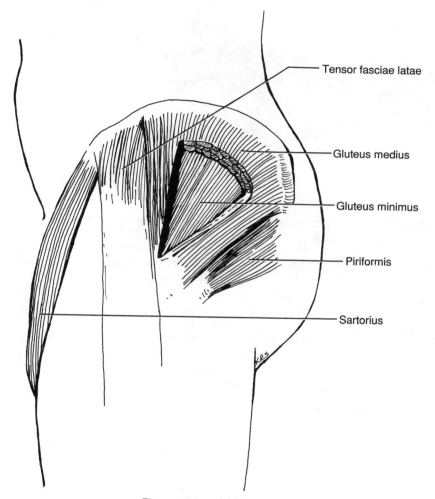

Tensor fasciae latae

Gluteus medius

Gluteus minimus

Piriformis

Sartorius

Figure 10.5 Hip abductors.

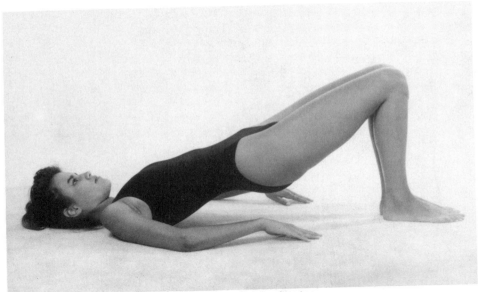

Figure 10.6 Pelvic elevator.

LUMBOSACRAL SPINE AND HIP EXERCISES

10.1. Pelvic Elevator (Fig. 10.6)

Description

From supine position with hands by sides (palms inferior), feet on the floor, and knees in flexion, elevate buttocks off the floor.
Exercise Format. Standard function 1.
Area Affected. Hip flexors and erector spinae.

Action Mode. Active stretching, isotonic.
Intent. Flexibility, mobility, strength.
10.1.1 Variant
Exercise format. Standard function 2.
Note. The closer the feet are to the buttocks, the easier the exercise is to perform.

10.2. Abdominal Strengthener (Fig. 10.7)

Description

Starting position is supine with the arms crossed on the chest and the head and

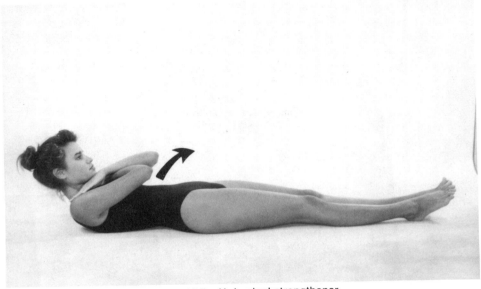

Figure 10.7 Abdominal strengthener.

DYNAMICS OF CLINICAL REHABILITATIVE EXERCISE

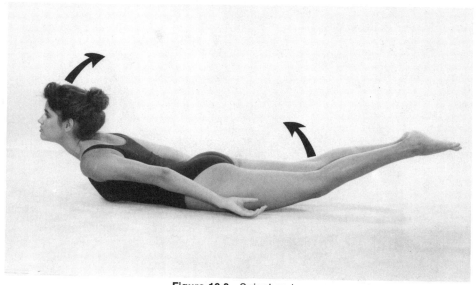

Figure 10.8 Spinal archer.

shoulders elevated off the floor. From this position, flex the trunk partially, then return to the starting position.

Exercise Format. Standard function 3.
Area Affected. Abdominal musculature.
Action Mode. Isotonic resistance.
Intent. Strength.

10.2.1 Variant

By emphasizing the eccentric phase over the concentric phase, the strengthening function will increase.

10.3. Spinal Archer (Fig. 10.8)

Description

From a prone position with arms at side, elevate head and legs, keeping them extended.

Exercise Format. Standard function 4.
Area Affected. Erector spinae musculature, hamstrings, gluteals, abdominals, cervical extensors.
Action Mode. Isometric, isotonic.
Intent. Strength.

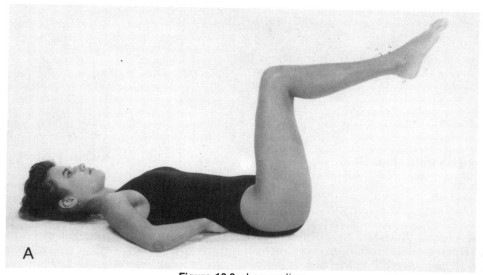

A

Figure 10.9 Leg cycling.

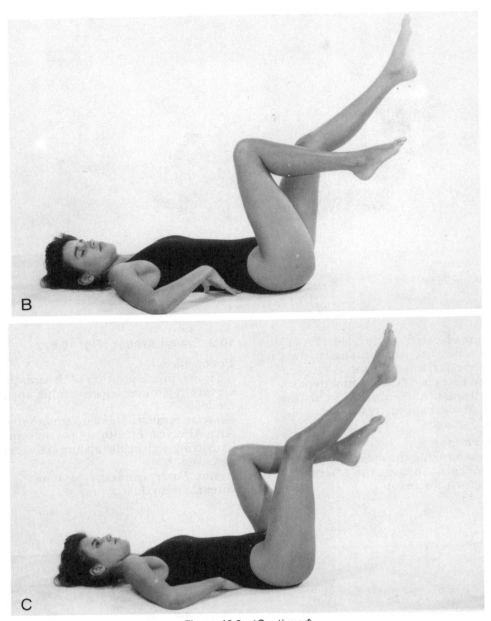

B

C

Figure 10.9 (Continued)

10.4. Leg Cycling (Fig. 10.9)

Description

From supine position with arms inferior, flex hip and knees 90° and begin cycling maneuver.

Exercise Format. Standard function 2.
Area Affected. Abdominal musculature, hip, hip flexors, sacroiliac joint.
Action Mode. Isotonic, isokinetic.

Intent. Flexibility, mobility, strength, endurance.

10.5. Full Knee Flexion (Fig. 10.10)

Description

Standing erect with arms extended anteriorly, flex knees while keeping spine erect. Avoid total flexion, so there is no rest position between phases, and to prevent exces-

DYNAMICS OF CLINICAL REHABILITATIVE EXERCISE

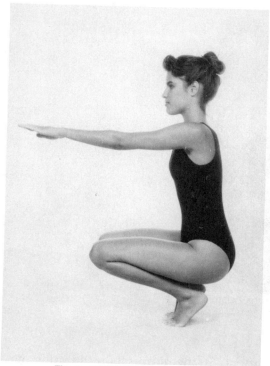

Figure 10.10 Full knee flexion.

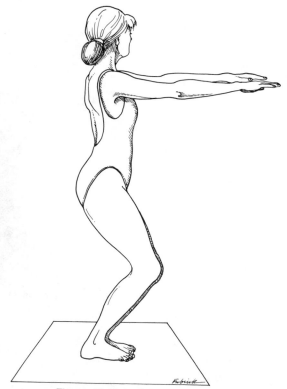

Figure 10.10.1 Full knee flexion.

sive tension on knee cruciate ligaments.
Exercise Format. Standard function 5.
Area Affected. Quadriceps, hip capsule, hamstrings, lower leg, and erector spinae.
Action Mode. Isotonic.
Intent. Mobility, strength, endurance.

10.5.1. Variant (Fig. 10.10.1)
Repeat position as above, keeping feet flat on floor to stretch Achilles tendon.
Precaution. Patients with more serious knee problems should not flex knees more than 45°.

10.6. Trunk Twister (Fig. 10.11)

Description
Stand erect with arms abducted 90° and hold feet and legs in position. Rotate hips and arms only first to the right side, return to center position, rotate to the left side, and return to center position.
Exercise Format. Standard function 2.
Area Affected. Obliquus externus abdominis, erector spinae, and tensor fascia lata.
Action Mode. Active stretching.
Intent. Flexibility mobility.

10.6.1 Variant
Have therapist restrict motion at a particular angle.
Exercise Format. Standard function 6.
Action Mode. Isometric.
Intent. Strength.
Note. Avoid lateral flexion.

10.7. Pelvic Twister (Fig. 10.12)

Description
From a supine position with arms at sides, palms pronated, and keeping shoulders and arms in place, first internally rotate left hip and adduct left thigh over the right leg. Return to the supine position, then internally rotate and adduct the right hip and thigh, as above.
Exercise Format. Standard function 1.
Area Affected. Hip flexors and external rotators, sacroiliac joint, pelvic girdle, tensor fascia lata, lumbar spine.
Action Mode. Active stretching, isotonic.
Intent. Flexibility, mobility, strength.

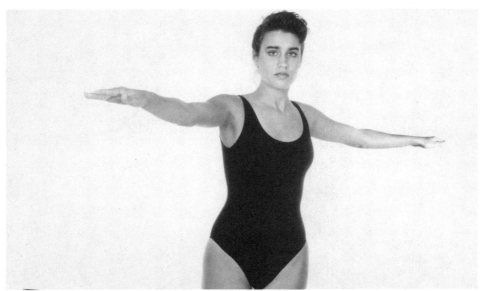

Figure 10.11 Trunk twister.

10.8. Pelvic Roller (Fig. 10.13)

Description

Standing erect with hands on hips, and keeping feet and hands in position, circumduct hips in a circular pattern clockwise 10 times as if you were using a hula hoop. Repeat counterclockwise 10 times.

Exercise Format. Standard function 2.
Area Affected. Lumbosacral musculature, sacroiliac joint, hip joint.
Action Mode. Isotonic.
Intent. Mobility, muscle skill, endurance.
Note. See "Knees and Ankles" for other effects.

10.9. Lumbar Spine Flattener (Fig. 10.14)

Description

Stand erect with back against a wall, arms at side, and palms against the wall. Press spine against the wall, making sure that the posterior occiput, shoulders, buttocks, and heels are in contact with the wall. Extend pelvis so as to bring the posterior superior iliac spine (PSIS) against wall.

Exercise Format. Standard function 8.
Area Affected. Postural muscles including the erector spinae, abdominal muscles, cervical muscles, shoulder, pelvis, and gluteals.
Action Mode. Isometric.

Intent. Strength, muscle reeducation, postural.

10.10. Abductor Strengthener (Fig. 10.15)

Description

Lying on right side with right arm under occiput, or utilizing a cervical spine pillow, and left arm lying across waist, keeping both legs extended and toes pointed caudad, abduct left leg as far as possible. Repeat while lying on left side.

Exercise Format. Standard function 2.
Area Affected. Hip abductors.
Action Mode. Active stretching, isotonic.
Intent. Strength.
Note. Above exercise may be performed with weights. Exercise format, action mode, and intent remain unchanged.

10.10.1 Variant

From starting position, raise leg to middle of motion (30 to 40°). Therapist applies resistance on the leg. Placement of the therapist's hand depends on the strength of the leg. The stronger the limb, the more distal the resistance. Resistance is applied laterally for abductors and medially for adductors.

Exercise Format. Standard function 6.
Area Affected. Hip abductors, hip adductors.

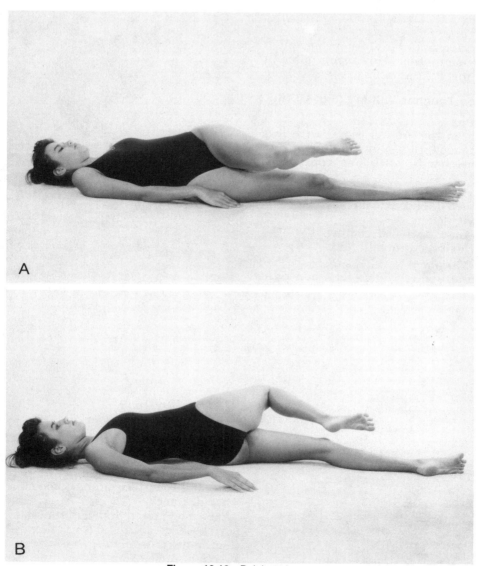

A

B

Figure 10.12 Pelvic twister.

Action Mode. Isometric.

Intent. Strength.

10.10.2 Variant

Proprioceptive neuromuscular facilitation is used for hip abductors and internal flexion.

10.10.3 Variant

Add flexion and/or extension component to abduction motion. This affects different fibers of involved muscles.

10.11. Toe Toucher—Sitting (Fig. 10.16)

Description

Sitting on the ground (floor) with legs fully extended, flex spine and touch toes with both hands, with one continuous motion.

Exercise Format. Standard function 1.

Area Affected. Hip extenders, erector spinae, pelvic flexors.

Action Mode. Active stretching.

Intent. Flexibility, mobility.

10.11.1. Variant

Touch alternately with left then right hands.

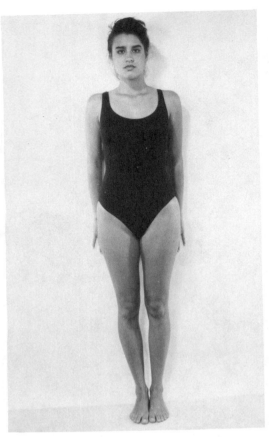

Figure 10.14 Lumbar spine flattener.

10.12. Lateral Trunk Flexor (Fig. 10.17)

Description

Standing with arms extended cephalad, flex laterally to the right, return to the center, and then flex laterally to the left. **Do not flex neck.**

Exercise Format. Standard function 1.

Area Affected. Lateral trunk flexors, intrinsic spinal musculature.

Action Mode. Active stretching, isotonic.

Intent. Flexibility, strength.

10.13. Spinal Stretcher (Fig. 10.18)

Description

From a kneeling position with knees and legs on floor, flex anteriorly, placing hands on floor at shoulder level and width. Hip joint is flexed 90°, and head is parallel to floor. Keeping arms extended, lower head and raise buttocks. For position 2, back is arched, head is extended, hips are flexed;

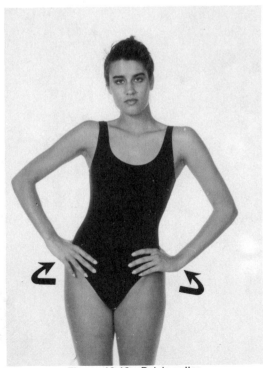

Figure 10.13 Pelvic roller.

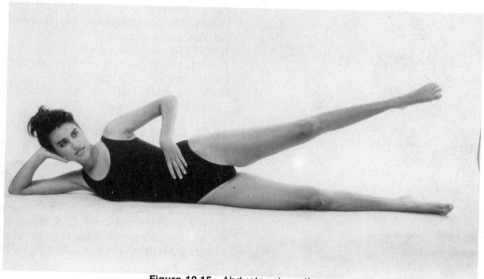

Figure 10.15 Abductor strengthener.

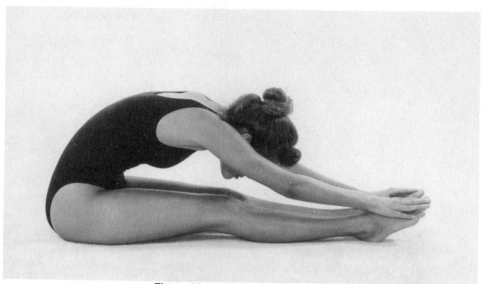

Figure 10.16 Toe toucher—sitting.

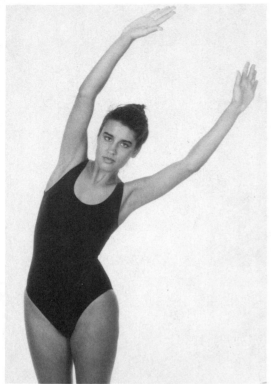

Figure 10.17 Lateral trunk flexor.

then return to starting position. For position 3, flex pelvis, flex hip joints, and flex neck.

Exercise Format. Standard function 1.

Area Affected. Abdominal musculature, paraspinal musculature, hip flexors, pelvic flexors and extensors.

Action Mode. Active stretching, isotonic.

Intent. Flexibility, mobility, strength, posture, muscle reeducation.

Note. Initially, all patients should be assisted for proper form.

10.14. Crawl Exercise (Fig. 10.19)

Description

From a kneeling position with knees and legs on floor, flex anteriorly, placing hands on floor at shoulder level and width. First move one knee cephalad as far as possible, turn head toward cephalad shoulder, and move the contralateral hand cephalward, as far as possible, keeping the hand on the floor.

Exercise Format. Standard function 2.

Area Affected. Paraspinal musculature, lateral trunk flexors, hip flexors.

Action Mode. Isotonic.

Intent. Mobility, postural, neuromuscular reeducation, coordination.

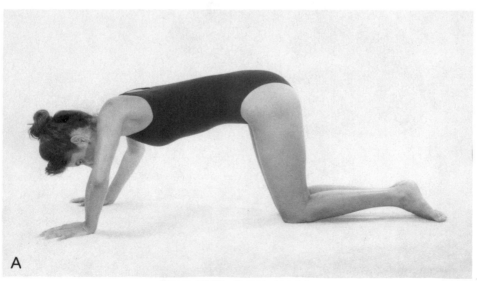

A

Figure 10.18 Spinal stretcher.

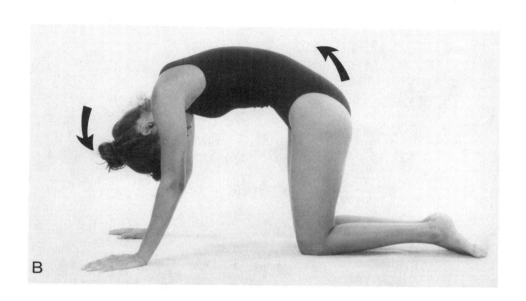

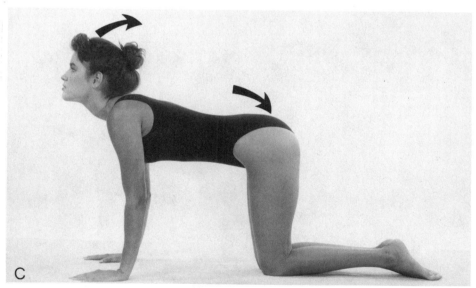

Figure 10.18 (*Continued*)

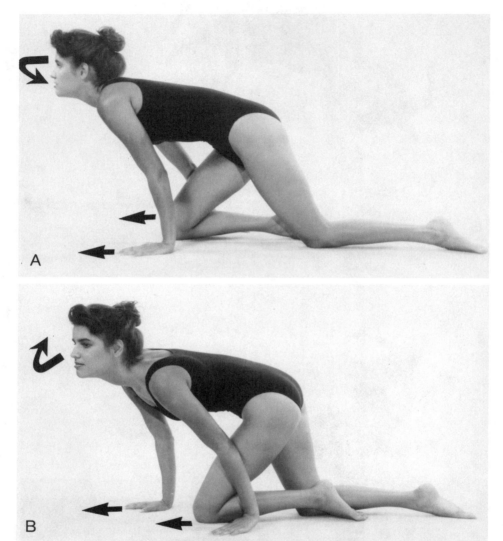

Figure 10.19 Crawl exercise.

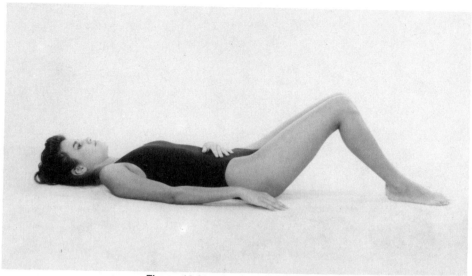

Figure 10.20 Abdominal contractor.

10.15. Abdominal Contractor (Fig. 10.20)

Description

For position A, from a supine position with one hand on abdomen and the other hand along side, flex knees equally, with feet on floor. Holding pelvis and thorax in position, contract abdominal muscles. Hold this position for 5 to 10 sec, then relax slowly.

For position B, maintaining same position as in A, place arms at sides. Contract gluteal muscles, holding pelvis and thorax in position. Hold this position for 5 to 10 sec.

Initially do A and B separately, then do together.

Exercise Format. Standard function 6.

Area Affected. Hip muscles, abdominal musculature, perineum, gluteals.

Action Mode. Isometric.

Intent. Muscle endurance, strength.

10.16. Supine Pelvic Rotation (Fig. 10.21)

Description

From a supine position with elbows flexed 90°, rotate pelvis posteriorly and elevate head, flexing chin toward chest.

Exercise Format. Standard function 4.

Area Affected. Paraspinal musculature, cervical flexors.

Action Mode. Active stretching, isometric.

Intent. Flexibility, mobility, strength.

10.17. Prone Pelvic Rotation (Fig. 10.22)

Description

For position A, from prone position, with arms extended cephalad, contract gluteal muscles. Hold position for 5 to 10 sec, then relax slowly.

For position B, beginning with the same position as above, contract abdominal muscles abruptly, then relax.

Combine A and B, while at the same time rotating the pelvis posteriorly. Hold this position for 5 to 10 sec.

Exercise Format. Standard function 6.

Area Affected. Gluteals and abdominal musculature.

Action Mode. Isometric.

Intent. Strength.

10.18. Pelvic Rotation/Hip Flexion (Fig. 10.23)

Description

For step A, from supine position with arms flexed cephalward, rotate pelvis posteriorly and flex the right hip and knee slowly up to the chest. Hold this position for 5 to 10 sec, and then slowly return the leg to the rest position.

For step B, repeat with left leg. Then repeat step A, flexing both hips and legs slowly up to the chest. Hold this position for 5 to 10 sec, then slowly return the legs to the rest position.

Exercise Format. Standard function 1.

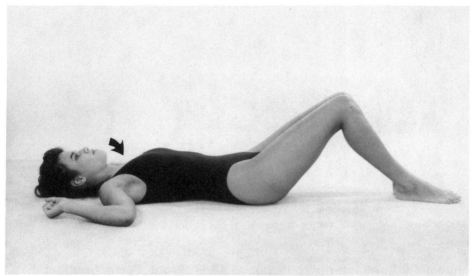

Figure 10.21 Supine pelvic rotation.

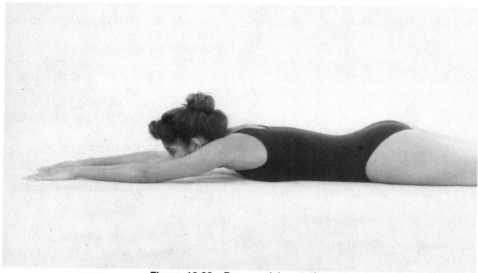

Figure 10.22 Prone pelvic rotation.

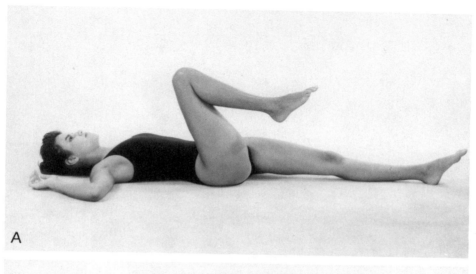

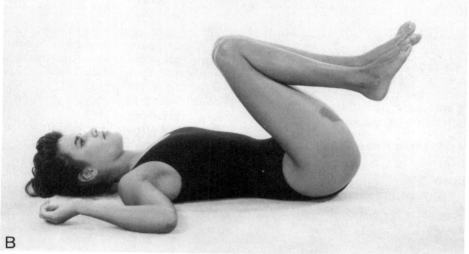

Figure 10.23 Pelvic rotation/hip flexion.

Area Affected. Hip flexors, paraspinal musculature, abdominal musculature.
Action Mode. Isotonic.
Intent. Mobility, strength.
10.18.1 Variant
Therapist applies resistance against hip flexion. The area affected will be the hamstrings, the action mode will be proprioceptive neuromuscular facilitation, and the intent will be for flexibility.

10.19. Pelvic Rotation/Leg Extension (Fig. 10.24)

Description
Assume supine position with arms flexed cephalward, slightly abducted from the midline, and knees flexed with feet on floor. Rotate pelvis posteriorly, and maintain position while extending hip and knee of right leg, and then the left leg, then both legs. Then slowly flex both knees and hips, returning to starting position.
Exercise Format. Standard function 2.
Area Affected. Abdominal muscles, sacroiliac, lumbar spine, hip flexors, hamstrings, quadriceps.
Action Mode. Isotonic.
Intent. Strength, mobility.

10.19.1 Variant
Do same exercise as above, not allowing patient to place feet on floor, then rest. Ac-

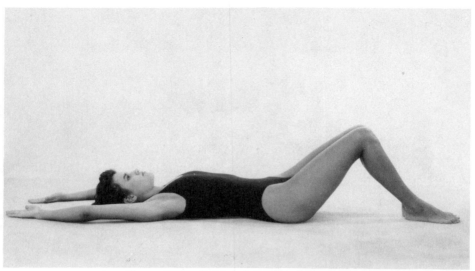

Figure 10.24 Pelvic rotation/leg extension.

tion mode is emphasized for abdominal musculature.

10.19.2 Variant

Do same as 10.19, but therapist resists both flexion and extension of joints, thus creating an isometric mode, emphasizing strengthening of leg muscles.

10.20. Hip Flexion/Knee Chest (Fig. 10.25)

Description

From a supine position with arms abducted 90° and hands cephalad, bilaterally flex hips, bring knees to chest, and then extend legs, maintaining hip flexion to maximum allowed. Hold this position for a while and then bilaterally flex knees and return to starting position.

Note. Maintain posterior pelvic tilt during knee extension.

Exercise Format. Standard function 1.

Area Affected. Hip flexors, abductors, hamstrings, knee extensors.

Action Mode. Active stretching, isotonic.

Intent. Flexibility, mobility, strength.

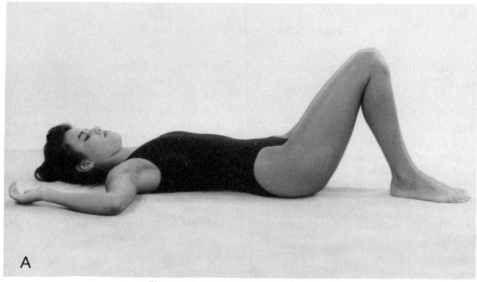

A

Figure 10.25 Hip flexion/knee chest.

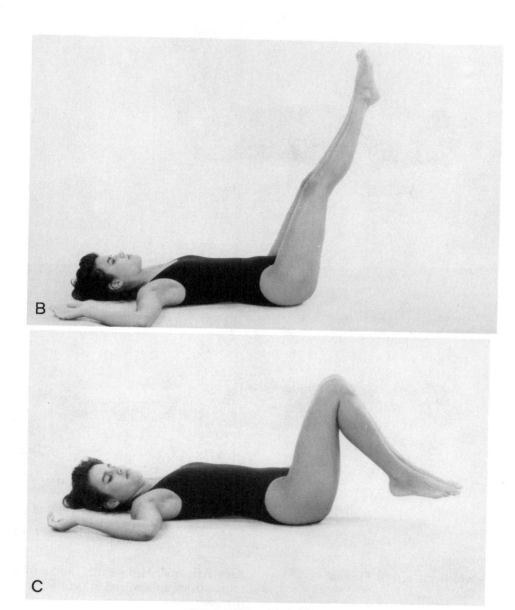

Figure 10.25 (*Continued*)

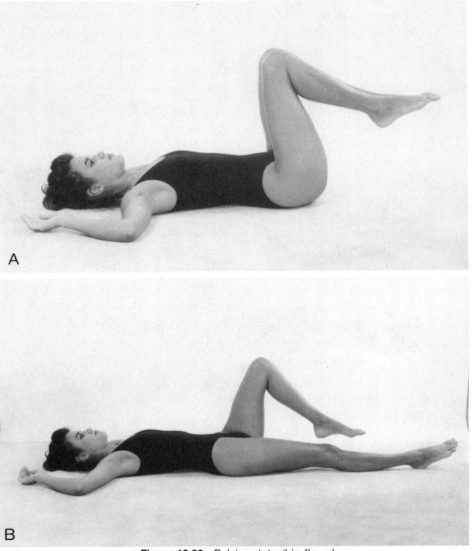

Figure 10.26   Pelvic rotator/hip flexed.

10.21. Pelvic Rotator/Hip Flexed (Fig. 10.26)

Description

Assume standard supine starting position, flexing both hip and knees. Rotate pelvis posteriorly. Unilaterally extend one hip and knee along table, while maintaining contralateral leg position. Repeat with opposite leg.

Exercise Format. Standard function 3 (frequency modified to 20 per minute).

Area Affected. Hip flexors, abductors, pelvic rotators, abdominal musculature, sacroiliac joint, lumbosacral joint.

Action Mode. Isotonic.

Intent. Flexibility, mobility, strength.

10.21.1 Variant

Assume position as above. Continually alternate extension and flexion without returning to starting position. Only use this variant as patient becomes more advanced. Weights may also be added, eventually.

Exercise Format. Standard function 2.

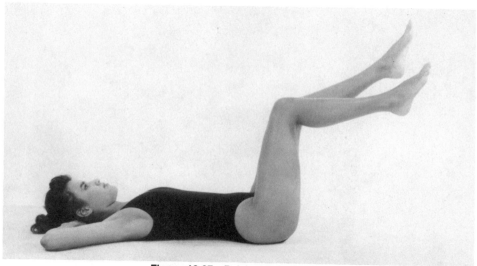

Figure 10.27 Pelvic rotator/cycling.

10.22. Pelvic Rotator/Cycling (Fig. 10.27)

Description

From a supine position with arms abducted 90° and hands cephalward, bilaterally flex hips and knees 90°. Gradually extend one leg at a time, initiating a "cycling" motion. Maintain to tolerance, and then return to starting position.

Exercise Format. Standard function 2.

Area Affected. Pelvic rotators, abdominal, paraspinal muscles, hip flexors, knee flexors and extensors.

Action Mode. Isotonic.

Intent. Flexibility, mobility, strength.

10.23. Prone Pelvic Rotator (Fig. 10.28)

Description

Assume a kneeling position with neck extended and lumbar spine flattened, with weight on knees and hands. Flex cervical spine, contract abdominal musculature, and flex at thoracolumbar junction. Rotate pelvis posteriorly. Hold end positions.

10.23.1 Variant (Fig. 10.28.1)

From same starting position, initially extend cervical spine and pelvis, relaxing abdominals, and increase lumbar lordosis. Alternate with flexion position above.

Exercise Format. Standard function 4.

Area Affected. Pelvic rotators, abdominal, paraspinal musculature, cervical flexors and extensors, lumbar extensors.

Action Mode. Active stretch, isometric.

Intent. Flexibility, mobility, strength, postural.

10.24. Prone Pelvic Extension (Fig. 10.29)

Description

From a prone position with arms flexed and elbows extended, rotate pelvis posteriorly. Unilaterally reach with each arm, forcibly stretching the hand cephalward. Hold for 5 to 10 sec, and slowly relax. Then repeat, bilaterally elevating arms. Hold for 5 to 10 sec, and slowly relax.

Exercise Format. Standard function 4.

Area Affected. Abdominals, pelvic rotators, paraspinal muscles, lateral thoracic muscles, shoulder girdle.

Action Mode. Active stretching, isometric.

Intent. Flexibility, mobility, strength.

10.25. Supine Pelvic Rotator—Sit Up (Fig. 10.30)

Description

From a supine position with arms at sides, knees flexed, and feet on table, rotate pelvis posteriorly. While flexing the neck and thorax until the lower borders of the scapulae are elevated, extend both hands toward the knees. Repeat with hands crossed on chest.

Exercise Format. Standard function 3 (modified to patient tolerance).

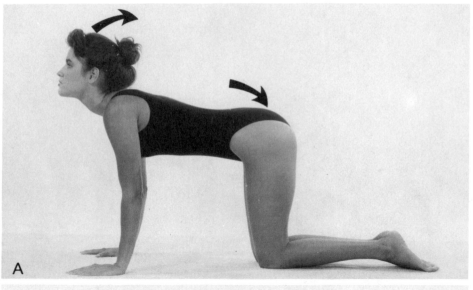

A

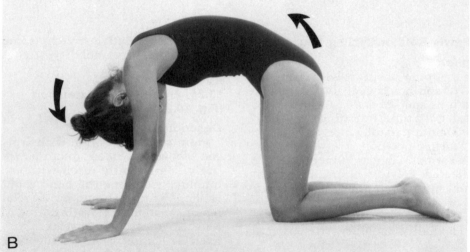

B

Figure 10.28   Prone pelvic rotator.

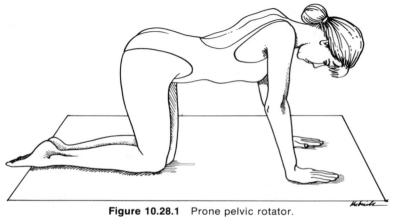

Figure 10.28.1   Prone pelvic rotator.

DYNAMICS OF CLINICAL REHABILITATIVE EXERCISE

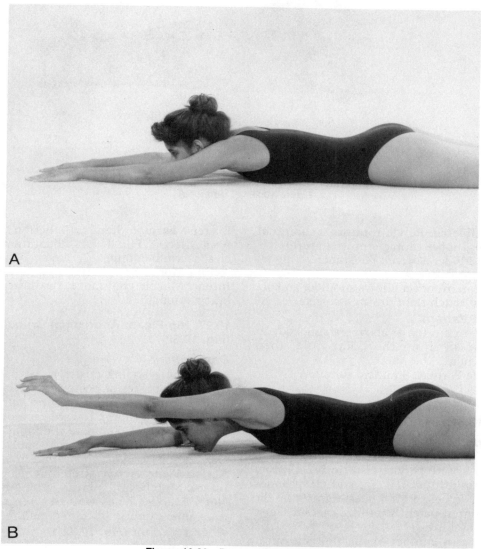

Figure 10.29 Prone pelvic extension.

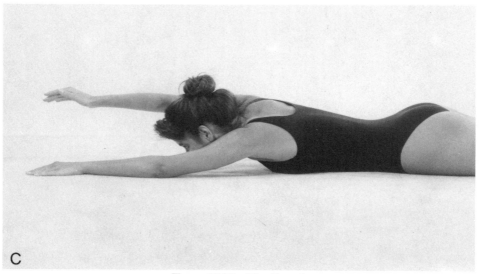

C

Figure 10.29 (*Continued*)

Area Affected. Pelvic rotators, abdominal muscles, upper thoracic musculature.
Action Mode. Isotonic resistance.
Intent. Mobility, strength.
Note. Patient never allows shoulder and occiput to touch floor during exercise.

10.25.1 Variant
Perform motion as above, raising body to at least 45° from the floor. Hold, then slowly relax.
Exercise Format. Standard function 1.

10.26. Lumbar Flexor—Hip Rocker (Fig. 10.31)

Description
Assume a supine position; flex hips and knees. Rotate pelvis posteriorly, contract abdominal musculature, and clasp hands around knees. Pull knees tightly to the chest, intermittently pulling knees to cause pelvic rocking.

Maintain contact of the thoracic spine and occiput against the table.
Exercise Format. Standard function 3.

10.26.1 Variant
Repeat above maneuver, unilaterally flexing one hip and knee, while keeping the other hip and knee in extension. Repeat with opposite leg.

10.26.2 Variant
Take position as above, but circumduct knees clockwise and counterclockwise in frontal plane.

Exercise Format. Standard function 2.
Area Affected. Hip flexors, abdominal muscles, sacroiliac joint.
Action Mode. Active stretching, isotonic.
Intent. Muscle endurance, flexibility, mobility, strength.

10.27. Hip Flexor/Abdominal Cruncher (Fig. 10.32)

Description
Assume a sitting position, with hands clasped on posterior occiput. Contract abdominal muscles and flex hips, one then the other, and thorax toward each other.
Exercise Format. Standard function 7.
Area Affected. Hip flexors, paraspinal muscles, sacroiliac joint, abdominal muscles.
Action Mode. Active stretching, isotonic.
Intent. Mobility, flexibility, strength.
Note. Exercise lends well to a progressive resistance exercise (PRE) regimen.

10.27.1 Variant (Fig. 10.32.1)
The same exercise is performed in the supine position.

10.28. Lumbar Extensor—Crouched (Fig. 10.33)

Description
From a kneeling position with forehead on table and arms flexed cephalad, lower chest against knees, and contract abdominal muscles.
Exercise Format. Standard function 1.

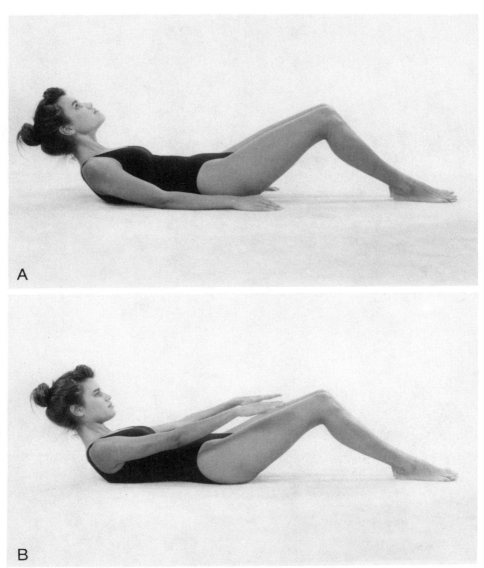

Figure 10.30 Supine pelvic rotator—sit-up.

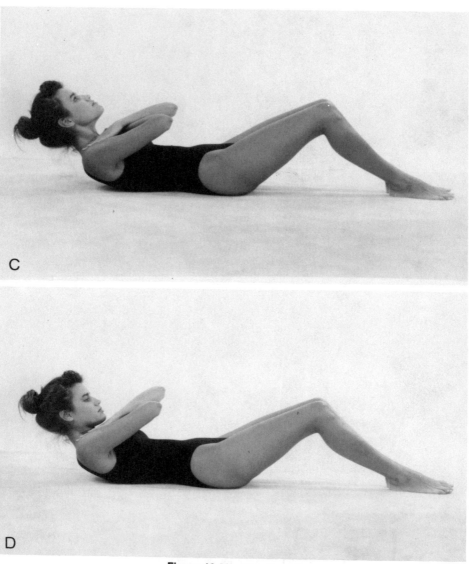

Figure 10.30 (*Continued*)

DYNAMICS OF CLINICAL REHABILITATIVE EXERCISE

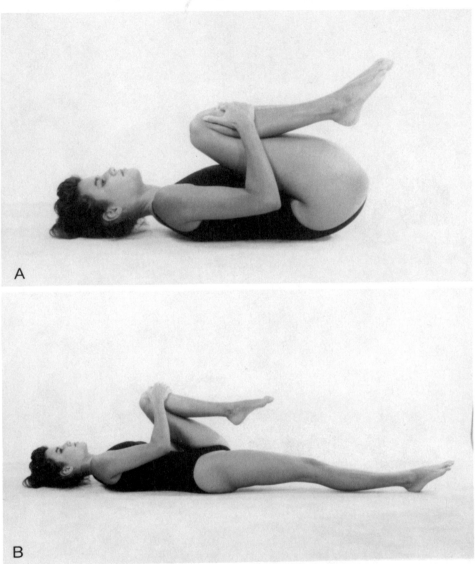

Figure 10.31 Lumbar flexor—hip rocker.

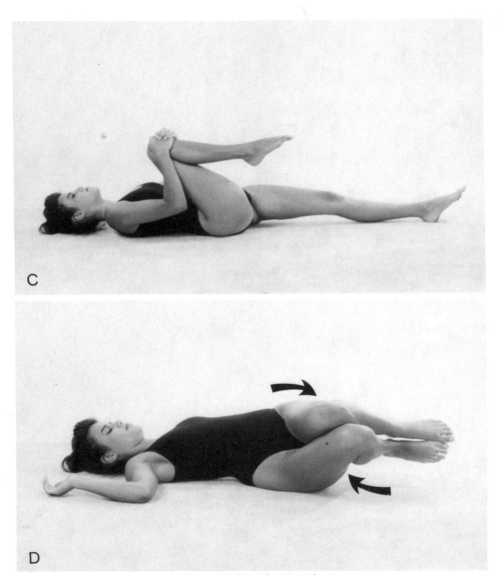

C

D

Figure 10.31 (*Continued*)

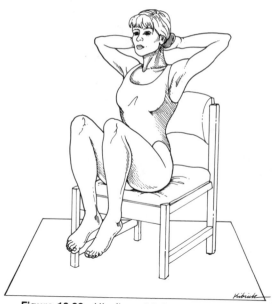

Area Affected. Paraspinal muscles, hip flexors, abdominal muscles.
Action Mode. Active stretching.
Intent. Flexibility, mobility.
Note. Patient will not receive maximum benefit until able to plantar flex ankle fully.

10.29. Lumbar Extensor—Thorax Rotation (Fig. 10.34)

Description

From a supine position with arms at sides and hands pronated, rotate pelvis posteriorly. Simultaneously deviate each leg, one at a time, laterally 10 to 30°, keeping pelvis in contact with floor, while reaching caudally toward that side with the contralateral arm. Repeat with right and left sides done successively.
Exercise Format. Standard function 4.

Figure 10.32 Hip flexor/abdominal cruncher.

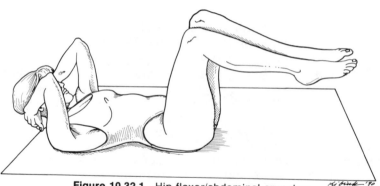

Figure 10.32.1 Hip flexor/abdominal cruncher.

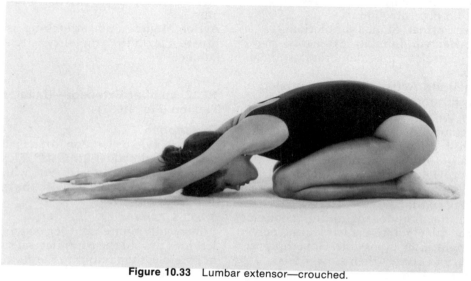

Figure 10.33 Lumbar extensor—crouched.

LUMBAR SPINE AND PELVIS

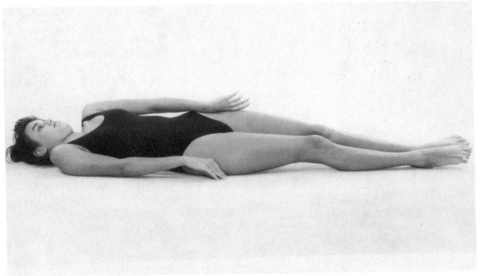

Figure 10.34 Lumbar extensor—thorax rotation.

Area Affected. Spinal rotators, lumbar and pelvic lateral flexors, shoulder girdle.
Action Mode. Active stretching, isometric.
Intent. Flexibility, strength.

10.30. Lumbar Extensor—Leg Rotation (Fig. 10.35)

Description

From a supine position with arms flexed 90° cephalward, rotate pelvis posteriorly. Internally rotate left arm and shoulder to the right as far as possible, without allowing the pelvis and lower extremity to move. Repeat on opposite side.
Exercise Format. Standard function 4.
Area Affected. Lumbar extensors, paraspinal muscles, hip abductors, and adductors.
Action Mode. Active stretching, isometric.
Intent. Flexibility, strength.

10.30.1 Variant

Continue above exercise at the end point, and allow the pelvis and left leg to rotate internally to the right side and across the other leg. Hold this position for 5 to 10 sec, then slowly relax.

10.30.2 Variant

With the shoulder maintaining contact with the table, rotate the left leg and pelvis to the right as far as possible. Hold this position for 5 to 10 sec, then slowly relax.
Intent. Flexibility, mobility, strength.

10.31. Lumbar Extensor—Knee Rotation (Fig. 10.36)

Description

From a supine position with arms abducted 45°, bilaterally flex knees with feet on table. Lower knees laterally to the right side, maintaining shoulder contact with the table. Return slowly to starting position, and repeat with other side.
Exercise Format. Standard function 2 (with frequency reduced as necessary).
Area Affected. Lumbar extensors, abdominal muscles, hip, pelvic, and lumbar muscles.
Action Mode. Active stretching, isotonic.
Intent. Flexibility, mobility, strength, endurance.

10.32. Lumbar Extensor—Unilateral Hip Flexion (Fig. 10.37)

Description

From a supine position, rotate pelvis posteriorly, and abduct arms 45°. Slowly flex hip and knee of right leg to 90°, while maintaining shoulder contact with the table. Repeat with other leg.

10.32.1 Variant

Internally rotate right leg, extending the left toes toward the contralateral side as far as possible, then return to the starting position, extend, and then relax.

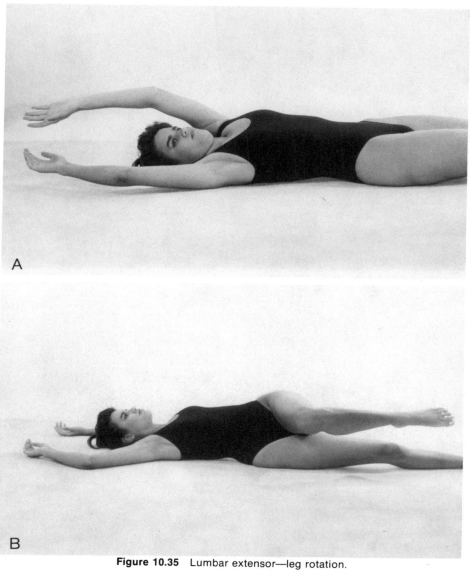

A

B

Figure 10.35 Lumbar extensor—leg rotation.

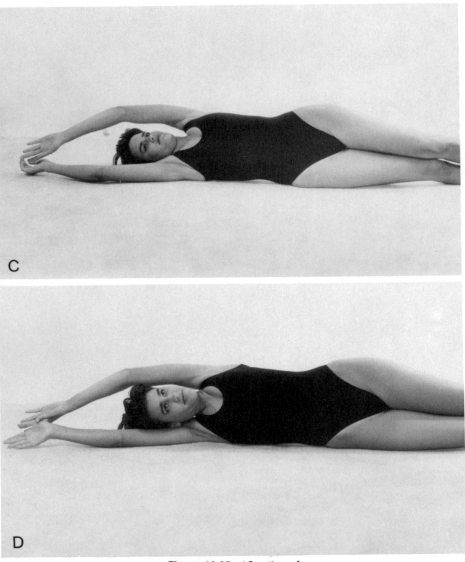

Figure 10.35 (*Continued*)

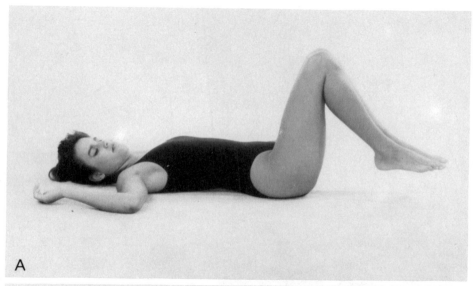

A

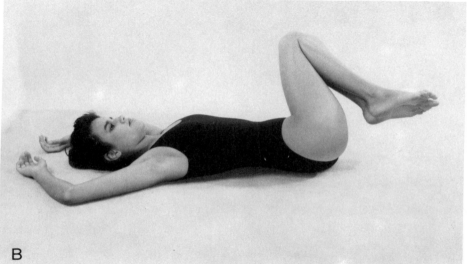

B

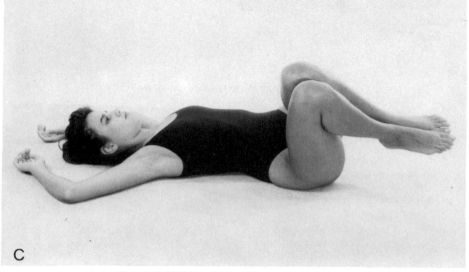

C

Figure 10.36 Lumbar extensor—knee rotation.

233

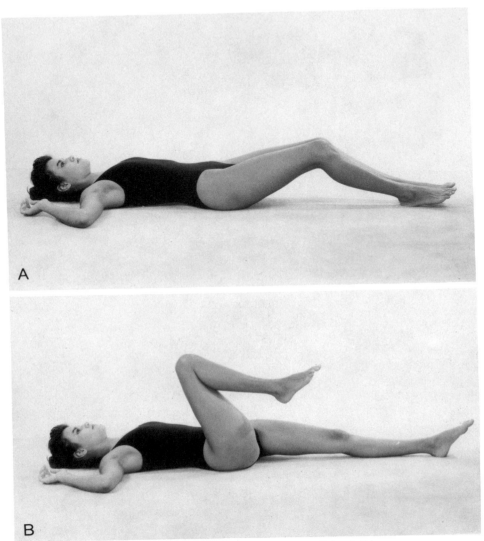

A

B

Figure 10.37 Lumbar extensor—unilateral hip flexion.

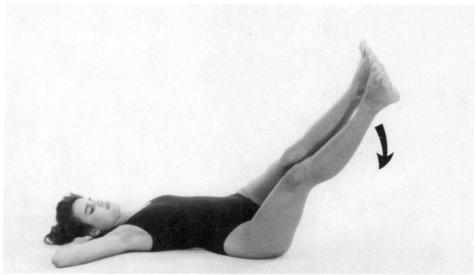

Figure 10.38 Lumbar extensor—bilateral hip flexion.

10.32.2 Variant

Use a towel across foot to assist holding leg in air.

10.32.3 Variant

Use proprioceptive neuromuscular facilitation to stretch hamstrings. Exercise format is standard function 9.
Exercise Format. Standard function 1.
Area Affected. Lumbar and pelvic muscles, abdominals, hip flexors and extensors.
Action Mode. Active stretch, isotonic.
Intent. Flexibility, mobility, strength.
Note. Patient may flex contralateral leg to facilitate exercise.

10.33. Lumbar Extensor—Bilateral Hip Flexion (Fig. 10.38)

Description

From a supine position with arms abducted 45°, rotate pelvis posteriorly. Bilaterally flex hips as much as possible, then extend knees fully. Bilaterally lower legs laterally toward each side as far as possible.
Exercise Format. Standard function 2 (frequency modified to 20 per minute).
Area Affected. Abdominals, pelvis, and hip.
Action Mode. Active stretching, isotonic.
Intent. Flexibility, mobility, strength, endurance.
Note. Patient may place arms, hands pronated, along side to facilitate exercise.

10.34. Hip Flexion/Abdominal Cruncher—Supine (Fig. 10.39)

Description

From a supine position, rotate pelvis posteriorly, clasp hands on posterior occiput, and flex the right hip, knee, and thorax to touch the knee to the left elbow. Repeat with left side.
Exercise Format. Standard function 5.
Area Affected. Abdominal muscles, hip flexors, paraspinal musculature.
Action Mode. Isotonic.
Intent. Mobility, strength.
Precaution. Patients with cervical disorders, should not clasp hands on neck. Instead hands should be placed gently on malar prominences.

10.35. Hip Flexors (Fig. 10.40)

Description

From a standing position, flex right hip and knee, maintaining contact with the floor, and extend left hip, then flex left knee and lower it to floor. Lean upper body anteriorly as far as possible, creating spinal extension. Repeat with opposite side.
Exercise Format. Standard function 4.
Area Affected. Hip flexors, extensors, lumbar muscles, gluteals.
Action Mode. Active stretching, isometric.
Intent. Flexibility, mobility, strength.

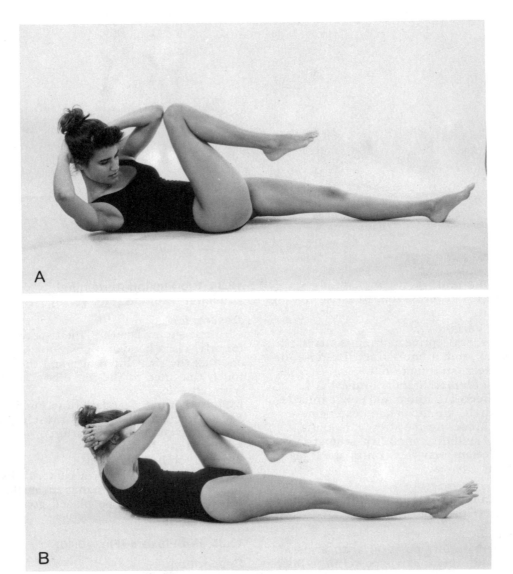

A

B

Figure 10.39 Hip flexion/abdominal cruncher—supine.

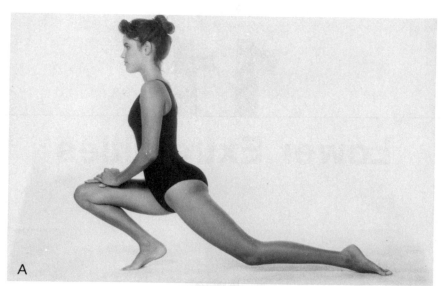

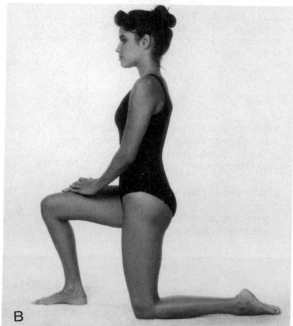

Figure 10.40 Hip flexors.

References

1. Cailliet R: Low Back Pain Syndrome. Philadelphia: FA Davis, 1968.
2. Kapandji IA: The Physiology of the Joints. 2nd ed. New York:Churchill Livingstone, 1982, vol 3.
3. Kendall HO, Kendall FP, Wadsworth GE: Muscle Testing and Function. 2nd ed. Baltimore:Williams & Wilkins, 1971.
4. Hoppenfeld S: Physical Examination of the Spine and Extremities. New York:Appleton-Century-Crofts, 1976.
5. Williams PL, Warwick R, Dyson M, Bannister LH, eds.: Gray's Anatomy. 37th ed. New York: Churchill Livingstone, 1989.

11

Lower Extremities

Knee

Action	Muscle	Exercise
Extension	Quadriceps, tensor fascia lata	10.4, 10.5, 10.5.1, 10.18, 10.19, 10.20, 11.1, 11.2, 11.2.1, 11.3, 11.4, 11.4.1, 11.4.2, 11.5, 11.7, 11.7.1, 11.8
Flexion	Sartorius, gracilis, popliteus, plantaris,[a] semimembranosus, semitendinosus, short head of biceps, long head of biceps, gastrocnemius[a]	10.4, 10.5, 10.5.1, 10.18, 10.19, 11.3, 11.6, 11.8.1
Lateral rotation[a]	Short head of biceps, long head of biceps	10.6, 10.8, 11.9
Medial rotation[a]	Sartorius, gracilis, popliteus, semimembranosus, semitendinosus	10.6, 10.8, 11.9

[a] With knee in flexion.

The knee is a ginglymus joint similar to the elbow with respect to range of motion. It is the largest joint and the most susceptible to injury, because of its limited motions and heavy weight-bearing functions (1, p. 100).

Knee flexion and extension are the result of a gliding movement of the tibia on the femur. During knee flexion, the lower leg rotates internally with the femur; in extension, the lower leg rotates externally (1, p. 100).

The complex configuration of the knee is supported by the cruciate ligaments, which assist in flexion. The posterior cruciate ligament prevents excessive internal rotation, and the anterior cruciate ligament prevents excessive external rotation. With the knee in extension, the collateral ligaments prevent rotation, adduction, and abduction. The medial and lateral menisci are attached to the tibia and femur, and move during flexion and extension (1, pp. 100–2).

The primary extensors of the knee are the quadriceps, which are innervated by the femoral nerve (L2,L3,L4) roots (Fig. 10.4). The primary flexors are the semimembranosus and semitendinosus, which are innervated by the tibial portion of the sciatic nerve (L5) root, and the biceps femoris, which is innervated by the tibial portion of the sciatic nerve (S1). These three muscles

DYNAMICS OF CLINICAL REHABILITATIVE EXERCISE

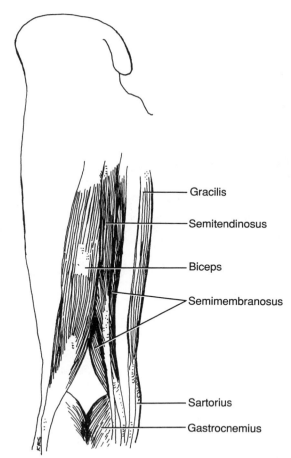

Figure 11.1 Hamstrings.

KNEE EXERCISES

11.1. Patellar Positioner (Fig. 11.2)
Description
From a supine position with knee extended, contract upper and lower leg muscles. Concentrate on patellar motion.
Exercise format. Standard function 6 (frequency modified to 1 per second).
Area affected. Patellar tendons.
Action mode. Isometric.
Intent. Strength, coordination.

11.2. Straight Leg Raise (Fig. 11.3)
Description
From a supine position, raise leg as high as possible, keeping knee in extension. Rotate pelvis posterior.
Exercise format. Standard function 1.
Area affected. Hamstrings, abdominals, quadriceps.
Action mode. Active stretching, isotonic.
Intent. Flexibility, mobility, strength.

11.2.1 Variant
Use proprioceptive neuromuscular facilitation with patient pushing down against resistance by therapist.
Exercise format. Standard function 9.
Note. Lumbosacral support may be needed for patient.

11.3. Knee Flexor/Extender (Fig. 11.4)
Description
Start in a supine position, with both legs extended. Flex knees approximately 90°, placing feet alternately on floor. Flex hip 90°, maintaining knee flexion, and slowly return to original position.
Exercise format. Standard function 2.
Area affected. Hip and knee flexors and extensors, abdominal muscles.
Action mode. Active stretching, isotonic.
Intent. Flexibility, mobility, strength.

make up the hamstrings (Fig. 11.1) (2, p. 189).

The ranges of motion of the knee are flexion, extension, and internal and external rotation. Table 11.1 describes the ranges of motion of the knee.

It is of primary concern in the rehabilitation of the knee to assure the development of the upper and lower leg musculature and to reduce stress on the knee joint itself.

Table 11.1 Knee Ranges of Motion (ROM)[a]

Motion	ROM	Anatomical	Cartesian
Flexion	135°	Sagittal	Positive θ_x
Extension	0°	Sagittal	Negative θ_x
Internal rotation	10°	Transverse	Positive/negative θ_y
External rotation	10°	Transverse	Positive/negative θ_y

[a] **Depending upon side of body.**

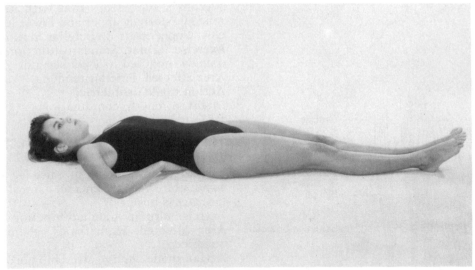

Figure 11.2 Patellar positioner.

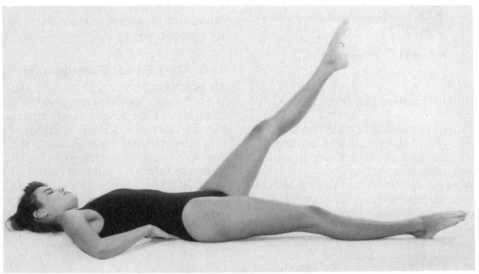

Figure 11.3 Straight leg raise.

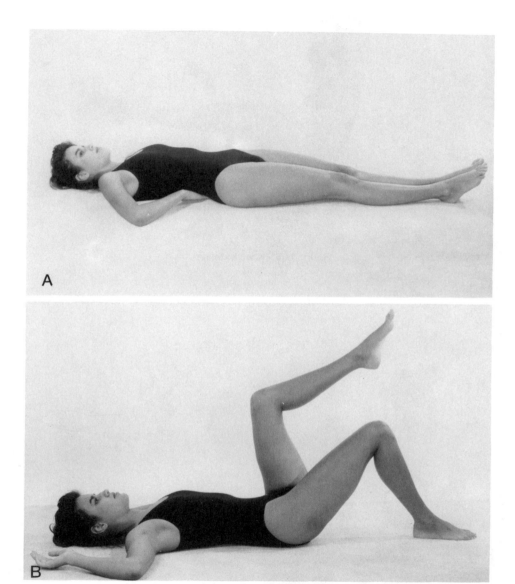

Figure 11.4 Knee flexor/extender.

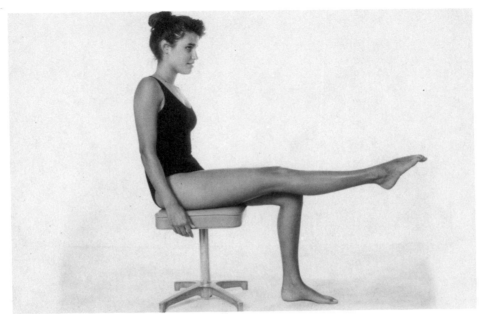

Figure 11.5 Knee extender.

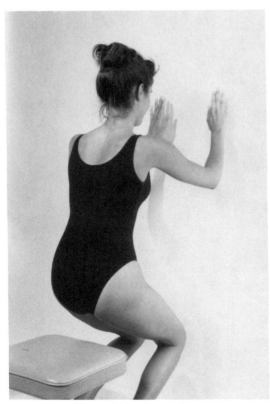

Figure 11.6 Knee raiser.

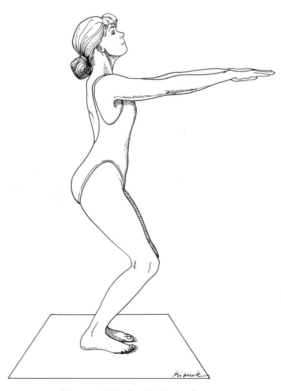

Figure 11.7 Partial knee flexor.

DYNAMICS OF CLINICAL REHABILITATIVE EXERCISE

11.4. Knee Extender (Fig. 11.5)
Description
From a sitting position with knees in flexion, slowly extend knee. Hold position for 5 to 10 sec, then slowly relax. Exercise is initially performed unilaterally, then bilaterally.

Exercise format. Standard function 1.
Area affected. Knee extenders.
Action mode. Isotonic.
Intent. Mobility, strength.

11.4.1 Variant
Repeat exercise 11.4 adding weights.
Exercise format. Standard function 1.

11.4.2 Variant
Therapist applies resistance to exercise 11.4.
Exercise format. Standard function 6.
Action mode. Isometric.

11.5. Knee Raiser (Fig. 11.6)
Description
From a sitting position with pelvis rotated posteriorly, arms extended with hands on wall at arms length, slowly raise up to an erect position, with knees slightly flexed.

Exercise format. Standard function 1.
Area affected. Knee extensors, gluteals.
Action mode. Isotonic.
Intent. Strength.

11.6. Partial Knee Flexor (Fig. 11.7)
Description
From a standing position with knees extended, partially flex knees approximately 45°, then extend 5 to 10°.

Exercise format. Standard function 5.
Area affected. Knee extenders.
Action mode. Isotonic.
Intent. Strength.

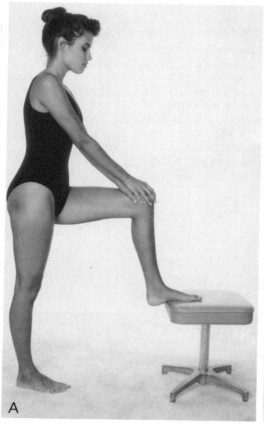
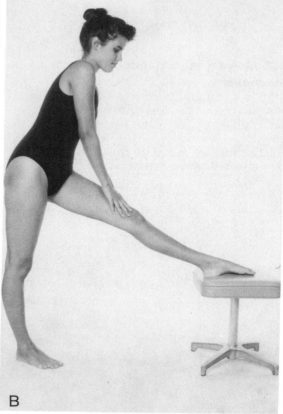

A
B

Figure 11.8 Active knee extender.

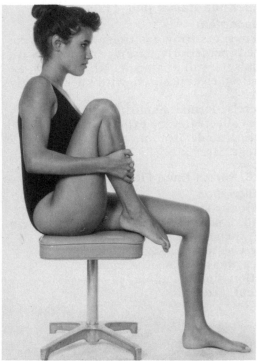

Figure 11.9 Active knee flexor.

11.7. Active Knee Extender (Fig. 11.8)
Description

From a standing position, place foot of affected leg on a stool. With knee in flexion, bilaterally grasp knee and force it into extension.

Exercise format. Standard function 4.
Area affected. Knee extensors.

Action mode. Active stretch.
Intent. Flexibility, endurance.

11.7.1 Variant

Repeat 11.7 with ankle in dorsiflexion. Area affected becomes the posterior leg muscles.

11.8. Active Knee Flexor (Fig. 11.9)
Description

From a sitting position with knee in flexion, grasp lower leg above ankle. Force leg into flexion, while attempting to extend the knee.

Exercise format. Standard function 6.
Area affected. Knee extensors.
Action mode. Isometric resistance.
Intent. Strength.
Note. Patient must hold back straight and try to eliminate extraneous movements of the body.

11.8.1 Variant

Therapist applies resistance to knee flexion.

11.9. Isometric Knee (Fig. 11.10)
Description

Assume a supine position with knees extended and legs held in position at the ankle. Internally and externally rotate knee against resistance.

Exercise format. Standard function 6.
Area affected. Primary: leg and ankle muscles; secondary: anterior thigh muscles.
Action mode. Isometric.
Intent. Strength.

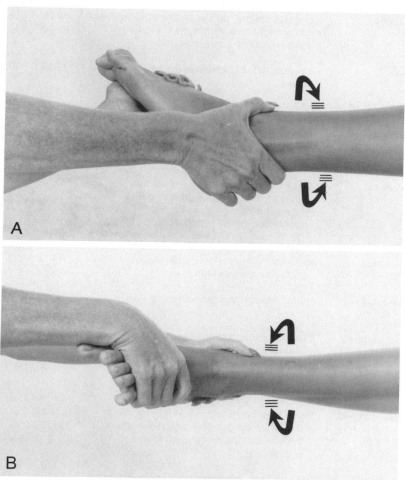

Figure 11.10 Isometric knee.

Ankle and Foot

Action	Muscle	Exercise
Ankle dorsiflexion	Tibialis anterior, extensor digitorum longus, peroneus tertius, extensor hallucis longus	10.5.1, 11.16, 11.16.1, 11.17, 11.18, 11.19
Ankle plantar flexion	Peroneus longus, tibialis posterior, plantaris, flexor digitorum longus, flexor hallucis longus, soleus, gastrocnemius	10.28, 11.18, 11.19
Foot eversion	Peroneus tertius, peroneus longus, peroneus brevis	11.10, 11.13
Foot inversion	Tibialis anterior, tibialis posterior	11.11, 11.14
Metatarsophalangeal extension	Extensor hallucis longus, extensor digitorum longus (2–5 digits), extensor digitorum brevis (1–4 digits)	11.12
Metatarsophalangeal flexion	Flexor hallucis brevis,[a] flexor hallucis longus,[a] flexor digitorum brevis (2–5 digits), flexor digitorum longus (2–5 digits), lumbricals, dorsal interosseus, plantar interosseus, flexor digitorum accessorius	11.12, 11.15
Metatarsophalangeal abduction	Abductor hallucis, dorsal interosseus, abductor digiti minimi	11.12
Metatarsophalangeal adduction	Plantar interosseus, adductor hallucis	11.12
Proximal interphalangeal extension	Extensor hallucis longus, extensor digitorum longus (2–5 digits), extensor digitorum brevis (1–4 digits), dorsal interosseus (2–4 digits), plantar interosseus (3–5 digits), lumbricals	11.12, 11.15
Proximal interphalangeal flexion	Flexor digitorum brevis (2–5 digits), flexor digitorum longus (2–5 digits), flexor hallucis longus, flexor digitorum accessorius	11.12, 11.15
Distal interphalangeal extension	Extensor hallucis longus, extensor digitorum longus (2–5 digits), extensor digitorum brevis (1–4 digits), lumbricals, dorsal interosseus (2–4 digits), plantar interosseus (3–5 digits)	11.12, 11.15
Distal interphalangeal flexion	Flexor hallucis longus, flexor digitorum longus (2–5 digits)	11.12, 11.15

[a] Only flexors in great toe.

The foot and ankle are the foundation for proper body mechanics. Consequently, any deviation in their stability has a negative effect on the biomechanical structure of the body. The ankle and feet act as a shock absorber during ambulation, and they must constantly adjust, as necessary, to maintain proper balance and coordination.

The foot is divided into three functional anatomical cells: anterior, medial, and posterior.

The posterior cell is the primary weight-bearing compartment, articulating superiorly with the ankle mortise and inferiorly with the calcaneus. The ankle mortise is formed by the articulation of the tibia and fibula with the talus. This union functions as a hinge joint, permitting dorsal and plantar flexion of the foot.

The middle cell consists of five tarsal bones, whose union forms the transverse and longitudinal arches. Accommodation of the foot to adapt to uneven surfaces during ambulation is accomplished by the mobility within the middle cell and through its articulations with the posterior cell.

The anterior cell begins with the articulation of the metatarsals with the tarsals.

The foot has four arches: the longitudinal arch and three transverse arches.

The dorsiflexors of the ankle are the tibialis anterior, innervated by the deep peroneal nerve (L4,L5 roots), the extensor hallucis longus, and the extensor digitorum longus, which are both innervated by the deep peroneal nerve (L5 root) (Fig. 11.11) (2, p. 227).

The plantar flexors of the ankle are the peroneus longus and brevis, innervated by the superficial peroneal nerve (S1 root), the gastrocnemius and soleus, innervated by the tibial nerve (S1,S2 roots), the flexor hallucis longus, the flexor digitorum longus, and the tibialis posterior, which are all innervated by the tibial nerve (L5 root) (Figs. 11.12 and 11.13) (2, p. 228).

Subtalar inversion of the foot is controlled by the tibialis anterior and tibialis

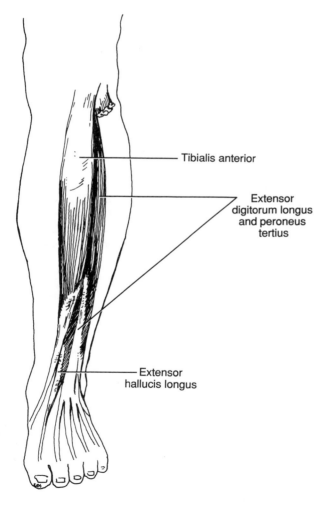

Tibialis anterior

Extensor digitorum longus and peroneus tertius

Extensor hallucis longus

Figure 11.11 Ankle dorsiflexors.

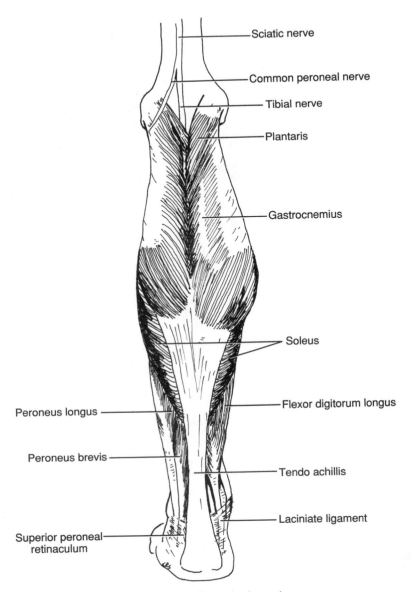

Sciatic nerve

Common peroneal nerve

Tibial nerve

Plantaris

Gastrocnemius

Soleus

Flexor digitorum longus

Peroneus longus

Peroneus brevis

Tendo achillis

Laciniate ligament

Superior peroneal retinaculum

Figure 11.12   Posterior lower leg.

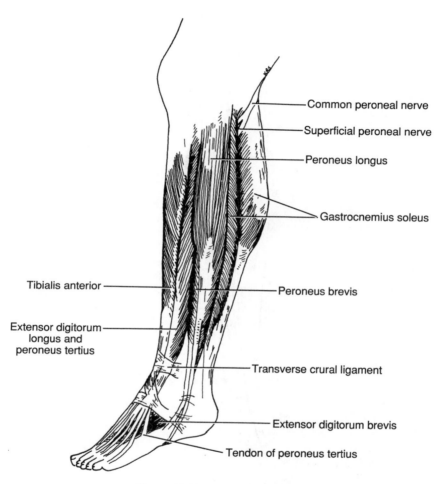

Common peroneal nerve

Superficial peroneal nerve

Peroneus longus

Gastrocnemius soleus

Tibialis anterior

Peroneus brevis

Extensor digitorum longus and peroneus tertius

Transverse crural ligament

Extensor digitorum brevis

Tendon of peroneus tertius

Figure 11.13 Lateral lower leg.

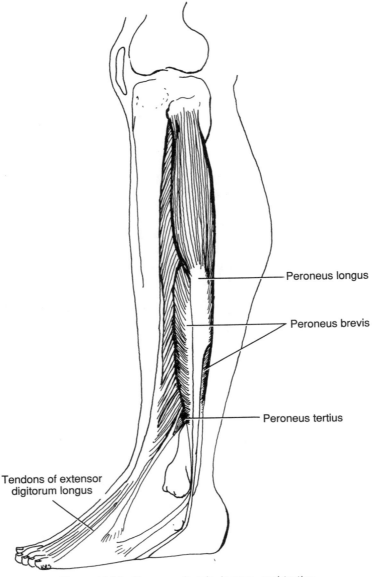

Figure 11.14 Peroneus brevis, longus, and tertius.

Peroneus longus

Peroneus brevis

Peroneus tertius

Tendons of extensor
digitorum longus

posterior. Subtalar eversion is a function of the peroneus longus, brevis, and tertius (Figs. 11.14 and 11.15) (1, p. 194).

Ranges of motion of the ankle and foot are ankle dorsiflexion and plantar flexion, subtalar inversion and eversion, midtarsal adduction and abduction, and flexion, extension, abduction and adduction of the toes. Table 11.2 describes the ranges of motion of the ankle and foot.

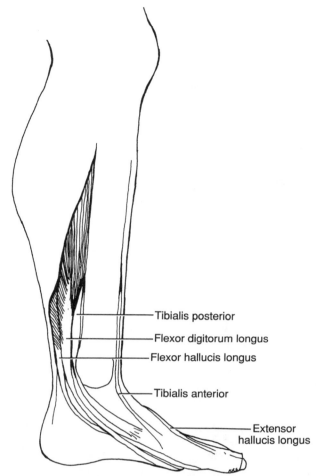

Figure 11.15 Lateral ankle.

Tibialis posterior
Flexor digitorum longus
Flexor hallucis longus
Tibialis anterior
Extensor hallucis longus

Table 11.2. Foot and Ankle Ranges of Motion (ROM)

Motion	ROM	Anatomical	Cartesian
Ankle dorsiflexion	20°	Sagittal	Negative θ_x
Ankle plantar flexion	50°	Sagittal	Positive θ_x
Subtalar inversion[a]	5°	Frontal	Positive/negative $\theta_z{}^b$
Subtalar eversion[c]	5°	Frontal	Positive/negative $\theta_z{}^b$
Forefoot adduction	20°	Transverse	Positive/negative $\theta_y{}^b$
Forefoot Abduction	10°	Transverse	Positive/negative $\theta_y{}^b$
First metatarsophalangeal joint			Positive/negative $\theta_x\theta_z$
Flexion	45°	Sagittal	Positive θ_x
Extension	70–90°	Sagittal	Negative θ_x

[a] Plantar flexion and internal rotation.
[b] Depending on side of body.
[c] Dorsiflexion and external rotation.

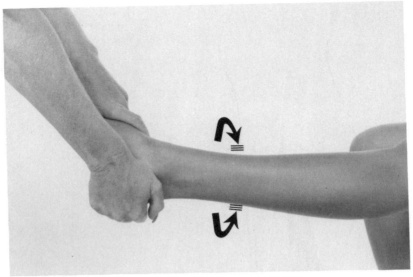

Figure 11.16 Eversion strengthener.

ANKLE EXERCISES

11.10. Eversion Strengthener (Fig. 11.16)

Description

From a sitting or supine position with leg in extension, grasp with one hand the posterior calcaneus, and with the other hand the metatarsals. With the patient attempting to evert, force the ankle into inversion.
Exercise format. Standard function 6.
Area affected. Ankle and foot inverters.
Action mode. Isometric.
Intent. Strength.

11.11. Inversion Strengthener (Fig. 11.17)

Description

From a supine position with leg in extension, grasp with one hand the posterior calcaneus, and with the other hand the metatarsals. With the patient attempting to invert, force the ankle into eversion.
Exercise format. Standard function 6.
Area affected. Ankle and foot everters.
Action mode. Isometric.
Intent. Strength.

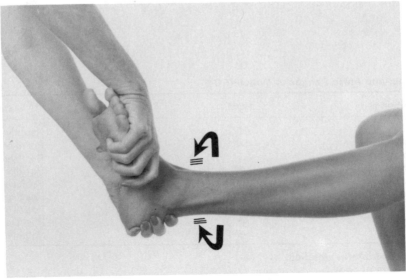

Figure 11.17 Inversion strengthener.

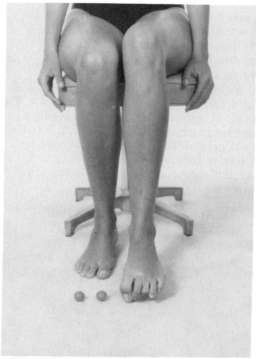

Figure 11.18 Metatarsal phalangeal mobilizer.

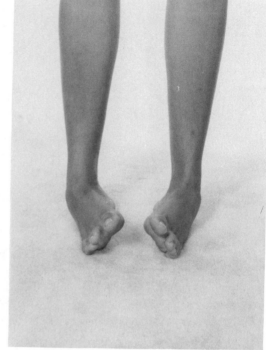

Figure 11.19 Eversion standing.

11.12. Metatarsal Phalangeal Mobilizer (Fig. 11.18)

Description

Assume a sitting position. Place a marble on the floor. Grasp the marble with the metatarsal phalangeal area of the foot.

Exercise format. Standard function 1.

Area affected. Metatarsal phalangeal flexors.

Action mode. Isotonic.

Intent. Mobility, coordination, strength, endurance.

11.13. Eversion Standing (Fig. 11.19)

Description

Standing with feet slightly apart and equally balanced, bilaterally evert both ankles, holding position for 5 to 10 sec.

Exercise format. Standard function 4.

Area affected. Ankle and foot everters.

Action mode. Isometric, active stretch.

Intent. Strength, flexibility, mobility.

11.14. Inversion on Toes (Fig. 11.20)

Description

Standing with feet slightly apart and equally balanced, raise up on toes and invert ankles.

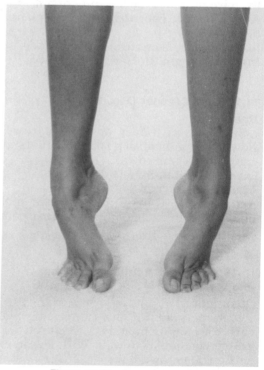

Figure 11.20 Inversion on toes.

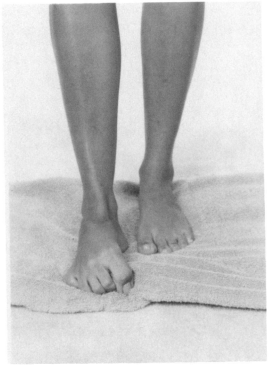

Figure 11.21 Toe crawler.

Exercise format. Standard function 4.
Area affected. Foot inverters and plantar flexors, digits.
Action mode. Isometric, active stretch.
Intent. Strength, flexibility, mobility.

11.15. Toe Crawler (Fig. 11.21)
Description
Standing with feet on a bath towel, slowly flex metatarsal phalangeal joints, attempting to grab towel.
Exercise format. Standard function 5.
Area affected. Foot.
Action mode. Active stretching, isotonic.
Intent. Flexibility, mobility, strength, coordination.

11.16. Standing Achilles Stretcher (Fig. 11.22)
Description
Assume standing position facing wall with toes approximately 2 feet from wall and perpendicular to wall. With legs in extension, lean toward wall against forearms. Keep heels on the ground.

Exercise format. Standard function 1.
Area affected. Achilles tendon.
Action mode. Active stretching.
Intent. Flexibility.

11.16.1 Variant
Assume standing position with one foot anterior and the other foot posterior. Flex knee of anterior leg, while keeping posterior leg in extension and foot in slight dorsiflexion. Motion is gentle slow rocking.
Exercise format. Standard function 2.
Action mode. Isotonic, active stretch.
Intent. Flexibility, strength.

11.17. Achilles Tendon Stretcher (Fig. 11.23)
Description
Standing with feet together and heels on ground, flex knees until there is tension on the Achilles tendon.

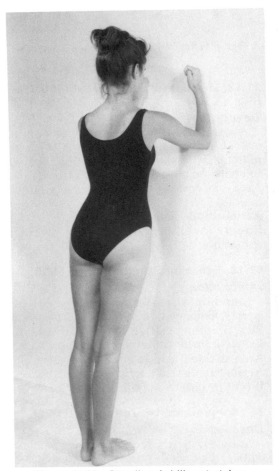

Figure 11.22 Standing Achilles stretcher.

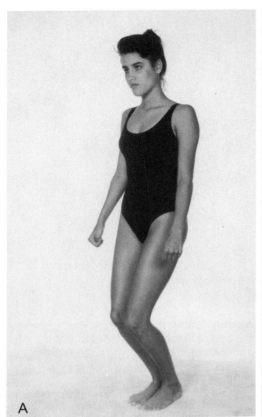
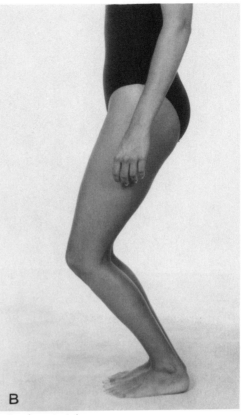

A B

Figure 11.23 Achilles tendon stretcher.

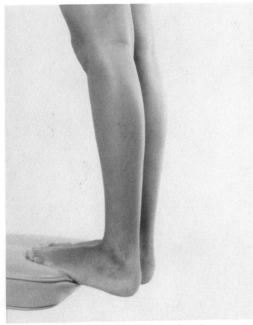

Figure 11.24 Achilles tendon drop.

Exercise format. Standard function 1.
Area affected. Achilles tendon, knee.
Action mode. Active stretching.
Intent. Flexibility.
Precaution. Patients with knee pathology may not be able to perform this exercise.
Note. Patients in early stages of trauma recovery may abduct legs and/or externally rotate feet to relieve pressure. This maneuver has a secondary gain in that quadriceps muscles are strengthened.

11.18. Achilles Tendon Drop (Fig. 11.24)
Description
Standing on a step with a tarsal/metatarsal contact, inferiorally drop calcaneus, keeping knee in extension.
Exercise format. Standard function 4.
Area affected. Achilles tendon, ankle plantar flexors.
Action mode. Active stretching, isometric.
Intent. Flexibility, endurance, strength.

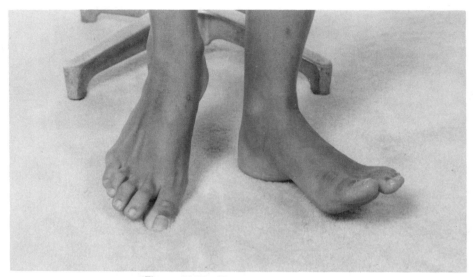

Figure 11.25 Plantar flexor/extensor.

11.19. Plantar Flexor/Extensor (Fig. 11.25)

Description

Sitting with knees flexed and feet on floor, elevate feet off floor, alternately plantar flexing one foot while dorsiflexing the other.

Exercise format. Standard function 2.

Area affected. Ankle plantar and dorsiflexors.

Action mode. Isotonic.

Intent. Flexibility, coordination, endurance, strength.

References

1. Basmajian JV: Primary Anatomy. 8th ed. Baltimore:Williams & Wilkins, 1982.
2. Hoppenfeld S: Physical Examination of the Spine and Extremities. New York:Appleton-Century-Crofts, 1976.

12

Aquatic Exercises

Many of the exercise principles that we have already discussed also apply to exercises done underwater. There are two main differences in these exercises, as opposed to those done out of the water. First, the person effectively weighs less in proportion to the amount of body mass that is submersed, due to the buoyant property of the water. Secondly, the water provides an even and continuous resistance to any motion undertaken within it, due to the relatively high specific gravity of water, especially when compared to that of air. Once again, exercises could be comprised of any of the modes discussed in Chapter 5. Furthermore, assistive mode exercises can be facilitated either manually or mechanically. It should be noted that exercises underwater are more difficult to perform, require more energy, and generate fatigue more quickly. The same goals, intents, and parameters apply as elsewhere, but they are generally performed more safely in the water because of its supportive features. Sometimes, more motion can be achieved when the identical exercise is performed in water rather than on land, for the same reason. Sometimes an arc of motion can be achieved in water that cannot be achieved without the water, due to the supportive nature of the water. Also, performing exercises in water causes them always to be executed against a measure of resistance. The interesting fact is that the harder and faster one tries to move, the greater the resistance to that motion.

Aquatic exercises have the same parameters to adjust as other exercises, with two notable exceptions. One still regulates the load, the velocity, the spatial and temporal configurations, the frequency, and the duration of the exercises. However, in water, one is concerned with the resistance to the motion, which is a conditional factor upon the load. One can employ devices affixed to the extremities whose shape causes more fluid turbulence, thus demanding greater resistance to movement. If a paddle-shaped attachment is used, the resistance is directly proportional to the surface area, provided the paddle is inflexible (1, p. 196). This means that an equal amount of resistance can be produced while moving in any direction of the arc, according to the force and velocity of the motion. Furthermore, angulation of the paddle face, with respect to the arc of motion, alters the resistance. As the paddle approaches a 90° angle with the arc of motion, the resistance is maximized. Similarly, as the paddle approaches a 0° or a 180° angle, the resistance reaches its minimum.

The second factor is the temperature of the water. The warmer the water, the more relaxing it is. The cooler the water, the more it soothes inflamed conditions, in general. The ideal temperature range for long-term hydrogymnastics is from 92 to 95°F, depending upon the quantity of muscular activity (1, p. 227).

After the two great wars, pioneering work was done in underwater rehabilitation in some of the great spas of Europe. This was of particular significance for neurological and rheumatic diseases at first, then for orthopedic cases that resulted from wartime traumas (1, p. 275). It was not long before European spas without hot springs began to develop and see the importance of water exercises.

The chief indication for aquatic exercises is a patient with sufficient injury and muscle weakness that air exercises are very difficult, but for whom one suspects that voluntary work will increase strength (1, p. 276). Patients with extensive dermatic burns, rheumatic disorders, neurological diseases, and joint injuries are good candidates for such programs. Some of the contraindications for this therapy (also called hydrogymnastics) are extremes of blood pressure, dermatic infections or open wounds, patients whose body temperature has been reduced to normal for less than 72 hr, and seriously debilitated patients (1, p. 276). Exercises should begin an appropriate amount of time after meals, and the patient should attempt to micturate prior to beginning.

Depending upon the amount of debilitation, one may alter intensity, frequency, or duration of exercise. Also, the more debilitated the patient is, the more assistive the exercises may need to be. Assistance can be provided by moving the body part in the direction it seeks when placed in water or by providing the body part with floats to increase its buoyancy. As the person becomes stronger, free weights or certain mechanized devices may be employed in the exercises, thus producing resistive type exercises. A corollary procedure to this is to vary the depth of the water in which one exercises. As the healing process accrues benefit, the patient can perform exercises in progressively more shallow water, either with weights or without.

Numerous types of devices and containers are employed in these exercises. They can be performed in anything from a small metal tub, called a Hubbard tank, large enough for one person, to a full-sized swimming pool. A paraplegic or seriously injured individual may be lowered into the tank and have exercises passively or assistively performed for him/her. The tank is large enough and has the proper shape to permit a large range of bodily motion. Often, systems of pulleys and lines of various materials (including material like Penrose tubing)

are implemented in the performance of certain exercises. There are not as many devices that can be so utilized in pool exercises, but one may also do exercises in pairs or in a group when working in a pool. Here, metal rails may be held by the hand or feet while the patient undertakes specific maneuvers. Sometimes, a bench, canvas hammock, or netting may be placed under the water, thus freeing the extremities to work in unison, without regard for the need to stay afloat. This is especially useful when weights are employed.

Of course, swimming itself can be among the best exercise procedures, provided that it is properly thought out and well controlled. There are many forms of swimming, each emphasizing different muscle groups, even though joints involved may be similar. There is clearly a difference in the specific motions, ranges of motion, and soft tissue elements involved in, for instance, the breast stroke, the butterfly stroke, and the back stroke. Modifications of these and other strokes can be used, and modified according to the parameters listed above, to provide a fairly good rehabilitative program. Such a program may need to be started in one's office setting, both because the patient may be that debilitated and in order to instruct the patient in proper techniques. Swimming is easily adaptable to home application for anyone who has regular access to a pool. However, as an exercise, swimming is often only good for generalized results, because it is such a complex activity when performed like one does in the sport. To overcome this, break down the particular stroke into its component parts, and utilize them separately, as necessary. If a certain portion of the stroke is performed with greater difficulty, it can be emphasized during the course of the exercises. Water exercises can be isotonic or isokinetic, but it serves no purpose to perform them isometrically.

The exercises listed below are examples of a set of exercises the authors have employed in aquatic environments. We have written their descriptions in a similar format to the land-based exercises within this text. This set is meant only to be suggestive of the potential for such exercising, not as an inclusive list, and variations of the exercises are not included.

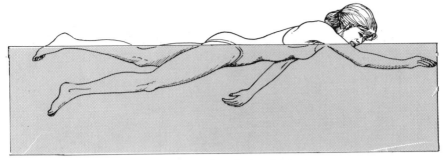

Figure 12.1 Swimming.

12.1. Swimming (Fig. 12.1)
Description
Have patient swim at a slow, even pace, avoiding any erratic muscular action.
Exercise format. Standard function 1.
Area affected. Cervical, thoracic, lumbar spine, shoulders, hips, and legs.
Action mode. Isotonic.
Intent. Strength, mobility, flexibility, endurance.

12.2. Shoulder Adductors and Abductors (Fig. 12.2)
Description
Standing in water with level above shoulders, slowly abduct arms 90°, with hands pronated and open. Slowly adduct arms back to starting position.
Exercise format. Standard function 1.
Area affected. Shoulder abductors and adductors.

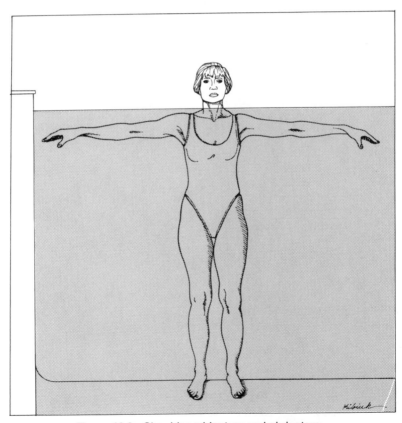

Figure 12.2 Shoulder adductors and abductors.

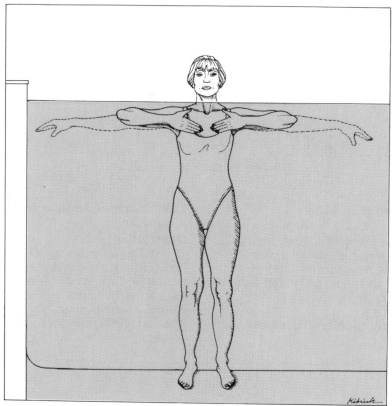
Figure 12.3 Elbow flexors and extenders.

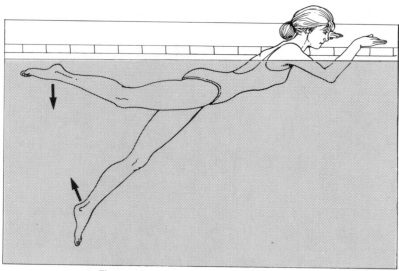
Figure 12.4 Hip flexors and extenders.

DYNAMICS OF CLINICAL REHABILITATIVE EXERCISE

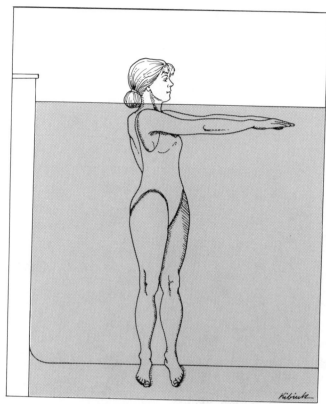

Figure 12.5 Lumbar rotators.

Action mode. Isotonic.
Intent. Strength, mobility, flexibility, endurance.

12.3. Elbow Flexors and Extenders (Fig. 12.3)
Description
Standing in water with level above shoulders, abduct arms 90°. Slowly flex and extend elbows, with fingers extended, palmar surface toward torso, and ulnar edge inferior. Move hands from midchest to full extension of elbows and back to chest again.
Exercise format. Standard function 1.
Area affected. Elbow flexors and extenders and anterior chest.
Action mode. Isotonic.
Intent. Strength, mobility, flexibility, endurance.

12.4. Hip Flexors and Extenders (Fig. 12.4)
Description
Lying prone in the water, floating, with hands grasping side of pool and legs extended, alternatively flex one hip while extending the other.
Exercise format. Standard function 1.
Area affected. Hip flexors and extenders, lumbosacral and pelvic areas.
Action mode. Isotonic.
Intent. Strength, mobility, flexibility, endurance.

12.5. Lumbar Rotators (Fig. 12.5)
Description
Stand in water with level above shoulders, shoulders abducted 90°, and elbows

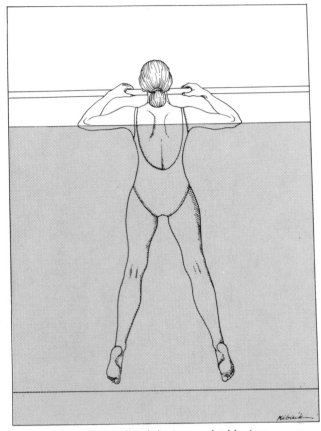

Figure 12.6 Hip abductors and adductors.

extended, palms inferior. Rotate torso to right, hold position for 5 to 10 sec, and return to center position. Repeat, rotating to the left side.

Exercise format. Standard function 4.

Area affected. Abdominals, anterior and posterior thorax.

Action mode. Isotonic.

Intent. Strength, mobility, flexibility, endurance.

12.6. Hip Abductors and Adductors (Fig. 12.6)

Description

Standing in water with level up to shoulders and feet not touching bottom, grasp side of pool to support body weight. Abduct legs, hold position, then adduct legs.

Area affected. Hip adductors and abductors.

Action mode. Isotonic.

Intent. Strength, mobility, flexibility, endurance.

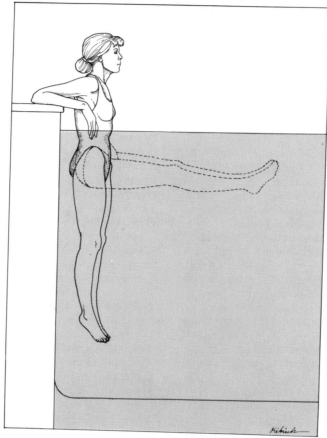

Figure 12.7 Hip flexors.

12.7. Hip Flexors (Fig. 12.7)

Description

Stand with back against side of pool and water level above the waist. Support weight with elbows on side of pool, and slowly flex hips. Hold position, then slowly return to starting position.

Exercise format. Standard function 1.

Area affected. Hip flexors and extensors, abdominals.

Action mode. Isotonic.

Intent. Strength, mobility, flexibility, endurance.

Reference

1. Basmajian JV, Wolf SL: Therapeutic Exercise. 5th ed. Baltimore:Williams & Wilkins, 1990.

GLOSSARY

Abduction. The act of moving outward.

Adduction. The act of moving toward the center.

Anterior. Situated in front of.

Archimedes. Principle stating that a body placed in a liquid is buoyed up by a force equal to the weight of the displaced liquid.

Asymptomatic. Without evidence of disease.

Avulsion. Tearing away of a part of structure.

Axonotmesis. Damage to nerve fibers resulting in complete peripheral degeneration.

Bilateral. Pertaining to both sides.

Buoyancy. Tendency to float in a liquid.

Caudad. Directed toward the tail, same as inferior.

Cephalad. Directed toward the head.

Circumduction. The active or passive circular motion of a limb.

Collateral. Secondary or accessory.

Concomitant. Accompanying; joined with another.

Condyloid. Resembling a condyle or knuckle.

Contraindication. Any condition that renders a particular form of treatment improper or undesirable.

Distal. Farther from any point of reference.

Dorsi-. Same as posterior in human anatomy.

Dorsiflexion. Backward flexion or bending.

Duration. The amount of time an exercise is performed. By increasing the duration, the exercise creates more intensity.

Endurance. The ability of a muscle or muscle group to contract repeatedly and to sustain tension over an extended period.

Evert. Turning outward.

Exacerbate. Increase the severity of a disease or condition.

Flexion. The act of bending.

Frequency. The number of repetitions of an exercise.

Frontal. Pertaining to the forehead.

Ginglymus. Synovial joint that allows movement in one plane, forward and backward.

Hydro-. Denoting relationship to water.

Hyperextend. Extreme or excessive extension of a limb.

Hyperkyphosis. Increase in the normal kyphotic curve.

Idiopathic. Unknown causation.

Impairment. Decrease in strength or function of a body part or process.

Inferior. Situated below or directed downward.

Insidious. Coming on in a slow and sly manner.

Inversion. Turning inward.

Isokinetic. Muscle contraction against a load, where the movement is maintained at a fixed rate of speed mechanically.

Isometric. Contraction of a muscle that remains the same length due to the resistance being equal to or greater than the force of the muscle. There is no movement.

Isotonic. Resistance applied to a muscle either manually or mechanically, maintaining the same tension, allowing the muscle to maintain the same tone. The joint is allowed to go through a normal range of motion.

Lateral. Pertaining to a position farther away from the midline.

Lordosis. Abnormally increased concavity in a curvature of the spine.

Medial. Pertaining to the middle.

Mobility. Susceptibility to being moved.

Mobilization. The process of making a fixed or ankylosed part movable.

Opposition. Antagonistic action of a muscle.

Overexertion. Exertion to the point of exhaustion or overstrain.

Overload. In order to increase strength, power, and endurance, the load used during the exercise must exceed the normal muscle capacity. It is the muscle's adaptation to this increased demand that produces the desired effects.

Palmar. Pertaining to the palm.

Passive. Movement by an external force within the unrestricted range of motion. There is no voluntary muscle contraction.

Plantar. Pertaining to the sole of the foot.

Plantar flexion. The act of bending the ankle downward.

Pronation. The act of assuming the prone position. Applied to the hand, the act of turning the palm posteriorly.

Prone. Lying with the face downward.

Protraction. To drag forth from a place.

Proximal. Nearest; closer to a point of reference.

Rehabilitation. The restoration of normal form and function after injury or illness.

Retraction. The act of drawing back.

Rotation. The process of turning around an axis.

Spondylosis. Ankylosis of a vertebral joint.

Strength. The ability of a muscle or muscle group to contract and sustain tension in direct relation to an opposing force.

Superior. Situated above or directed upward.

Supination. The act of assuming a supine position. Applied to the hand, the act of turning the palm anteriorly.

Supine. Lying on the back, face upward.

Therapeutic. Pertaining to the art of healing.

APPENDIX
Scoliosis

As much as there is written on scoliosis, there is surprisingly little agreement as to why it occurs and exactly how to treat it. Scoliosis is usually defined as a lateral curvature, of abnormal and constant nature. However, it is useful to think of it in biomechanical terms as well. We could say that it is an abnormal deformation between and within vertebrae, an excess frontal plane curvature and vertical (y axis) rotation, in the wrong direction (1 p. 94). Cailliet (and others) say that ". . . exercises per se will not deter a curvature that is progressing in a growing child, but will maintain flexibility and improve posture." (2, p. 722). However, in another source, Cailliet stated that "With current concepts of treatment, bracing and exercise is considered for any curve of 20° or more," also mentioning the need to account for the rotary components of such curves (3, pp. 432–3). The normal versus abnormal coupling motions of spinal vertebrae are important in understanding scoliosis, its etiology and management (1, pp. 72, 76, 93). This coupling again underscores the necessity for three-dimensional complex type motions, as soon as allowed. Kisner and Colby state that nonoperative treatment is almost always indicated for curves between 18 and 40° (4, p. 501). Others suggest that stretching, muscle reeducation, and strengthening may be effective in retarding the development of scoliosis (1, p. 577).

Some sort of immobilization is often recommended as well, such as Risser or Milwaukee type braces. However, even after such bracing has occurred, there is a great need for subsequent rehabilitation, usually in proportion to the amount of atrophy present. LeGrand-Lambling stated his case for exercise as ". . . object will be to avoid the reappearance of the deviation in the standing position by progressive reeducation of automatic and reflex mechanisms. . ." (3, p. 475). For such reeducation to occur, a vigorous and well-supervised exercise program must be instituted, so that both the patient and the muscles can relearn proper behaviors (1, p. 104). In scoliosis, the main needs are usually to restore strength and endurance to scapular adductors, the erector spinae, and the abdominal musculature (1, p. 650). Other muscle areas which often need attention paid to them are sacrospinalis, quadratus lumborum, hamstrings, tensor fascia lata, and thoracic cage musculature, due to weakness, tightness, or incoordination (1, p. 577). Additionally, contractures in the anterior and posterior longitudinal ligaments, ligamentum flavum, and interspinous ligaments may be factors in limiting symmetrical spinal movements (4, p. 500).

It is most important that home exercises be repeated often and regularly by the patients, if exercise is to be effective at all. Because we are usually dealing with children in this condition, it is important to have parental cooperation and involvement to ensure compliance. Sometimes, a home cervical traction unit is helpful to support the exercises, and we have often used gravity inversion devices in the same manner (3, p. 371). One last objective of rehabilitation for scoliosis is to restore or improve respiratory function (3, p. 435). Patients with thoracic curves measuring 50° or more, especially with significant rotation, often present with respiratory difficulties (3, p. 446). Improvement in respiratory function may be accomplished, in part, by use of those exercises suggested in that portion of this text. As a final note here, we generally suggest that the expiratory phase of respiration be about twice the duration of the inspiratory phase (3, p. 448). This more closely approximates the normal breathing cycle and promotes relaxation as well.

Scoliosis exercises are often performed with the trunk perpendicular to the gravity field, so as to minimize the effects of the pull of gravity on the unbalanced musculoskeletal system. The three main positions to provide such exercises are dorsal reclining (i.e., supine), abdominal reclining (i.e., prone), and quadruped horizontal (i.e., crawling) (1, p. 520) (Fig. A1). The patient will have a sense of relationship of body parts to each other (statesthesia) and of dynamic positioning of the body parts (kinesthesia). There are a number of specific exercise programs based upon this typing, but in this text the authors discuss only the composite set of movements. Additionally, body tone is monitored, both segmentally and generally, by the patient, and assisted by the therapist. The tone is regulated in order to affect relaxation. Exercises are first applied in such a manner as to mobilize any fixated segments. Later exercises are designed to strengthen chronic hypotonic areas, so that they may hold their proper positions. The number of

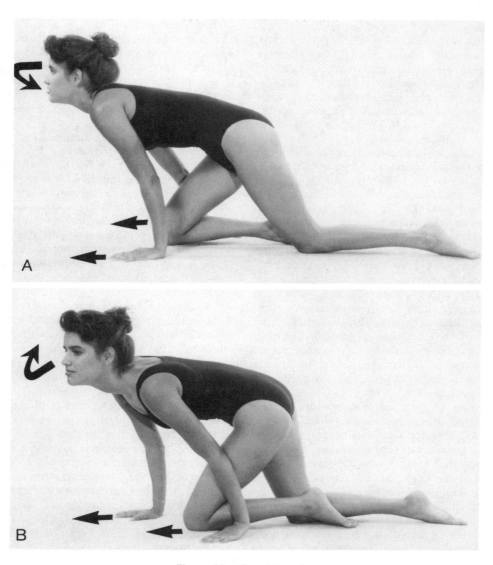

Figure A1. Crawl exercise.

combinations of positions and segmental exercise movements available is limited only by the doctor's imagination and the patient's flexibility and conditions.

Furthermore, the number of seconds each position is held and the number of repetitions are variables that must be controlled. The idea to hold foremost is to implement those exercises that will effect the necessary outcome and that are appropriate to the patient's level of dysfunction. Therefore, one varies the exercise structures, as well as the parameters of exercise, in order to meet the structural contingencies encountered. A cervical curve is not directly affected by a set of exercises in which the most stretched segments are in the thoracolumbar area, such as trunk rotations and flexions. Similarly, if the convexity of the curve is on the left side, it stands to reason that left lateral flexion is diminished, as compared to that motion to the right. Therefore, the rightward motion would be easier and favored, but the leftward motion would need to be accentuated. Even more specifically, one may need to highlight a portion of a segment of the spine.

Exercises that can be effectively performed in the quadruped horizontal position are the cross-crawl maneuvers of Dolman and Delgato (5). However, stretching, mobilizing, and strenthening exercises are also available for this position. In fact, there are mechanical devices designed to allow the patient to ambulate in place in the quadruped horizontal position. In performing the exercises on this device, the two main categories would be cross-crawl and homolateral-crawl (refer to Fig. 4.7). The choice depends upon the necessary effect. The position and the exercise that best neutralize the abnormal spinal curves are the ones chosen. Additionally, electromyographic studies can help pinpoint the hypertonic elements that need stretching and the hypotonic elements that need toning and strengthening.

Many of the exercises recommended for scoliosis rehabilitation can be performed as well, or better, in water, and even by adaptations of various normal swimming strokes. There has been reported about a 90% favorable reaction to therapeutic exercises in functional scolioses, ones in which structural changes have not occurred (1, p. 535). The hallmark of the functional curves is that they usually diminish or disappear completely in the Adam's position of forward flexion while standing. This comports with our concept of performing the exercises in the postures we have suggested, since the Adam's position simulates the orthogonality with the gravity field. At any rate, the success of any of these programs is dependent upon the proper choice of exercises and full compliance of the patient in following them regularly. Full compliance also implies complete attention to the exercise and engaging the full muscle power required to obtain adequate results, especially in building strength.

A caveat for a scoliosis patient would be the avoidance of asymmetrical activities, especially such sporting activities as tennis, golf, and bowling. Activities that require considerable bending and twisting, such as ice hockey, bicycling on certain bicycles, gardening, and baseball, would all have the same warning, (1, p. 533). The exception here would be if the doctor could utilize the asymmetry or flexion motions specifically to exercise against the unbalanced pattern(s), or if the activities that were asymmetrical were performed in an ambidextrous manner. Similarly, patients should not go unsupported into any position that may worsen the curve. This is another aspect of patient compliance and requires patients to pay full attention to their daily activities at work and play. Do they work at a desk and face slightly to the right for long periods of time while typing at a computer work station? When they run for their track team, do they always circle the track in the same direction? If activities do occur in this asymmetrical manner and their actions are such that the curves are enhanced, inform patients of this and help them to rearrange their activities. Patients who like to lie in a fetal position or on their abdomen in bed, or who tend routinely to carry heavy objects, like shoulder bags and school books, on the same side need to be warned against such indiscretions. You may need positional x-rays to convince the patient of the correctness of this attitude. On a proper bicycle, prohibited motions can be avoided or grossly minimized, especially by altering the relative heights of the handlebars, the seat, and the pedals, as well as their anteroposterior relationships. Special precautions evolve out of special patient conditions. Although swimming is deemed to be the most effective general exercise treatment for scoliosis, it may be contraindicated temporarily in someone with current or potential upper respiratory, optic, or otic infections (1, p. 534).

When there is greater than one lateral curve in the spine, one of the curves is deemed to be primary and the other(s) deemed to be secondary or even tertiary (both others being only compensatory). When this primary curve can be surely identified, the treatment should be aimed at it initially (1, p. 544). If another curve exists after such treatment, either the primary curve was identified incorrectly or there were more than one of them. When there is more than one primary curve, this is referred to as a double major curve, and this usually only occurs if they are structural in nature (4, p. 496). If there is any doubt, in the presence of a triple curve, we suggest beginning with more symmetrical type exercises. This gives an idea of the detail needed in the proper approach to correction by nonsurgical means.

It should be noted that in organic (or structural) scolioses, some sort of osteoarticular lesion(s) tends to fixate the abnormal curve, thus making it much less amenable to correction through therapeutic exercise. In fact, in larger curves, there may be deformation of osseous structure and considerable stress placed upon discoid tissues. However, one may be able to arrest development of such abnormalities if one is very specific in designing the exercises to mobilize and strengthen the areas of maximum tension upon the spinal column. This normally occurs at the apical vertebrae or the transitional vertebrae, within the curve. X-rays may be useful to establish the positions and ranges of motion necessary to accomplish such activities. In fact, cineroentgenology may be a formidable tool in assisting in the design of such exercises. With this medium, one can evaluate the form and result of a chosen exercise, both qualitatively and quantitatively. Of course, the studies need to be performed in the positions in which the exercising will occur. For those without access to such sophisticated equipment, palpation and motion palpation, in position, and sequential static films, either postural or in position, will have to suffice. These latter procedures have two drawbacks—they are not as quantitative and they provide less feedback to the patient— but an astute physician can make them work reasonably well. One other type device which may be useful for such treatment is either an electrogoniometric instrument or an infrared computerized device to document actual movement at specific levels of the spine. These data, in three dimensional space, are even more useful, when very carefully accumulated, as quantitative information. This information facilitates the decision in determining exactly how far to flex, extend, or rotate and exactly what should be the starting and finishing positions. Both types of devices mentioned here are expensive and their usage is time consuming. Also, one needs to consider the dosage in the case of the radiologic approach. Whether the gain in therapeutic advantage justifies the cost of service must be evaluated. Whichever method of analysis is utilized, it is important that a reliable measurement be regularly accomplished. If the exercises are not designed or executed in such a way as to focus precisely upon the segments where the stress and deformity are greatest, there is a potential for exacerbation of the curve (1, p. 541). Standard radiographic measurements for lateral flexion and rotatory deformity can assist in the decisions (6).

We do not mean to imply that scoliosis treatment should be restricted to the spine. On the side of hip adduction, adductor muscles will be contracted and tight and the abductor muscles will be stretched and weak. The opposite may be true for the contralateral extremity. Whether or not the spinal imbalance preceded that in the extremity, they are both current problems which synergistically maintain an abnormal curve of the spine. If every time the patient walks, due to extremity imbalances, he or she reinforces the spinal curvature, how effective will be the spinal exercises just performed? If, on the other hand, we reinforce the former with appropriate extremity exercises, our chances of success are much higher. Think about the muscles that affect the balance of the hips and pelvis, from the iliopsoas and quadratus lumborum, to the gluteus and external rotator groups, down to the long thigh muscles. They affect the motion and balance of the pelvis within the three planes of allowable motion. Since the spine is seated upon the sacrum, which is interrelated with the pelvis, it does not take much imagination to envision the multiplicity of events that can cause or worsen spinal curves. Stretching and relaxation exercises for the hypertonic sides and toning and strengthening exercises for the hypotonic sides are certainly in order. In the presence of scoliotic curves, simply test the muscles of the lower extremities (the upper ones are not weight bearing and are less likely to be involved) to determine such imbalances. As a last point, we need not stop at the hip, because joint disease, structural imbalances like a short leg, and pedal abnormalities like unilateral pes planus can all affect the spine grossly. When viewing the patient from the posterior, if one looks caudad from the scoliotic spine down to the

Achilles tendons, often one finds a lateral or medial deviation that is greater on one side than the other. Whether the foot is a cause or an effect in this case is not yet relevant. Treat the malcontracted Achilles tendon, at least initially, to support hoped for spinal corrections. In fact, by the principle of leverage, the further away from the spine the distal abnormality is, the larger the likely complication in the spine. Therefore, when applicable, utilize the appropriate exercises for the involved extremity in patients with scoliosis, simultaneous to the spinal exercises.

Exercises may be performed while in a bracing device or without the device. If the curve has been regarded as being sufficient to demand such a support, it is wise not to remove it during postural exercising, but it may be proper to remove it during the horizontally positioned exercising. If the brace is too restrictive to allow sufficient movement, you might switch to an isometric mode, at least temporarily. The advantages of exercising with the brace are 2-fold. First, the supporting nature of the device protects the patient from accidental postures and the ravages of fatigue. Secondly, the structure can provide feedback as to the direction and location of the necessary exercise stresses. The pads in a Milwaukee brace cause a shift of the spinal column, at a specific location and in a specific direction. This can only help reinforce to the patient what is trying to be accomplished. Once the memory of the routine is established, the patient may enact the same exercises, without the brace feedback, at later times after its removal. For patients in a brace, only contact sports are contraindicated (4, p. 508). Bracing is considerably easier on all involved and is chosen sometimes when compliance demands it, even though the curve is not so severe that one could not expect good results from exercise alone.

Every action that attempts to straighten or maintain scoliotic curves has a good effect on the evolution of ventilatory deficit (1, p. 545). This normally refers to large curves in which respiratory function has been significantly depressed or altered. However, if one does not think in digital terms, but, instead, in the analog continual functioning that is the life process, why wouldn't all curves diminish respiratory function to some extent? Therefore, when we rehabilitate for respiratory function we look very closely for spinal curvature variations that can be exercised and improved. This is another main functional disadvantage of corsets, supports, and braces. Their primary disadvantage is that they end up reducing muscular function and thereby causing some atrophy. The secondary disadvantage is that respiratory function is automatically depressed to that same degree. On the other hand, increased respiratory function, independent of muscular exertions, will cause overoxygenation and fatigue, because the physiological need for that oxygen was not produced. Therefore, we recommend applying both types of exercises sequentially (and, eventually, simultaneously) for maximum efficiency. After all, in normal functioning, don't we automatically perform both tasks in synchrony? Anything less is inefficient and energy depleting.

Before prescribing exercises for scoliosis patients, take a very careful history and evaluate their lifestyle as to needs, activities, and time spent in each. Then explicitly delineate for them (and their parents, when necessary) which activities are not to be done, which need not be altered, which need to be modified, and in what way. Obviously, one will accentuate the activities and postures that encourage correction and decrease those that exacerbate the curve. The doctor also needs to consider how performing activities in different media, such as in the air, in water, or on the ground, will affect the instructions. The usual decisions in terms of exercise parameters must be made, including the number of sessions per week with the therapist and the number of sessions per week (and per day) at home. The duration of the program should be from 4 to 6 weeks initially, depending upon the severity of the curve(s), the age of the patient (and the age of onset of the condition), and any underlying conditions that may adversely affect the progress of the exercise regimen. Always challenge the patient to augment the program, but always in a gradual enough manner so as not to provoke fatigue. A weary patient will perform in a slovenly manner, which may be counterproductive. The estimate of the initial course of treatment is just that, and it should be updated with regular evaluations of progress, including serial x-rays. Also, one must remember that patient enthusiasm varies, according to the person and the day, and each program must be tailored to that amount of need for prodding or dampening the intensity of performance. Additionally, if the patient is wearing a supportive device, the doctor needs to decide if and when the exercises are performed without the device in place. For structural (organic) forms of scoliosis, a valuable result can only be obtained by hours of training each day (1, p. 549).

Conservative care, other than bracing, for the scoliotic patient includes unilateral exercises to strengthen the musculature on the convex side and stretch the musculature on the concave side. This is especially important for more mature patients (ages 17 to 25) in whom curve progression is no longer a current factor, even with curves up to 40°, and who are not candidates for bracing (7).

Since it was pointed out that most of the deformity in scoliosis resides in the intervertebral disc(s), it is reasonable to study them and develop exercises that mobilize and strengthen them before any other exercises are performed (8). Cox's unilateral distraction office techniques would wisely be followed up by the types of home or office exercises that have been suggested here. Similar effects can be produced with judicious exercising in an antigravity position.

References

1. White AA, Panjabi MM. Clinical Biomechanics of the Spine. Philadelphia:JB Lippincott, 1978.
2. Kottke FJ, Stillwell KG, Lehman JF: Krusen's Handbook of Physical Medicine and Rehabilitation. 3rd ed. Philadelphia:WB Saunders, 1982.
3. Basmajian JV, Wolf SL: Therapeutic Exercise. 5th ed. Baltimore:Williams & Wilkins, 1990.
4. Kisner C, Colby LA. Therapeutic Exercise: Foundations and Techniques. Philadelphia: FA Davis, 1987.
5. Stevenson RW. Cross crawl pattern: an adjunct to other exercise programs. Dig Chiropract Econ, Jan/Feb, 1977; 9, 114.
6. Aragona RJ. Lateral bending lumbar x-rays. American Society of Biological Engineers course notes, Lumbar Section, 1987; 70.
7. Tuthill AR. Scoliosis: making a case for conservative care. Am Chiropract, Oct 1988; 24–5.
8. Cox JM. Unilateral distraction in scoliosis, subluxation and disc protrusion. Dig Chiropract Econ, Nov/Dec 1981; 18: 46–9.

INDEX

Page numbers in *italics* denote figures; those followed by "t" denote tables.

Biceps brachii, 154, 164, *164, 165*
Biceps femoris, 238, *239*
Bilateral, defined, 264
Biofeedback, 67
Biological task equivalents, 64
Blisters, 112
Bones. *See* Skeletal system
Bouyancy, 257
  definition of, 264
Brachial plexus, 143–144, 154
  injuries of, 136
Brachialis, 164, *164*
Brachioradialis, 164, *164, 165*
Breathing exercises, 70–72, 75
  aim of, 70
  conditions where useful, 71
  easing congestion for, 75
  environment for, 70
  forced expiration and, 71
  modifications of, 125
  muscles for, 71
  patient instruction for, 71–72
  patient preparation for, 70
  posture and, 124
  principles for, 124–125
  reducing asthmogenicity of, 124
  relaxation for, 71–72
  for thoracocostal facet syndrome, 125
Breathing patterns, 70–71
BRIME technique, 80, 106
Bursae, *54*
Bursitis, 54
  rehabilitation principles for, 115
  of shoulder joint, 137

Calcium, role in muscle contraction, 21
Calluses, 112
Capsular tears, 53
Cardiovascular rehabilitation, 72–73
  aims of, 72
  cardiovascular stress in water, 73
  endurance and, 72
  for fitness, 72–73
  principles of, 123–124
    National Athletic Health Institute recommendations, 123
    program parameters, 123–124
    proper diagnosis for, 124
Carpal bones, 7, *8*
  fractures of, 137
  joints of, 172
Carpal metacarpal joint, 172
Cartesian geometry, 10–16
  Cartesian axes, 10
    human body on, 10–12, *11*
  to describe 3-dimensional body motion, 12–13, *13*
  example of application of, 14
  to express nonlinear motion, 12
  resolution of vectors, 13

right-hand screw rule, 12, *12*
scalar vs. vector quantities in, 12
spatial configuration of exercise and, 74
Cartilage injuries, 52–53
  of knee, 53, 117
  rehabilitation principles for, 116–117
  of spine, 53
  of temporomandibular joint, 53
Caudad, defined, 264
Causalgia, 56, 122
Center of gravity, 27
Center of mass, 27
Central artery, 14
Cephalad, defined, 264
Cerebral vascular accidents, 121
Cervical curve, 3, 118
Cervical plexus, 143, 156
Cervical spine
  musculature of, 142–143, *143*
  ranges of motion of, 142, 143t
Cervical spine exercises, 142t, 142–153
  cervical flexion and extension, 144, *144*
  cervical flexion resistance, *152,* 153
  cervical hand resistance, *147,* 147–148
  cervical lateral flexion, 145, *145*
  cervical lateral flexion resistance, *153,* 153
  cervical mobilizer, 148, *148*
  cervical rotation, 145, *146*
  cervical towel resistance, *148,* 148–151
  cervico-occipital glide, 145–147, *147*
  head and neck motions and, 142
  purposes of, 142
  sitting, hands on posterior occiput, *151,* 152
  sitting cross-legged, *150,* 151–152
  standing, hands on head, *152,* 153
  supine, cervical rotation, *149,* 151
  supine, occipital stretch, *149,* 151
Cervical spine injuries, 132–136, 133t
  acute cervical sprain syndrome, 132
  brachial plexus injuries, 136
  hyperextension injury, 132
  hyperflexion injury, 132
  lateral flexion injuries, 132, 136
  rehabilitation principles for, 117–118
  rotation injuries, 132
  scalenus anticus syndrome, 136

torticollis, 136
Chest conditions, 134t, 138
  asthma, 138
  emphysema, 138
  Cheyne-Stokes respirations, 70–71
Chondroitin sulfates, 127
Chondromalacia patellae, 139
  progressive resistive exercise for, 117
  rehabilitation principles for, 117
Cicatrization, 66
Circuit training, 106
Circumduction, defined, 264
Clothing for exercising, 88
Coccyx, 1–3, *3, 5, 5*
Collateral, defined, 264
Collateral ligaments, 238
Colles' fracture, 137
Comcomitant, defined, 264
Concentric contractions, 37–38, 99, 100
Conditioning, 72, 75–76
  intensity of exercise for, 90
  vs. rehabilitation, 89–90
Condyloid, defined, 264
Conjoint tendon, 199
Connective tissues
  effect of immobilization on, 110
  elasticity of, 65–66
Conservation of momentum
  angular, 27
  linear, 27
Constrictor muscles, inferior, *143*
Contractures, 55, 65
  exercise precautions for, 110
  heat or cold for, 65
  passive stretching of, 65, *65*
Contraindications
  definition of, 264
  to exercise, 110–112
  during pregnancy, 127
Coordination, 69–70
  causes of problems with, 69
  definition of, 69
  engram production and, 69, 77
  exercises for, 76–77
  genetic part of, 69
  neuromuscular reeducation for, 69, 76–77, 107
  principles for development of, 70
Coracobrachialis, 154
Coracohumeral ligament, 154
Countermovement jump, 100
Coupling, 74
Cramps, 112
Cranium, 5, *6*
  development of, 5
  sutures of, 5
Cross-crawl exercises, 78, *79,* 128
Crossed extensor reflex, 43
Crossed reflex, 45
Cruciate ligaments, 238
  rehabilitating injuries of, 114